Intermediate and Continuing Care: Policy and Practice

Edited by

Brenda Roe
Professor of Health Sciences,
Liverpool John Moores University

Roger Beech
Reader in Health Services Research, Keele University
and Academic Lead for Research, Central Cheshire
Primary Care Trust

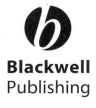

Blackwell
Publishing

Editorial offices:
Blackwell Publishing Ltd, 9600 Garsington Road, Oxford OX4 2DQ, UK
   Tel: +44 (0)1865 776868
Blackwell Publishing Inc., 350 Main Street, Malden, MA 02148-5020, USA
   Tel: +1 781 388 8250
Blackwell Publishing Asia Pty Ltd, 550 Swanston Street, Carlton, Victoria 3053, Australia
   Tel: +61 (0)3 8359 1011

First published 2005 by Blackwell Publishing Ltd

Library of Congress Cataloging-in-Publication Data
Intermediate and continuing care : policy and practice/edited by Brenda Roe, Roger Beech.
   p. ; cm.
Includes bibliographical references and index.
ISBN-13: 978-1-4051-2033-3 (alk. paper)
ISBN-10: 1-4051-2033-9 (alk. paper)
1. Older people–Intermediate care–Great Britain.   2. Older people–Long-term care–Great Britain.   3. Intermediate care (Nursing care)–Great Britain.   4. Long-term care facilities–Great Britain.   5. Continuum of care–Great Britain.
[DNLM: 1. Intermediate Care Facilities–organization & administration.   2. Ambulatory Care–Aged.   3. Health Planning.   4. Health Services for the Aged–organization & administration.   5. Home Care Services–Aged.   6. Housing for the Elderly.   WT 27.1 I61 2005]   I. Roe, Brenda H. II. Beech, Roger.

RA998.G7I58 2005
362.16′0941–dc22
2005016455

ISBN-10: 1-4051-2033-9
ISBN-13: 978-1-4051-2033-3

A catalogue record for this title is available from the British Library

Set in 10/12.5 pt Palatino
by Graphicraft Limited, Hong Kong
Printed and bound in India
by Gopsons Papers Ltd. Noida

For further information on Blackwell Publishing, visit our website:
www.blackwellnursing.com

This book is dedicated to

Pearl Roe (1920–2004) and Esme Elsden
and Izan, Hebba and Alice Beech

Contents

Foreword

When I first became a consultant I shared responsibility with a colleague for a 40-bed 'half-way home' sited in a large Victorian mansion in a leafy suburb. It was devoid of facilities, needed refurbishment and the onward move to home for clients was often delayed for months. Such units were not unusual and this unit like most others of its kind were closed as the emphasis switched to improving services for older people in the acute hospital. Twenty-five years later, as part of the Department of Health's *National Service Framework for Older People*, we have seen the opening of similar types of units in the community established as part of what are now called intermediate care services. Whilst recognising that not all people presently admitted to an acute hospital need to be (this includes younger people as well as older individuals), and that hospital has dangers of its own, it is important that alternatives are patient-orientated, effective, sustainable in the long term and not just used as a way of meeting government targets on waiting times and waiting lists. One hopes that the cycle does not repeat itself!

The greater emphasis on primary care, in both its commissioning and providing roles requires re-engineering of what often seems like the dividing wall between the hospital and the community. This is particularly so when it comes to the continuing care of older people, many of whom suffer from chronic diseases. Bringing the expertise to where the person lives requires training for primary health care and social care teams and much more flexible referral arrangements. This is particularly important in care homes, where numerous studies have described the inadequacies of the present health care systems. It is interesting to reflect that the Certificate of Additional Qualification in Geriatrics in the USA is equally open to family physicians as it is to those who have first trained in internal medicine in hospital.

Thus, this book is extremely timely. Brenda Roe and Roger Beech are to be congratulated on assembling a team of policy makers, researchers and practitioners whose expertise and clarity of thought will be of benefit to all those interested in this area. I can thoroughly recommend it.

Peter Crome
Professor of Geriatric Medicine, Keele University
President-Elect, British Geriatrics Society

Introduction

Intermediate care is a key standard within current UK health policy, and local services have been developed since the early 1990s with little strategic planning. Recently social services and health services have been working together in partnership with local voluntary organisations and stakeholders to develop strategy and services. To date, there has been little empirical evidence available to shape the development of these services, despite evaluation and user and consumer involvement being explicit within government policy. There is an emerging body of knowledge on the development, organisation and evaluation of intermediate care but there remains insufficient evidence of economic evaluation.

Intermediate care is not a universal term and does not feature in the international literature, which therefore makes comparison between countries and services difficult. For example, many different terms are used in the UK for services which come under the umbrella of intermediate care, such as hospital at home, rapid response teams, rehabilitation and recovery teams, acute medical trauma or early discharge, and 'nurse-led beds' in care homes. In the USA, intermediate care is taken to mean ambulatory urgent medical care similar to 'walk in' or 'out of hours' general practice centres in the UK. 'Subacute care' would be a more comparable term in the USA to our understanding of intermediate care in the UK.

The purpose of this book is to draw together what we know about intermediate care services. Main reference is given to UK services although, where possible, reference to international literature and studies is provided. Intermediate care services are being developed with no reference or national debate on how they relate to continuing care in the community. There is a long history of continuing care provision within the health and social welfare literature, which this book also draws upon. Continuing care is developing with care in the community, by the community or closer to home, as opposed to large long-stay institutions. The development of assisted living, retirement communities and extra care housing is also emerging in the UK, having already been established in the USA. Intermediate and continuing care form part of the 'care continuum' and should be viewed together as part of a whole system. This book advocates such a whole system approach to the development, organisation and evaluation of intermediate and continuing care, including policy and context. Essential to this are carers and the involvement of users and the public in the development and evaluation of services. End of life issues also form part of the 'continuum of care' and require consideration within the whole system approach.

This book is aimed at health and social care providers as well as managers, researchers and academics. It comprises three parts and involves contributing authors who have knowledge and experience of policy, management and research in health and social care. Part 1 looks at intermediate care, with some chapters forming 'how to guides' on the development and organisation of services. Part 2 looks at continuing care, while Part 3 considers the involvement of carers and consumers. All chapters provide a current 'state of the art' and include a summary with recommendations for services and care, as well as for future research.

In Chapter 1, Jenny Cowpe sets the policy and context for intermediate care, looking at past policy and history within a national and local context. She goes on to look at current and future developments including success factors as well as outstanding policy and implementation issues. In Chapter 2, Roger Beech identifies the need and scope for intermediate care using performance indicators to support planning and the use of utilisation review as a particular technique. In Chapter 3, The Balance of Care Group, comprising Tom Bowen, Paul Forte and Chris Foote, look at the management and planning of services for intermediate care. The authors argue for developing a whole systems perspective using the Appropriateness Evaluation Process as part of a methodology involving surveys and workshops. They provide an illuminating case study looking at alternatives to acute admission and discharge planning.

In Chapter 4, Wanda Russell considers the coordination of intermediate care, addressing key questions of whom services are aimed at, what is offered and who provides them. She discusses who the users of the services are and how they are referred, processes and systems of implementation and delivery, monitoring, public involvement and evaluation. In Chapter 5, Brenda Roe goes on to look at service development and evaluation in intermediate care. She includes the development of services and professionals and argues for a whole system integrated approach. The role of evaluation for service monitoring and development is also discussed. Brenda identifies barriers and constraints to the delivery of intermediate care and concludes by describing the range of schemes and services available.

Chapter 6 involves another group contribution from Anne Marriott, Gaynor Reid, Kathy Jones, Rae de Villiers and Christine Kennedy. They look at interdisciplinary working within intermediate care and argue for generic working as the key to a person centred approach. The development of interdisciplinary working and how it compares to multidisciplinary working is discussed. The authors use the development of their own Rehabilitation Link Team and service within East Cheshire Primary Care Trust as a case study. They consider care management and processes along with the benefits and limitations of interdisciplinary working. In Chapter 7, Julie Howden builds on her own experience of running courses on interdisciplinary training and development for intermediate care. She considers interdisciplinary joint working and training compared with the multidisciplinary approach, interprofessional education and curricula, and some common learning programmes. Learning styles and teaching strategies, along with the gains and benefits of interdisciplinary training and development, are also included.

The final two chapters in Part 1 consider the evidence underpinning intermediate care. In Chapter 8, Roger Beech looks at the evidence on effectiveness, which includes both quantitative and qualitative empirical evidence from systematic reviews and local evaluations. Implications for current services and directions for future research are considered. In Chapter 9, Richard Little presents a guide to economic evaluation, commencing with some basic economics and evidence. He goes on to look at key questions and potential methods for comparison, costs and benefits.

In Part 2, David Challis and Ann Netten set the scene for continuing care, its policy and context. To mirror Part 1 they include past policy and history, looking at long-term commitment to community based care, past developments and the modernisation of social care services. They also consider workforce issues, the acute and continuing care interface, performance, regulation, best value, commissioning of services, funding of long-term care and future demand. In Chapter 11, David Challis and Jane Hughes look at service delivery and the development and evaluation of community care. The chapter includes service development, delivery, coordination and continuity, locations and care packages, information needs and systems to support continuing care.

In Chapter 12, Robin Darton and Ann-Marie Muncer consider alternative housing and care arrangements. This includes sheltered housing and private retirement housing and their provision, and more recent developments in extra care housing and assisted living. Costs and funding issues of these alternatives, the characteristics and needs of residents, and staffing issues are discussed. Finally, the authors look at retirement communities and extra care housing, using two developments in the UK as examples. The chapter concludes by identifying future research needed to fill the gaps in current knowledge. Care homes and continuing care are the focus of Chapter 13 presented by Ann Netten, Robin Darton and Jacquetta Williams. They begin by identifying the supply and characteristics of homes, their funding, their costs and their prices. Quality of care and quality of life are also included, as are lengths of stay and resident outcomes. Areas where more research is required are identified and conclusions and recommendations drawn.

Part 2 is completed by Chapter 14 by Abigail Masterson and Sian Maslin-Prothero. The chapter discusses interprofessional care and interdisciplinary working in the context of community care and continuing care, with specific reference to people living with continuing care needs and chronic conditions. The authors start out by looking at policy, then go on to consider interdisciplinary working and education, competence and regulation. This chapter builds on Chapter 7 in Part 1, by taking a specific focus on continuing care.

Part 3 comprises two chapters looking at the involvement of carers and consumers. Chapter 15 by Diane Seddon and Catherine Robinson looks at carers and caregiving in the context of intermediate and continuing care. The authors begin by looking at the challenges of caregiving and set this into a policy context. They then go on to include carers' experiences of services and support. The valuable roles of consultation and working in partnership to deliver intermediate and continuing care are also explored. In Chapter 16, Bie Nio Ong and Geoff Wood look at patient and public involvement in service development and evaluation. They define what involvement is, the challenges and tensions in receiving and giving care, how to judge quality of care and how individuals can have meaningful influence over service provision.

In Chapter 17, Brenda Roe and Roger Beech summarise the book by drawing together what is known about intermediate and continuing care, identifying areas for future research and reflecting on implications for policy and practice.

We are indebted to the contributing authors who shared our vision for this book and who made it possible, despite the competing demands of heavy workloads and schedules. We should also like to thank Beth Knight at Blackwell Publishing for appreciating the scope and value of this book.

Brenda Roe and Roger Beech

Contributors

Roger Beech is a Reader in Health Services Research in the Centre for Health Planning and Medicine, University of Keele, and the Academic Lead for Research for Central Cheshire Primary Care Trust. He is also an honorary member of the Faculty of Public Health Medicine. His research can be categorised as having four main but overlapping themes: the economic and organisational aspects of health services, in particular services for elderly people, for intermediate care, and for patients with stroke; the development and application of methodologies for planning health services, in particular services for intermediate and emergency care; health needs assessment, particularly needs for renal services; and the use of modelling techniques to evaluate changes in the delivery of health care.

Tom Bowen is an independent consultant and lead member of The Balance of Care Group (www.balanceofcare.com). He has an extensive background in the fields of health care planning and information systems spanning two decades. Following analytical and management posts in both the Department of Health and the NHS, for the past nine years he has been operating in consultancy for the NHS and in other European countries. UK projects have ranged from national policy work and key infrastructure projects to extensive work with local Trusts, health authorities, Primary Care Trusts, local authorities and partner organisations on a variety of planning and informatics issues. Tom has extensive experience of developing service plans for patient groups with chronic care needs, in particular services for older people.

David Challis is Professor of Community Care Research and Director of the Personal Social Services Research Unit (PSSRU) at the University of Manchester. He was responsible for a series of evaluations of the effectiveness and efficiency of intensive care management for older people, which were influential in the development of community care services in the UK. He has also acted as an advisor on care management to a number of governments and service providers in the USA, Canada, Australia and Japan. Current areas of activity include a range of studies on assessment of older people and patterns of service provision.

Jenny Cowpe is a Senior Fellow in the Centre for Health Planning and Management at Keele University and Associate Director of the Centre's Clinical Management Unit. Jenny's previous professional experience was as a General Manager and Trust Chief Executive within the National Health Service, where she worked in teaching hospital, district general hospital, community and mental health organisations. At Keele, she both manages, and teaches on, the national Clinical Leadership Programmes, provided previously for the NHS Leadership Centre and now for the Institute for Innovation and Improvement. She also jointly leads the extensive range of Specialist Registrar and Consultant programmes offered by the Clinical Management Unit.

Robin Darton is a Research Fellow in the Personal Social Services Research Unit at the University of Kent. He has a background in psychology and statistics, and research interests in health and social services provision for elderly people and in methodological issues relating to the design and analysis of studies of health and social care. He has been involved in a number of major surveys of care homes, and is currently working on studies of care homes, home care and extra care housing.

Chris Foote is an independent consultant undertaking work to facilitate integrated care across a wider population base and is a lead member of The Balance of Care Group (www.balanceofcare.com). For 23 years he worked as a consultant physician in general hospital settings developing services for the elderly population. He has been working for the past 15 years on developing integrated care systems that put older people and their carers at the heart of the process, work which has been commended by the Audit Commission. He has been facilitating similar models in both Sweden and New Zealand and has networks with the Institute of Health Care Improvements in Boston, USA. He was previously a member of one of the working parties for the *National Service Framework for Older People*.

Paul Forte is an independent consultant in health planning and management and is a lead member of the Balance of Care Group (www.balanceofcare.com). He is also a senior lecturer at the Centre for Health Planning and Management, Keele University, where he teaches on MBA and diploma courses for managers and clinicians. He previously worked in health services research at the University of Leeds and in the Department of Health Operational Research Service. Throughout his career Paul has focused on the development and application of management decision support systems in health services, particularly services for older people. He has extensive experience of working with NHS and local authority organisations at national and local levels, and has also undertaken overseas projects for WHO and the World Bank.

Julie Howden is a Head Occupational Therapist working for Mid Staffordshire General Hospitals NHS Trust and has been an occupational therapist for the past 20 years. She has taken a particular interest in continuing professional development of staff and set up and coordinated a strategy for CPD within therapy services between 1998 and 2001. Julie became the Project Leader for the Intermediate Care Training and Development Team at Staffordshire University between 2001 and 2002. She was part of a steering group instrumental in the development and implementation of a part-time in-service Occupational Therapy degree course at Staffordshire University in 2002 and has also been involved in the development of a Masters degree in Occupational Therapy at Staffordshire University between 2003 and 2004.

Jane Hughes is a Lecturer in Community Care Research in the Personal Social Services Research Unit (PSSRU) at the University of Manchester. She has previously worked as a practitioner, service manager and policy manager in social services departments in England. Her current area of activity includes studies of the impact of assessment processes for older people, hospital discharge and balance of care.

Kathy Jones works as a Social Worker Rehabilitation Coordinator in the Rehabilitation Link Team of East Cheshire Primary Care Trust. Previously she has worked as a hospital social worker and carried out group work within psychiatric services. She has also worked as a social worker in the Rapid Response Team at the same Trust and played a part in developing this service.

Christine Kennedy is the Team Manager of the Rehabilitation Link Team in East Cheshire Primary Care Trust. She has worked as a social worker for several different local authorities. For the past 14 years she has worked in Cheshire, originally within Social Services, moving to manage the Rehabilitation Link Team three years ago. She plays an active part in local single assessment developments, sharing the lessons learned within the Rehabilitation Link Team.

Richard Little is a Senior Research Fellow in Health Economics at the Centre for Health Planning and Management at Keele University. His interest is in promoting applied health economics through research and teaching, with a particular focus in supporting decision making, especially to public health. Richard has extensive experience in the NHS and Department of Health, especially with public health and NHS information which he uses in applied health economics. Richard has undertaken modelling analysis for the National Screening Committee evaluating screening options for Down's syndrome and diabetic retinopathy, programme budgeting and marginal analysis for cancer services and has been extensively involved in applying health economics to areas of public health including health impact assessment, intermediate care and health promotion. Richard teaches health economics in various programmes and is Director of the International Health Economics module at the Centre.

Anne Marriott is the Intermediate Care Manager for East Cheshire Primary Care Trust and set up the Rehabilitation Link Team in East Cheshire in May 2000. She has experience of working in physical rehabilitation and mental health fields. She was Head Occupational Therapist for Psychiatric Services in East Cheshire from 1991 to 1999. During this time she managed the Psychiatric Day Hospital for three years and had the lead role in setting up the Eating Disorder Service and Rosemount Day Care Service. She has a particular interest in clinical effectiveness, staff development, user/carer involvement and team approaches to change.

Sian Maslin-Prothero is Professor of Nursing at Keele University School of Nursing and Midwifery. She has worked in academia, education, clinical nursing and midwifery in a variety of settings in both the United Kingdom and overseas. Her research interests include policy and practice in the NHS, the recruitment of women to breast cancer clinical trials, and user and carer involvement in health and social care.

Abigail Masterson is an independent health care consultant. She works with many local, national and international health care organisations carrying out research, developing innovative educational programmes and reviewing services. Abi has postgraduate degrees in nursing and management, and has published widely in the areas of health policy and new role development in health care.

Ann-Marie Muncer is a Research Officer in the Personal Social Services Research Unit at the University of Kent. She has a background in psychology and has worked in rehabilitation units for adults with enduring mental health problems and children with behavioural difficulties. Current research interests include housing and care options for older people and how transitions into different care environments are mediated by psychological factors.

Ann Netten is Professor of Social Welfare at the University of Kent. She joined the Personal Social Services Research Unit in 1987 and has been Director of the Kent branch of the Unit since November 2000. Her research interests include cost estimation and economic evaluation of health and social welfare interventions (including criminal justice), care of older people, developing theoretical approaches to the evaluation of community care and measuring quality and outcomes in social care.

Bie Nio Ong is Professor of Health Services Research at the Primary Care Sciences Research Centre, Keele University. She has published research on health policy, health needs assessment, musculoskeletal pain, and user and community involvement and is interested in combining qualitative and quantitative methods in health research. She is also the Chair of Central Cheshire Primary Care Trust.

Gaynor Reid is a Lecturer in Occupational Therapy at The University of Liverpool teaching on the BSc(Hons) Occupational Therapy Programme. Over the years she has gained experience of working with adults and children with physical and learning disabilities, in a variety of settings in health and social care, education and the private sector. In recent years she has carried out evaluative and qualitative research within intermediate care, which has entailed collaborative working with users, carers and providers.

Catherine Robinson is a Senior Research Fellow in the Institute of Medical and Social Care Research. She is responsible for the North Wales section of the

All Wales Alliance for Research and Development in health and social care and is the National Convenor. Her research interests relate to social care and the interface with health. Catherine is involved in a number of research projects related to carers.

Brenda Roe is Professor of Health Sciences at Liverpool John Moores University, and formerly Senior Lecturer in Social Gerontology at Keele University. She has a background in nursing, health visiting, education, research and health services management. Her research interests focus on the development and evaluation of health care and health systems for people with continuing care needs in the community, such as older people, young disabled people or those living with chronic conditions. She is a Fellow of the Royal Society for the Promotion of Health, and a Fellow and Member of Council of the Queens' Nursing Institute.

Wanda Russell is a Lecturer in Health Services Research at the Centre for Health Planning and Management at Keele University. Wanda has a background in epidemiology and her key research interests include research methods (both quantitative and qualitative) with an emphasis on health status measurement and health-related quality of life, and health care issues amongst elderly groups.

Diane Seddon is a Research Fellow at the Institute of Medical and Social Care Research, University of Wales Bangor. Diane's research interests include family caregiving, older people with dementia, assessment and care management, and nursing and residential care home provision. Diane is involved in a number of research studies, looking at the effects of the National Strategy for Carers across England and Wales, and with work that aims to develop services to support carers of people with mental health problems.

Rae de Villiers works as Falls Coordinator at East Cheshire Primary Care Trust. She has worked in South Africa, Spain and England. Rae's other work experiences include being a lecturer, assessing and providing aids and adaptations, implementing the Manual Handling Regulations and working as a Rehabilitation Coordinator in the Rehabilitation Link Team for three years.

Jacquetta Williams is a Research Officer at the Personal Social Services Research Unit at the University of Kent. She has conducted research in the areas of care homes for older people and social care regulation. Prior to this she worked in the field of education research. Jacquetta is currently completing doctoral research on the process of closure of voluntary independent care homes for older people. The focus of her current research interests includes new forms of housing and care, as well as residential care, councils' powers and duties, and regulation.

Geoff Wood is Patient and Public Influence Manager for Central Cheshire Primary Care Trust. He has worked in the public sector for many years with long-standing interests in public health, health promotion and community development. Recent areas of work include helping to change and modernise NHS organisations based on the experiences of patients and views of local people.

Part 1
Intermediate Care

Chapter 1

Intermediate Care: Policy and Context

Jenny Cowpe

Introduction

The term 'intermediate care', as applied to elements of the British health and social care systems, emerged in the mid-1990s. Initially ambiguous, with its origins predating adoption as formal government policy, it was first recognised officially in the National Beds Inquiry consultation document (Department of Health, 2000a). Department of Health policy on this subject is now contained in the 2001 Health and Local Authority circular, HSC 2001/01: LAC (2001)1 (Department of Health, 2001a) and in Standard 3 of the *National Service Framework for Older People* (Department of Health, 2001b).

What is intermediate care? Its short history is peppered with attempted definitions, reflecting the evolutionary process by which the services now bearing this description have developed over recent years. Some essential common elements have emerged: these services are locally based, providing 'care closer to home' (Department of Health, 2000a, p. 13); they are focused on maintaining or restoring independence and are rehabilitative in nature; they are of short term duration. A key feature is the multiprofessional nature of the delivery teams, which are drawn from both health and social care. For the sake of clarity, a more comprehensive definition is attempted here:

'Intermediate care, when fully developed, comprises networks of local health and social care services, which deliver targeted, short term support to individual patients or clients, in order to prevent inappropriate admission to NHS acute inpatient or continuing care, or long-term residential care, facilitate earlier discharge from hospital and, most importantly, maximise people's ability to live independently within their communities.'

At present, most intermediate care services are focused on providing support for older people and will generally be provided in service users' own homes, or in community based settings, although, in some instances, they may be provided in discrete facilities on acute hospital sites. 'Social care' is provided by statutory, voluntary and independent agencies and also local authority housing departments.

The growth of intermediate care since the mid-1990s is a fascinating example of a grassroots response to local service pressures (albeit within a developing national 'consciousness'), which has dramatically influenced the direction of Government policy. However, its early history, one of local initiatives, usually small scale and established on short-term funding (and thus lacking stability), has resulted in a wide diversity of models: 'a thousand flowers have bloomed' (Department of Health, 2002b, p. 5). There has been no consistent approach across the country; while local initiative has been a strength, the proliferation of schemes has also led, in some areas, 'to confusion and fragmentation, in turn resulting in inequality of provision and access, duplication of effort, reduced cost effectiveness, and loss of impact' (Department of Health, 2002b, p. 5). In addition, until recently, there has been little robust evaluation of the effectiveness of intermediate care, and therefore no real guidance for investment decisions.

In this chapter the following themes are explored:

- The context within which intermediate care has evolved.
- The development of government policy on the subject.
- Some of the key policy and implementation issues which require resolution in order to embed intermediate care firmly into mainstream services.

Context

Whilst the term 'intermediate care' is relatively new, the underlying concept of inter-agency cooperation to maximise independent living, particularly for older people, clearly is not. Indeed, as Swift has recently argued in his article on the *National Service Framework for Older People*, 'in successful departments (providing specialist medical care for older people) excellent partnerships with other agencies (particularly primary and social care) and with other specialties have been axiomatic' (Swift, 2002). That being the case, why has there been such interest in 'intermediate care' in recent years?

The answer to this question lies in the complex interaction of a number of contextual factors, which coalesced in the 1990s to create a health and social care climate where increased demand, and changes in supply, produced service pressures which, allied with financial incentives, led to a search for alternative delivery methods, both at a local and national, level which made more intensive and appropriate use of health and social care resources. Thus, while local communities explored the potential benefits which a closer partnership between health and social care might bring, particularly at the interface between acute hospital care and community NHS and social care, at a Governmental level there was a developing interest in international experience of alternative systems, which also coincided with a greater focus on individual patient care. These contextual factors are examined in more detail below.

Changes in demand

A number of factors fuelled an increase in demand for health and social care services in the late 20th century. These included demographic trends, technical advances, and consumer awareness and expectations.

Demographic trends

In the latter years of the 20th century, demographic trends were continuing to change the underlying structure of the UK population. Between 1981 and 1997, total population increased by just 5%; interestingly, there was a drop in those aged between 65 and 74 but, and notably, those aged between 75 and 84 increased by 18% and those over 85 increased by 80% (Audit Commission, 1997). In addition, recent estimates have predicted that, from the mid-1990s, the number of people in England aged 65 and over will rise by almost 57% until the third decade of the 21st century and the number of people over 85 will rise by 79% over the same period (Vaughan and Lathlean, 1999). These trends have significant resource implications for both the health and social care sectors, since, as is well known, older people are major consumers of these services.

In its 1997 publication *The Coming of Age: Improving Care Services for Older People*, the Audit Commission noted that, while those over 65 constituted 14% of the population, they accounted for 47% of Department of Health expenditure and 48% of local authority social services expenditure (Audit Commission, 1997). In 2000, the National Beds Inquiry found that people aged over 65 occupied two-thirds of general and acute hospital beds and accounted for over half the recent growth in emergency admissions (Department of Health, 2000a). In addition to increased pressure on acute services, older people tend to recover more slowly than younger people and this places more pressure on both transitional and social care services.

Technical advances

In addition to demographic changes, technical advances in the late 20th century created a greater demand for chronic care support. These advances improved life expectancy generally, but also enabled people with serious disabilities to extend their lifespan. They also allowed more intensive therapies to be delivered at home, making home based care options feasible.

Increasing consumer awareness and expectations

Increasing consumer awareness, knowledge and expectations have created a demand for better rehabilitation services. Consumers also have a natural preference to be at home rather than in hospital or institutional residential care. As Steiner has noted, one of the attractions of intermediate care is that it 'focuses on the transition away from the status of "patient" towards the restoration of "person"' (Steiner, 1997, p. 5).

Changes in supply

Within the NHS, the second half of the 20th century saw a dramatic reduction in the number of NHS staffed beds for acute, general and maternity care, which peaked at around 250 000 in 1960 but had reduced to 147 000 by the end of the 1990s (Department of Health, 2000a). In addition, and particularly relevant to this debate, geriatric bed numbers fell from 56 000 to 30 000 over the same period (Vaughan and Lathlean, 1999). This trend was taking place at the same time as an increase in general hospital admissions and particularly admissions of older people: the National Beds Inquiry found that 'year on year, there has been continuous growth in the proportion of older people requiring overnight stays in hospital' (Department of Health, 2000a, p. 8). Importantly, the Inquiry also found that 'for older people around 20% of bed days were probably inappropriate if alternative facilities were in place' (Department of Health, 2000a, p. 8).

While the acute sector's ability to manage an increasing number of admissions through reducing numbers of beds has been partly attributable to the growth in day cases, it has also been managed through a sharp decline in the average length of time patients spend in hospital. From 1981 to 1996/97, average acute length of stay (per finished consultant episode) decreased from 9.3 to 5 days, while the average length of stay for people over 65 decreased from 66.1 to 18.6 days (Vaughan and Lathlean, 1999). Although this decline slowed towards the end of the decade, its impact had considerable implications for older people, who need longer to recover, creating pressures both within the acute health service (bed blocking) and on transitional and social care support, at a time when there had also been considerable changes in the availability of these latter services.

Before 1983, most publicly funded social care was provided directly by the public sector, through local authority social services residential, day and home care and housing departments. In the early 1980s, the availability of social security payments for care in private and voluntary sector residential and nursing homes for anyone qualifying for supplementary benefit, irrespective of need, (rising to £2.5 billion a year by 1993), led to a rapid expansion of this market, with independent sector nursing and residential beds increasing by 242% between 1983 and 1996. By contrast, the number of local authority residential beds fell by 43%, and the provision of home care to those aged 75 and over fell by 25%.

In parallel, the availability of social security monies in the 1980s enabled many health authorities to reduce their provision for long-term care, closing old and outdated geriatric and psychogeriatric wards and freeing revenue for use elsewhere (Audit Commission, 1997). Thus, during the 1990s, demand, particularly from older people, increased at a time when capacity within local authority-provided services was reducing. Expansion was taking place in the independent and voluntary sector, but at considerable cost to the taxpayer.

Changes in financial incentives

The 1980s and 1990s in the NHS were marked by a constant search for greater efficiency and productivity, as health organisations attempted to respond to increasing demand within a resource limited framework. As a result, there were considerable incentives to encourage more economical use of existing services and to develop new options which might reduce overall costs. The introduction, under the Thatcher Government, of the purchaser/provider split intensified pressures to provide health services at the lowest possible cost, whilst the advent of general practitioner and total fundholding created interest in service innovation and a focus on reducing hospital stays and expanding community care.

In social services, the 1990s were characterised by a number of pressures: supply side changes (as indicated previously); changes in funding arrangements (specifically, the capping of funds previously available through the social services system and their transfer to local authorities through the Special Transitional Grant); and the requirement, under the NHS and Community Care Act 1990 (introduced 1 April 1993) to act as lead agency for arranging comprehensive packages of social care. These combined to create a climate of incentives to prevent premature admission to long-term residential community care and maximise people's ability to live (relatively) independent lives within their communities for as long as possible.

A new UK government

The newly elected Labour Government in May 1997 focused renewed attention on the operation of the increasingly pressured health and social care systems. Major early policy documents such as *The New NHS: Modern, Dependable* (Department of Health, 1997b) and *Modernising Social Services* (Department of Health, 1998b) addressed the need to modernise service delivery through greater responsiveness to patients' and clients' needs, and by improving the partnership between, in particular, the health service and social services, in order to provide 'seamless' care. Later policy documents have placed greater emphasis on the delivery of services 'closer to home' (Department of Health, 2000a).

In addition, and for the same reasons, there was increasing interest in international developments in hospital bed utilisation. The National Beds Inquiry noted, for instance, 'a number of healthcare systems in the USA operate on hospital bed days (per 1000 population) that are roughly half the current England average and below the rate of even the lowest health authority. Their admission rates and average lengths of stay are both one-third lower than in England.' The Inquiry also noted that, in contrast to England, in some countries, notably the Netherlands, Canada and the USA, hospital admission rates for older people had been 'flat or falling for many years. In these countries, increasing pressures for emergency care are dealt with in the community or in ambulatory or outpatient facilities' (Department of Health, 2000a, p. 10). Of particular interest to the UK Government was the conclusion that 'health systems with low hospital bed utilisation appear to be characterised by a large range of ambulatory and intermediate care facilities and/or strict control on hospital services and expenditures' (Department of Health, 2000a, p. 10), and there has been much recent discussion and analysis of the benefits of organisations such as Kaiser Permanente in the United States (Light and Dixon, 2004).

Net effect

Thus, by the mid to late 1990s, the coalescence of the factors outlined above created an environment in which both health and social care organisations had an interest in exploring alternative service options, both to relieve pressure on acute and residential care and to make more efficient use of resources. In creating local responses to service pressures, 'intermediate care' was developed out of local necessity.

Policy development

As indicated earlier, the development of intermediate care is an interesting example of a grassroots service response to local pressures which has become mainstream policy. Its history demonstrates the important interplay between local service initiative and Government interest in stimulating an effective response to perceived service problems. The development of Government policy is traced below.

Although its formal history is short, three phases of policy development concerning intermediate care are already visible:

- *The early phase*, characterised by the search for a meaningful definition and ad hoc service developments.
- *The second phase*, when the requirement to develop intermediate care services became mainstream Department of Health policy and additional funding for both health and social services stimulated growth and expansion.
- *The current phase*, when Government policy is focusing on more effective coordination and integration – at professional, service and agency level – to create a 'whole systems' approach.

The early phase: mid-1990s to 2000

In the late 1980s and early 1990s, a number of experimental schemes, aimed at rehabilitation after hospital care, and often to support earlier discharge from acute hospitals, emerged on an ad hoc basis in the United Kingdom. In October 1996, a King's Fund seminar drew attention to these developments and to their potential to address some of the critical system pressures faced by both the health and social service sectors (Steiner and Vaughan, 1996).

During the later 1990s and in 2000, a number of other agencies and bodies commented on the potential of rehabilitation services to help to address service pressures, including the Department of Health, the (then) NHS Executive, the Social Services Inspectorate, the House of Commons Health Select Committee, the Royal Commission on Long Term Care for the Elderly and the British Geriatric Society. In addition, the Audit Commission published three reports: *United They Stand* (1995), *The Coming of Age* (1997) and *The Way to Go Home* (2000), which drew

Box 1.1 Intermediate care: early policy questions.

- What is it?
- Is rehabilitation the same as intermediate care?
- Is intermediate care a separate system or level within the total care structure?
- Is intermediate care an alternative to acute care or supplementary?
- Which types of service can be categorised as intermediate care (e.g. is rehabilitation on an acute site to be considered in this category)?
- Who are the target audience (i.e. older people only or should intermediate care cover those with serious and chronic disabilities)?
- What is the proper location for intermediate care services (i.e. 'a bridge between hospital and home' that is, not including home, or excluding services on an acute hospital site)?

---

attention to the shortcomings in the way in which health and social services worked together to develop services that would offer alternative options to unnecessary hospital, residential care or nursing home admission, or which could help vulnerable patients to recover greater independence following discharge.

In parallel, the Government issued a number of policy documents, particularly *Better Services for Vulnerable People* (Department of Health, 1997a) and *Better Services for Vulnerable People: Maintaining the Momentum* (Department of Health, 1998a), which emphasised the contribution that rehabilitation could make to the management of demand across the health and social care economy; the requirement for health and social services to work in partnership was also emphasised by section 31 of the Health Act 1999.

The evolution of thinking about intermediate care services during this early phase was marked by the search for a viable definition of the subject, which sought to answer a series of policy questions set out in Box 1.1. The questions themselves are an indication both of the terminological difficulties (compounded by different perceptions within different agencies, organisations and professional groups) and of the variety of models being developed. Although interest was growing, there was no formal Government policy statement about 'intermediate care'.

The second phase: 2000 to 2004

The year 2000 marked a watershed: for the first time, the description 'intermediate care' was given formal recognition in the National Beds Inquiry (Department of Health, 2000a). The second phase is therefore characterised by increasing certainty about definition and the emergence of a clear Government strategy and dedicated funding, albeit with a particular focus on older people as the target audience.

The key policy milestones in this phase are:

- *Shaping the Future NHS: Long-term Planning for Hospitals and Related Services.* The National Beds Inquiry (Department of Health, 2000a).

- *The NHS Plan: A Plan for Investment, A Plan for Reform* (Department of Health, 2000b).
- *Intermediate Care* HSC 2001/01: LAC (2001)1 (Department of Health, 2001a).
- *National Service Framework for Older People* (Department of Health, 2001b).
- *Securing our Future Health: Taking a Long-term View*. The first Wanless Report (HM Treasury, 2002).
- *Delivering the NHS Plan: Next Steps on Investment, Next Steps on Reform* (Department of Health, 2002a).
- *National Service Framework for Older People – Supporting Implementation. Intermediate Care: Moving Forward* (Department of Health, 2002b).

The contributions of each of these policy documents are briefly outlined below.

The National Beds Inquiry: 2000

The National Beds Inquiry examined recent trends in acute hospital activity, comparing bed usage in the UK with international experience. For the UK it 'found evidence of significant inappropriate or avoidable use of acute hospital beds', and in particular 'for older people, around 20% of bed days were probably inappropriate if alternative facilities were in place' (Department of Health, 2000a, p. 8). Arising from these findings, the Secretary of State consulted on three scenarios for the future development of care:

- Maintaining current direction, with no attempt to transfer services from hospital into community settings.
- Active development of acute bed focused care, where a wider range of services, including rapid assessment and rehabilitation, would be provided mainly in a hospital setting.
- Care closer to home, where there would be a major expansion of community health and social care to support the development of intermediate care services in order to avoid unnecessary admissions to acute care and to facilitate earlier discharge and a return to functional independence. Under this scenario acute hospital services would be focused on rapid assessment, stabilisation and treatment.

Option 3 was accepted, and subsequently developed as part of the NHS Plan.

The NHS Plan: 2000

The NHS Plan (Department of Health, 2000b), issued in July 2000, contained, amongst many developments, proposals for a major new programme to promote the independence of older people through developing a range of intermediate care and related services. It suggested a number of service models, with the stated aims of:

Box 1.2 Intermediate care: expected outputs.

- At least 5000 additional intermediate care beds and 1700 non-residential intermediate care places, together benefiting around 150 000 more older people each year
- Rapid response teams and other avoidable admission prevention teams benefiting around 70 000 more people each year
- 50 000 more people enabled to live at home through additional home care and other support
- Carers' respite care services extended to benefit 75 000 carers and those they care for compared with the 1999/2000 base line

All compared with the 1999/2000 base line.
From *Delivering the NHS Plan: Next Steps on Investment, Next Steps on Reform* (Department of Health 2002a). Crown copyright. Reproduced with permission from the Controller of HMSO and the Queen's Printer for Scotland.

- Helping people to recover and regain independence more quickly.
- Enabling easier discharge from acute care.
- Avoiding unnecessary long-term care.

The Plan explicitly provided for an extra £900m investment by 2003/4 to support these developments in the health and social care sectors. The NHS would receive approximately £405m, the balance relating to resources provided to local government, mostly for the personal social services. Tangible outputs expected by March 2004 from this investment are shown in Box 1.2.

The expectation from these intermediate care developments was that inappropriate acute admissions and avoidable delays in discharge would be dramatically reduced.

The Plan identified intermediate care as a key test of improved partnership between health and social services, and the Commission for Health Improvement, the Audit Commission and the Social Services Inspectorate were given responsibility for monitoring both progress towards the targets and the operation of effective joint working between the agencies.

Health and Local Authority Circular HSC 2001/01: LAC (2001)1

This circular was the first detailed statement of Government policy on intermediate care and provided 'initial guidance' on:

- The definition of intermediate care and appropriate service models.
- Responsibility for intermediate care and the role of the independent sector.
- Funding for intermediate care and community equipment services and charges for local authority services.

With regard to definition, the circular was prescriptive in stating that intermediate care should be regarded as describing services which meet all the following criteria:

Box 1.3   Intermediate care models.

- *Rapid response*: designed to prevent avoidable acute admissions by providing rapid assessment and diagnosis for patients referred from GPs, A&E, NHS Direct or social services and, if necessary, rapid access on a 24-hour basis to short-term nursing or therapy support and personal care in the patient's own home.
- *Hospital at home*: intensive support in the patient's own home.
- *Residential rehabilitation*: a short-term programme of therapy and enablement in a residential setting (e.g. a community hospital, rehabilitation centre, nursing home or residential care home) for people who are medically stable but need a short period of rehabilitation to enable them to regain sufficient physical functioning and confidence to return safely to their own home.
- *Supported discharge*: a short-term period of nursing and/or therapeutic support in a patient's home, to enable the patient to be discharged from acute care and to allow a patient to complete his/her rehabilitation and recovery at home.
- *Day rehabilitation*: a short-term programme of therapeutic support, provided at a day hospital or day centre.

Adapted from Health and Local Authority Circular HSC 2001/01: LAC (2001)1. Crown copyright. Reproduced with the permission of the Controller of HMSO and the Queen's Printer for Scotland.

- Focused on preventing unnecessary admission to health or social care facilities, and facilitating earlier discharge from hospital.
- Involving a comprehensive assessment and individual care plan, designed to maximise independence.
- Time-limited, normally lasting no longer than six weeks.
- Involving multi-agency input, but with a single assessment framework and record, and shared protocols.

It contained a specific framework of service models as shown in Box 1.3.

Critical to the effective functioning of intermediate care was the role of the care coordinator, who would have responsibility and accountability for developing care pathways and protocols for access to services, and for ensuring that intermediate care was integrated across primary care, community health services, social care, housing and the acute sector. The circular advised local NHS bodies and councils to appoint jointly one coordinator in at least each health authority area initially.

The National Service Framework for Older People: 2001

The *National Service Framework for Older People* encapsulated the Government's determination to deliver real improvements for older people and their families. In particular, Standard 3 was devoted to a detailed description of intermediate care services. The Standard is as follows:

'Older people will have access to a new range of intermediate care services at home, or in designated care settings, to promote their independence by providing enhanced services from the NHS and councils to prevent unnecessary

hospital admission and effective rehabilitation services to enable early discharge from hospital and to prevent premature or unnecessary admission to
long term residential care.' (Department of Health, 2001b, p. 41)

The *National Service Framework* defines the aim of intermediate care as 'to
provide integrated services to promote faster recovery from illness, prevent
unnecessary acute hospital admissions, support timely discharge and maximise
independent living' (Department of Health, 2001b, p. 41). The use of the term
'integrated services' is interesting, reflecting the Government's concern to move
forward from the fragmented approach which characterised the early phase
and to avoid the confusion over definition, a strategy further emphasised by the
later statement in the document that 'the key to this next phase of intermediate
care development is integrated and shared care, including primary and secondary
health care, social care, and involving the statutory and independent sectors'
(Department of Health, 2001b, p. 42).

In contrast, it is interesting to note recent decisions in Scotland, where, in
March 2003, the Scottish Executive made clear that they had decided not to pursue
the label 'intermediate care', arguing that it was unclear what distinguished
intermediate care from 'good, patient-centred mainstream services' and prefer-
ring the words 'integrated care' (Petch, 2003).

Standard 3 indicated that intermediate care services should focus on three key
points in the pathway of care: responding to or averting a crisis; active rehabilitation following an acute hospital stay; and where long-term care is being
considered.

Fundamental to the successful and effective delivery of intermediate care was:

- An open and effective partnership between health and social care agencies,
  involving a commitment to joint planning and joint investment.
- The requirement for providers to ensure that patients offered intermediate
  care support had guaranteed access to specialist assessment, diagnosis and
  treatment if required.
- The provision of care by a coordinated team, including, as appropriate,
  general practitioners and hospital doctors, nurses and physiotherapists, occupational therapists, speech and language therapists and social workers, with
  support from care assistants and administrative staff.

Other policy documents

Government policy on the development of intermediate care has been further
emphasised in both the first Wanless Report (HM Treasury, 2002) and in the
second report on the NHS Plan (Department of Health, 2002a). The former report,
highly influential in persuading the Government to announce, in the April 2002
budget, investment of an additional £40 billion for the health service up to
2007/8, together with a 6% increase in funding over three years for the personal
social services, stated 'the review believes the current balance between health

and social care is wrong: in particular, care is too focused on the acute hospital setting' (HM Treasury, 2002, p. 106). The latter document, while re-emphasising the requirement 'to prevent hospital admission and to provide more rehabilitation', stated that 'although progress has been made towards breaching the "Berlin Wall" between health and social care, there are still too many parts of the country where a failure to cooperate means that older people fail to get the holistic services they need' (Department of Health, 2002a, p. 32).

This last point was re-emphasised in the National Audit Office Report *Ensuring the Effective Discharge of Older Patients from NHS Acute Hospitals*, published in 2003, which commented on the 'mixed results to date' on joint working between health and social services to reduce delayed discharges (National Audit Office, 2003).

Finally, in the paper *Intermediate Care: Moving Forward* (Department of Health, 2002b), an assessment of progress to date was made, the guiding principles for intermediate care were explored, a series of useful practical case studies was presented (together with a list of success factors to guide implementation), and a useful review of research evidence to date was included.

Thus, the second phase of policy development was marked by a rapid and prolific production of policy statements. The reality in terms of implementation, however, did not meet Government expectations. Many examples of good practice had emerged, but there were still numbers of health and social care systems where services were less well developed, and where fragmentation and poor integration with other services were evident.

The current phase

The year 2004 marked another watershed in the development of intermediate care services. As indicated above, several major targets outlined in the NHS Plan were to be achieved by March 2004; if met, much needed extra service capacity will have been created. In addition, three major research projects on intermediate care, commissioned by the Policy Research Programme at the Department of Health, jointly with the Medical Research Council, are nearing completion. These projects involve:

- A national evaluation of the costs and outcomes of intermediate care services for older people.
- A comparative case study and national audit of intermediate care expenditure.
- A multi-centre study of the effectiveness of community hospitals in providing intermediate care for older people.

Their results will provide important information, and evidence, about the development of intermediate care across the country, its effectiveness and comparative costs, and the outcome for both service users and carers, and for the health and social care systems as a whole.

As the 2002 Department of Health paper *Intermediate Care: Moving Forward* stated: 'In many ways . . . intermediate care is still in its infancy and it depends on new ways of working within complex partnerships' (Department of Health, 2002b, p. 4). The early, and to some extent the second, phases of development have been marked by innovation but also, in some places, by inconsistency and fragmentation. There is a now a need, taking into account reliable, evaluative evidence, to create more coherent services, integrated across local health and social care systems. Intermediate care services are 'quintessentially, about partnership between organisations and professions' and yet 'one of the reasons that people have yet to enter into effective partnerships is that they may not know who all the partners are, or should be, and how they interact with each other. There is a need to understand system dynamics – components and interactions – both conceptually and in quantifiable terms' (Department of Health, 2002b, p. 6). The current phase of development will hopefully be marked by both a greater investment in effective, inter-agency, partnerships and by the creation of coherent local networks providing intermediate care services, where these services can clearly be recognised by their function of providing targeted, short-term care to prevent avoidable admission to hospital or long-term care, of facilitating earlier discharge, and above all, of enabling vulnerable people (be they older people or people with a variety of chronic disabilities) to maximise their independence.

Unresolved policy and implementation issues

A number of major policy and implementation issues remain to be resolved before the full potential of intermediate care can be realised, and some of the key questions are outlined below.

In terms of policy:

- Is the concept and definition of intermediate care sufficiently well understood, and, if understood, accepted generally, to provide a robust platform for moving forward?
- Which patient or client groups should be the beneficiaries of intermediate care support? Most focus to date has been on the needs of older people, but people with chronic physical disabilities and people with mental health problems may equally benefit.
- Is there good evidence to suggest that intermediate care services are:
  - delivering better outcomes for patients or clients than more traditional models?
  - accepted and supported by patients or clients and by their carers (do we understand the demand placed on carers by intensive support at home)?
  - cost effective?
- How is the question of charging for services (in relation to social care) to be resolved?

- What guidance, if any, is necessary to ensure that the principle of ensuring timely access to the appropriate levels of specialist care is implemented for all users of intermediate care services?
- What guidance is necessary to develop appropriate clinical governance mechanisms within intermediate care?
- Critically, will local health and social care systems be able to fund, and then sustain, the levels of investment required for effective intermediate care interventions or will this require further Government support?

In terms of implementation key concerns are:

- The action required to support effective partnership arrangements in areas of the country where joint working has not been effective in delivering intermediate care.
- The need to ascertain which models of single assessment work best and how they can be disseminated.
- The training and development implications of intermediate care services.
- The mechanisms likely to be most effective in disseminating examples of good practice.
- The most appropriate arrangements for commissioning intermediate care.

Funding remains a major hurdle to the development of coherent local services. Although both the NHS and the social services are now receiving the considerable extra funds promised in the April 2002 Budget, the issue of their allocation remains: will appropriate sums be allocated to these services, thus relieving pressures elsewhere, or will other targets and policy imperatives take precedence? Once again, it will be interesting to observe the interplay between local initiatives and developments and Government policy.

Summary

Intermediate care must be carefully defined in order to make sense to those who are interested in developing these services locally. A general definition is suggested in the Introduction to this chapter and the range of services now recognised under this title are included in Box 1.3. In its early development phase, intermediate care emerged as a grass roots response to local service pressures; it was only later (from 2000 onwards) adopted as mainstream government policy. The major policy statements on intermediate care are contained in the National Beds Inquiry consultation document (Department of Health, 2000a), the NHS Plan (Department of Health, 2000b), the Health Service and Local Authority circular issued in January 2001 (Department of Health, 2001a) and the *National Service Framework for Older People* (Department of Health, 2001b).

    The context in which intermediate care developed was shaped by a number of factors, including changes in demand for, and supply of, health and social care, financial pressures which created incentives for greater efficiency in resource use, and the election of a new Labour Government in May 1997. To work effectively, intermediate care networks require commitment and effective partnerships between health and social care agencies and the provision of care by coordinated teams of health and social care practitioners.

A number of key policy questions remain to be answered in order to obtain the maximum benefits for patients. Particularly important is the allocation of appropriate funding to develop coherent local networks capable of delivering the targeted services required.

References

Audit Commission (1995) *United They Stand: Co-ordinating Care for Elderly Patients with Hip Fractures*. London: Audit Commission.

Audit Commission (1997) *The Coming of Age: Improving Care Services for Older People*. London: Audit Commission.

Audit Commission (2000) *The Way to Go Home: Rehabilitation and Remedial Services for Older People*. London: Audit Commission.

Department of Health (1997a) *Better Services for Vulnerable People*. London: Department of Health.

Department of Health (1997b) *The New NHS: Modern, Dependable*. London: Department of Health.

Department of Health (1998a) *Better Services for Vulnerable People: Maintaining the Momentum*. London: Department of Health.

Department of Health (1998b) *Modernising Social Services*. London: Department of Health.

Department of Health (2000a) *Shaping the Future NHS: Long-term Planning for Hospitals and Related Services*. National Beds Inquiry. London: Department of Health.

Department of Health (2000b) *The NHS Plan: A Plan for Investment, A Plan for Reform*. London: Department of Health.

Department of Health (2001a). HSC 2001/01: LAC (2001)1 *Intermediate Care*. London: Department of Health.

Department of Health (2001b) *National Service Framework for Older People*. London: Department of Health.

Department of Health (2002a) *Delivering the NHS Plan: Next Steps on Investment, Next Steps on Reform*. London: Department of Health.

Department of Health (2002b) *National Service Framework for Older People – Supporting Implementation. Intermediate Care: Moving Forward*. London: Department of Health.

HM Treasury (2002) *Securing our Future Health: Taking a Long-term View. Final Report*. London: HM Treasury (The Wanless Report).

Light, D., Dixon, N. (2004) Making the NHS more like Kaiser Permanente. *British Medical Journal* **328**, 763–5.

National Audit Office (2003) *Ensuring the Effective Discharge of Older Patients from NHS Acute Hospitals*. London: National Audit Office.

Petch, A. (2003). *Intermediate Care: What Do We Know about Older People's Experiences?* York: Joseph Rowntree Foundation.

Steiner, A. (1997) *Intermediate Care: A Conceptual Framework and Review of the Literature*. London: King's Fund.

Steiner, A., Vaughan, B. (1996) *Intermediate Care: A Discussion Paper Arising from the King's Fund Seminar held on 30th October 1996*. London: King's Fund.

Swift, C. (2002) The NHS English National Framework for Older People: opportunities and risks. *Clinical Medicine* **2** (2), 129–43.

Vaughan, B., Lathlean J. (1999) *Intermediate Care: Models in Practice*. London: King's Fund.

Chapter 2
Identifying the Need and Scope for Intermediate Care
Roger Beech

Introduction

The National Inquiry into the use of acute beds throughout the National Health Service of the United Kingdom acted as a springboard for the policy to expand services for intermediate care (Department of Health, 2000a). This inquiry had been convened because of the difficulties that patients were facing in gaining access to services for acute inpatient care. These difficulties included long 'trolley' waits in casualty departments while patients waited for a hospital bed to become available, and the cancellation of elective admissions because beds for these admissions were being 'borrowed' by emergency patients (Beech, 2003).

The Inquiry concluded that a lack of overall capacity for inpatient care was, in part, a cause of such difficulties. It also concluded that a shortage of service alternatives to acute care was a cause and this meant that some acute beds were being used by patients whose care needs could be met in other settings. This conclusion was based on the findings of previous studies which had estimated that the prevalence of 'avoidable' bed use by adult medical patients ranged from 15–50% and that amongst older people at least 20% of bed use was 'avoidable' (McDonagh et al., 2000). As a result, the expansion of services for intermediate care was included as a core component of the UK Government's long-term plan of investment in and reform of the NHS (Department of Health, 2000b).

Intermediate care services have been defined as those 'designed to prevent avoidable admissions to acute care settings, and to facilitate the transition from hospital to home and from medical dependence to functional independence' (Department of Health, 2000a, p. 13). The types of scheme promoted in the NHS Plan include: multidisciplinary rapid response teams for preventing avoidable acute admission by providing care in patients' homes; for those patients who do require hospital admission, the use of 'step-down' beds in non-acute institutions or integrated home care teams to facilitate their timely acute hospital discharge; intensive rehabilitation services to help patients regain their independence more quickly; and one-stop clinics to improve patient access to services for health and social care (Department of Health, 2000b).

Such national policy directives need to be interpreted locally to ensure that when services for intermediate care are introduced they are in keeping with the needs of local patients. If not, either an inappropriate match between the care needs of potential users and the skill mix of service providers, or an inappropriate match between the capacity of the service and the potential number of service users, might result (Audit Commission, 2000; Department of Health, 2001). In other words, local health and social care professionals need to plan the introduction of services for intermediate care to ensure that the 'right' services are set up for the 'right' people in the 'right' place.

In a report prepared for the King's Fund, Stevenson and Spencer described the following 'cycle of change' surrounding the introduction of services for intermediate care: 'agreeing the future direction of intermediate care development'; 'making practical plans'; 'putting intermediate care into practice'; 'evaluation' of those services introduced (Stevenson and Spencer, 2002). This chapter describes analytical approaches that can be used to generate information to support planning activity during the first two elements of this planning cycle. In particular, whether the 'avoidable' use of acute beds currently exists and, if so, why does it exist. The answers to these questions help to identify whether or not an expansion of services for intermediate care is relevant locally and who the potential users of such services might be. The planning approaches described in this chapter were identified as a result of a study undertaken for the former Research and Development Directorate of the NHS Executive West Midlands (Beech and Cropper, 2001). The analytical framework that was developed was based upon a review of the scientific and grey literature and discussions with professionals involved in the development of services for intermediate care.

The following section of the chapter discusses the ways in which routinely available performance indicators can be used to undertake an initial assessment of whether or not the avoidable use of beds might be a problem in an acute hospital. Performance indicator analysis can also be used to highlight the types of patients who might be causing avoidable bed use and to provide a baseline against which to judge the impacts of any expansion of intermediate care services. However, to confirm the existence, nature, and scale of avoidable acute bed use, a more detailed approach is required. The subsequent section of the chapter describes the ways in which Utilisation Review, the systematic audit of the use of acute beds through the interrogation of clinical records, can be used to provide this additional information (Bristow et al., 1998). Indeed, studies which used Utilisation Review techniques were probably most influential in the National Beds Inquiry reaching its conclusion that an expansion of services for intermediate care was a key means of tackling problems surrounding patient access to NHS acute beds (Department of Health, 2000a; McDonagh et al., 2000).

If potential for an expanded role for services for intermediate care is identified, planning will then shift to the design of these services. The final section of the chapter summarises the key issues that will need to be explored in planning activity. In particular, information will be needed to ensure that there is an appropriate match between the care needs of potential users and the nature of those services provided to supply intermediate care. This aspect of planning is developed further in chapters 3 and 4.

Using performance indicators to support the planning of services for intermediate care

Focusing planning activity

The 'avoidable' use of acute beds might be linked to: the 'avoidable' admission of patients; delays in the acute management of patients; and delays in the acute discharge of patients. Performance indicator analysis aims to maximise the potential of readily available data to undertake an initial assessment of whether or not the avoidable use of acute beds might exist within a hospital and, if so, amongst which types of patients. Performance indicator analysis therefore helps to focus subsequent planning activity that is based on more sophisticated and time-consuming techniques and the use of non-readily available data.

Box 2.1 describes the ways in which performance indicators have been used to explore the possible existence of problems surrounding the avoidable acute admission or re-admission of patients, and Box 2.2 indicates potential problems surrounding their timely acute discharge (Audit Commission, 1997; Department of Health, 2000a; 2001; National Audit Office, 2000). Local performance in terms of, for example, acute admission rates per head of population or acute lengths of stay can be compared with an agreed benchmark: the national or regional norm, the norm for similar types of locations, or a locally agreed target. When undertaking this analysis, it is helpful to subdivide patient groups in terms of their diagnosis and/or age. Relatively high admission rates might suggest a shortage of service alternatives to acute care and relatively long lengths of stay might suggest delays in the acute management and discharge of patients.

Performance indicators can also be used to monitor internal hospital performance, regardless of performance elsewhere. For example, a high proportion of patients with a length of stay of less than two days might indicate that some admissions are avoidable. Alternatively, possible delays in acute management or discharge can be investigated by examining the proportion of patients with an acute stay longer than 15 days (an arbitrary cut-off point) and by comparing the lengths of stay of patients over and under 65 years of age: if older patients have longer lengths of stay this might be because of difficulties surrounding their discharge. Again, when performing this analysis it is helpful to subdivide patient groups by diagnosis.

Finally, rather than generating hypotheses about the existence of avoidable acute bed use, performance indicator analysis can be used simply to focus subsequent planning activity. Rankings can be generated in terms of, for example, those specialties and age groups which generate most admissions and/or occupied bed days. This helps to prioritise subsequent efforts surrounding the development of schemes for delivering intermediate care.

Box 2.1 Performance indicators for highlighting possible problems surrounding avoidable admissions to acute inpatient beds.

Performance indicator	Its role

Emergency admission rate per head of population:
• Overall
• For over 65s
• For over 75s
• By specialty
• By diagnosis
• By GP practice
• By locality
	Relative to a chosen benchmark (e.g. the national rate, the rate for similar populations, a locally agreed target), a high rate might indicate that a high proportion of current admissions could be cared for in non-acute settings.
	  Subdividing the analysis by clinical diagnosis/specialty helps to highlight specific issues surrounding particular patient groups. Ongoing analysis might then focus on these groups.
	  Similarly, analysis by GP practice or locality might indicate variations in referral policies and admission rates. Spatial mapping packages provide an additional means of visually illustrating and exposing such geographical variations (Clarke and Clarke, 1997).

Number of admissions from A&E as a proportion of A&E attendances: • Overall • By time of day	The rate would need to be compared with a benchmark. Research suggests (Duffy et al., 1998) that a high rate is associated with an increased proportion of avoidable admissions. Subdividing the analysis by time of day might expose problems; for example, during the night when a lower proportion of senior clinical staff may be available.
Proportion of emergency admissions with a length of stay less than 2 days, either: • Overall • By age band • By specialty or diagnosis	A high proportion of short-stay patients might indicate the existence of avoidable admissions. The hypothesis to be explored is that short stay reflects either a lack of alternative care options or difficulties in providing timely access to services for assessing the care needs of patients.
Number of re-admissions as a proportion of total emergency admissions, either: • Overall • Within 28 days • By age band • By specialty or diagnosis	The issue to be explored is whether or not such re-admissions are potentially preventable. A high proportion might indicate premature discharge from previous acute care or inadequate follow-up after acute care.

As indicated above, the analysis of performance indicators represents an initial assessment of whether or not the avoidable use of acute beds might exist and, if so, amongst which types of patient. However, performance indicator analysis cannot confirm the existence of avoidable bed use. For example, differences in the complexity of its case mix rather than deficiencies in the organisation of its services might be the cause of a hospital having relatively long lengths of stay. In addition, the use of readily available data might be regarded as a weakness of performance indicator analysis as professionals might have concerns about the quality of the data. Hence, to confirm the existence and scale of problems surrounding the avoidable use of acute beds, and to assess why such problems exist, a more sophisticated planning methodology is required.

Box 2.2 Performance indicators for highlighting possible problems surrounding the timely discharge of patients from acute beds.

Performance indicator	Its role
Rankings of acute occupied bed days by: • Specialty • Diagnosis • Age band	An initial step that might be used to identify the focus of analytical activity. A way of identifying the main users of beds.
Occupied beds for emergencies per head of population: • Overall • For over 65s, 75s	A way of focusing ongoing analytical activity. Relative to a chosen benchmark a high figure might indicate scope for a shift in the balance of care away from the acute sector.
Length of stay of emergency admissions by: • Specialty • Diagnosis, e.g. stroke, fractured neck of femur • Age band	Relative to a chosen benchmark (e.g. the national stay, or the stay for similar hospitals), a relatively long stay might indicate organisational problems surrounding the delivery of care.
Ratio of length of stay of emergency admissions over and under 65 by: • Specialty • Diagnosis • Age band	Over 65s having a longer stay might indicate that non-acute factors are the cause. Such non-acute care needs might be suitable for intermediate care.
Proportion of emergency admissions with a length of stay over 15 days	15 days is an arbitrary cut-off point. The assumption is that stays beyond this figure are primarily due to non-acute care needs.
Number of patients awaiting discharge to community hospitals and residential homes	A high number relative to a benchmark indicates a shortage of step-down beds.
Number of re-admissions as a proportion of total emergency admissions, either: • Overall • Within 28 days • By age band • By specialty or diagnosis	A high proportion might indicate premature discharge from previous acute care or inadequate follow-up after acute care.

The ways in which Utilisation Review, the systematic audit of the uses of acute beds, can be used to supply this more detailed information is discussed later in this chapter.

Generating commitment to change

Performance indicator analysis can generate an awareness that further investments in schemes for intermediate care might be necessary. Further support for this argument can be gained by combining performance statistics with local population projections. In the supporting analysis for the National Beds Inquiry

(Department of Health, 2000a), age banded data covering population size, admission rates, lengths of stay and the proportion of elective admissions treated as day cases were used to examine three scenarios surrounding the future needs for acute beds within a health authority serving a population of 500 000 people. The scenarios differed in terms of their assumptions regarding the supply of services for non-acute based care.

In scenario 1 the current balance of acute and community based services remained largely unchanged, in scenario 2 there was an expansion of acute based services and in scenario 3 there was an expansion of care closer to home services. From a 2003/4 baseline of 5760 acute beds, projected bed requirements for 2019/20 were estimated as 6020 under the maintain current balance of acute and community based services scenario, as 6290 under the expand acute care scenario, and as 5820 under the expand care closer to home scenario. These results were used to demonstrate that an expansion of services for intermediate care might be the most feasible way of meeting future demands for health care. Within a locality, similar analysis could be used to indicate the importance of exploring the role that an expansion of services for intermediate care might play in meeting a population's future demands for health care.

Using utilisation review to support the planning of services for intermediate care

History and development of the approach

Interest in whether or not the care needs of users of acute beds could be met in other ways or settings is not new. McDonagh et al. (2000) systematically reviewed a number of studies, dating back to 1988, which had examined the extent to which acute bed use by older people was 'avoidable'. The studies varied in terms of the levels of avoidable bed use that they identified but their combined results led McDonagh et al. to conclude that approximately 11% of emergency admissions amongst older people were avoidable and at least 20% of acute days of care. More intensive ways of supplying outpatient care and the use of non-acute beds were seen as the main ways of preventing avoidable admissions whilst schemes that offered moderate nursing care or long-term care were typically seen as ways to reduce avoidable days of care. McDonagh et al. emphasised that more research was required to identify the precise ways of reducing levels of avoidable bed use. This is because the main aim of studies which review the utilisation of acute beds is to quantify current levels of avoidable bed: they offer only preliminary guidance on the ways in which this problem might be tackled.

Many of the studies reviewed by McDonagh et al. had used clinical opinion to assess whether or not care delivered in an acute bed was avoidable. This approach can be regarded as being too subjective so it is preferable for the review of acute bed utilisation to be undertaken using a screening tool that incorporates criteria which aim to define care that can be delivered only in an acute setting (McDonagh et al., 2000). The use of a criteria based tool increases the validity and reliability of the utilisation review process. Validity is a measure of the extent to which there will be general agreement about how adequately the instrument's criteria describe care that can be delivered only in an acute setting. Reliability is a measure of the extent to which the same judgement about a patient's need for care in an acute setting is reached when two or more reviewers consider the case notes of the same patient.

Criteria based screening tools that have been used in the NHS include the Appropriateness Evaluation Protocol (AEP) (Gertman and Restuccia, 1981; O'Neill and Pearson, 1995), the Intensity Severity Discharge Adult criteria (ISDA) (Jacobs and Lamprey, 1992; Coast et al., 1996), and the Oxford Bed Study Instrument (OBSI) (Anderson et al., 1988; Fenn et al., 2000). The AEP and ISDA originated in the United States and the OBSI in the United Kingdom. Both the AEP and ISDA have been tested for validity and reliability and are regarded as superior to other instruments (Strumwasser et al., 1990). However, it is the AEP that has become the most widely developed and used tool both in the NHS and elsewhere in Europe (McDonagh et al., 2000).

In mainland Europe, the need for a valid, reliable and consistent way of analysing and comparing avoidable bed use across and within countries acted as a springboard for the development of a European version of the AEP (Lorenzo et al., 1999). This research need demonstrates that the avoidable use of beds is not only a problem that affects NHS hospitals. In Spain, reported levels of avoidable acute admissions have ranged from 2.1% to 44.8% and of avoidable days of care from 15.0% to 43.9%. Delays in the transfer of patients to settings for follow-on care and the conservative management of patients by physicians were seen as the main causes of this avoidable bed use (Lorenzo and Sunol, 1995). Similarly, studies in Italy have found levels of avoidable acute admission ranging from 25% to 38% and levels of avoidable days of care ranging from 28% to 49%. Causes of avoidable bed use included delays in access to tests and investigations and delays in transfer to long-term care (Fellin et al., 1995).

A modified version of the AEP, for use in NHS hospitals, has also been developed and re-tested for validity and reliability (Bristow et al., 1997). Box 2.3 lists the criteria used by this modified AEP to define care appropriate for an acute inpatient setting on a patient's day of admission or on any subsequent day of their care. Relative to the original AEP, most of the criteria are the same although the process of modification did 'anglicise' the language used to describe them. However, on studying the original AEP's day of admission criteria, the clinicians involved in the modification process thought: that one extra criterion was required ('overdoses waiting for psychiatric opinion'); that three of the original criteria could be removed (because they described care for which an acute admission was no longer required); and that the time allowed for pre-operative assessment could be reduced from 24 to 18 hours. These changes were seen as being required so that the modified AEP better reflected current NHS practice at that time. Similarly, four of the original AEP's day of care criteria

Box 2.3 Modified AEP criteria for defining adult care appropriate for an acute inpatient setting.

Adult day of admission criteria
(1)   Procedure in theatre within 18 hours
(2)   Monitoring of cardiac rhythm, blood pressure, pulse, temperature or respiration every 2 hours for at least 2 observations
(3)   Intravenous/subcutaneous/naso-gastric fluid replacement (includes new gastrostomy/does not include access previously established), intravenous/subcutaneous medications
(4)   Any form of artificial ventilation or respiratory support (new or changing)
(5)   Severe electrolyte/acid-base abnormality
(6)   Acute loss of ability to move a limb or other body part within 48 hours prior to admission
(7)   Acute impairment of sight or hearing within 48 hours prior to admission
(8)   Recent acute internal bleeding (except haematuria unless requiring catheterisation)
(9)   Acute rupture of recent surgical wound
(10) Pulse rate < 50 or > 140 per minute
(11) Systolic blood pressure < 90 or > 200, diastolic < 60 or > 120 mm Hg
(12) Acute confusional state/coma/unresponsiveness (excluding simple inebriation)
(13) Electrocardiogram evidence of acute ischaemia (including unstable angina with suspicion of acute myocardial infarction)
(14) Overdoses waiting for psychiatric opinion

Adult day of care criteria
(1)   Any major operative procedure that day
(2)   'Extraordinary' pre-operative consultation/evaluation for theatre the next day
(3)   On diet for test requiring strict dietary control
(4)   New/experimental treatment under medical officer supervision
(5)   Close medical officer monitoring at least 3 times per day
(6)   Any major invasive procedure within past 24 hours
(7)   Any form of artificial ventilation or respiratory support (new or changing)
(8)   Parenteral therapy
(9)   Vital sign monitoring < every 30 minutes for at least 4 hours
(10) Intramuscular and subcutaneous injections > 2 per day (including diabetic newly diagnosed)
(11) Input/output measurement and/or daily weighing
(12) Major surgical wound and drainage care
(13) Close nurse monitoring, medically directed, 3+ times per day
(14) Bowel obstruction, ileus and acute retentions (in past 24 hours)
(15) Transfusion or serial transfusions for acute conditions in past 48 hours
(16) Dysrythmias causing acute dynamic disturbance or acute ischaemia in past 48 hours
(17) Fever of at least 38°C within past 48 hours
(18) Episode of coma/unresponsiveness in past 24 hours (exclude patients with epilepsy)
(19) Acute confusional state in past 48 hours
(20) Acute haematologic disorders with signs and symptoms within past 48 hours
(21) Progressive acute neurological difficulties during past 48 hours

---

were dropped because they related to care that could now be delivered on a day case basis.

As Box 2.3 indicates, the criteria are not linked to the diagnosis of the patient. The 14 criteria for defining care appropriate to an acute inpatient setting on a patient's day of admission reflect the medical status of the patient or the intensity of the care that they require. Similarly, the 21 day of care criteria reflect a patient's need for medical or nursing/life support services, or their clinical condition.

Using the modified AEP to review the utilisation of acute beds

The key stages in undertaking a utilisation review process using the modified AEP have been described by Bristow et al. (1998). Initially, the patient group whose notes are to be screened must be determined. The utilisation review could focus on a sample of all adult acute emergency admissions. However, to streamline the process and make it more efficient, it might be better to target a patient group identified by previous analysis using performance indicators, for example groupings based upon age band and/or specialty and/or diagnosis. When identifying the need for investments in intermediate care, a review focusing on older people would probably be most beneficial.

Next, the mechanism for generating the sample of case notes to be screened needs to be agreed. One approach is to generate a retrospective sample, covering patients who have already been discharged from acute care, for example a random sample of all admissions over the previous year (Bristow et al., 1997). Alternatively, the sample of case notes to be studied can be generated prospectively. Here, the review focuses on the care of patients who are currently located in hospital beds. Point prevalence studies can be used to generate the sample, for example a review covering the care received by all occupants of beds on a particular day or days (Stevenson and Spencer, 2002; see also Chapter 3). Alternatively, the review period could be extended to ensure that every day of the week is included at least twice (Bristow et al., 1997). Retrospective sampling usually means that the care of a larger number of cases, admitted over longer time horizons, can be reviewed more quickly. Seasonal effects can also be studied more easily. However, a review based on prospective sampling might be considered more reliable because all of the documentation and other information to support review decisions are likely to be available.

The number of case notes to be reviewed also needs to be agreed. McDonagh et al. (2000) described a number of studies which had examined levels of avoidable bed use amongst older people. Sample sizes ranged from 146 to 1170 patients. In local audits, pragmatic rather than statistical considerations might determine the sample size.

Subsequent stages in the utilisation review process are indicated in Fig. 2.1. First, the case notes of those patients sampled are screened using the modified AEP. Screening might focus on the care received by patients on their days of admission and/or subsequent days of care. Both types of day are relevant when exploring the potential for an expansion of services for intermediate care. In this way the utilisation review will highlight the extent to which there are avoidable days of admission and avoidable days of care.

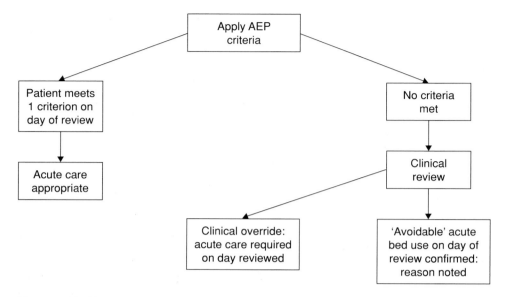

Fig. 2.1   Modified AEP review process.

If information in patient case notes indicates that at least one of the AEP's criteria are met, acute inpatient care on the day being reviewed is considered to be appropriate. If not, the case notes are subject to further clinical review. This subjective phase of the review process reflects the fact that it is not possible to have a list of criteria that cover all eventualities surrounding a patient's need for acute based care. The clinical review can be undertaken in conjunction with the clinicians responsible for the care of patients within the target group. Ideally, however, a multidisciplinary and 'whole system' panel of reviewers is used. Such a panel is likely to have a more complete understanding of the types of care that can be delivered beyond the acute inpatient setting and, in particular, in the community.

The clinical review phase might identify additional factors, which were not picked up by the AEP's criteria, that mean that acute care on the day screened is appropriate. This is termed 'clinical override'. Such additional factors should be linked to the clinical characteristics or care needs of patients and not to restrictions that existing custom and practice places on the delivery of care. For example, 'waiting for test results' would not be considered a valid reason for override if it was possible to reduce either admission rates or lengths of stay by providing results more quickly. Alternatively, clinical review might confirm that acute inpatient care on the day screened is avoidable. In this way, the residual proportions of avoidable days of admission and avoidable days of care are generated.

The next phase of the review process is to note the reasons why a day of admission or day of care has been classified as avoidable. Care on the day of an admission might be classified as avoidable because a patient has been admitted prematurely, for example a long pre-operative stay for an elective procedure. Alternatively, an avoidable admission day might also indicate that a patient's complete admission is avoidable, for example a patient admitted for social care following a fall. It is this latter group of patients and reasons that are of most interest when developing services for intermediate care. Similarly, an avoidable day of care might exist in the middle of a patient's stay (for example, delays in the supply of information to guide the continuing acute care of a patient) or towards the end of a patient's acute stay (for example, when a patient continues to receive care in an acute bed but does not require that intensity of care). Again, in the context of planning for intermediate care, the main focus will be on those factors that are generating avoidable bed use towards the end of a patient's stay.

The final aspect of the review process is to undertake a preliminary assessment of the types of action or service initiatives that are required to reduce levels of avoidable bed use. This again represents a subjective element of the review process and it is termed 'preliminary' because, up until now, relatively few professionals will have been involved in the review process. A much wider range of professionals will need to be consulted before any final decisions are reached on the best ways of tackling problems surrounding the avoidable use of beds. In this sense, the results of the utilisation review exercise represent the start of this consultation process.

Concerns about the utilisation review process

Concerns have been expressed about whether or not the results generated by the utilisation review process represent a valid measure of the extent to which there is avoidable bed use within a hospital (Coast, 1996; Vetter, 2003). Critics argue that it is not appropriate to classify a day of admission or day of care as avoidable if no alternative to acute based care currently exists. For example, a patient cannot be discharged to a multidisciplinary team for home based care if no such service exists. Clearly, professionals need to be aware of such limitations in order to avoid false planning assumptions about how much it might be possible to reduce levels of avoidable bed use in the short term. However, it is important that classifications of avoidable bed use continue to be based on the care needs of the patient rather than the service options that currently exist. If not, it will not be possible to use the results of a utilisation review exercise to guide decision making surrounding the future development of services for intermediate care.

Critics have also noted that, although the problem of avoidable bed use occurs within a hospital, the ways of tackling this problem may require actions beyond the boundaries of the hospital (Vetter, 2003). In other words, hospital staff might feel that they are being blamed for problems that are beyond their control. Clearly, hospital staff might become frustrated if they think that they have limited ability to respond to problems. However, the drive to develop services for intermediate care is a recognition that whole systems solutions to the problem of avoidable bed use are required (Department of Health, 2000a).

It has also been argued that, until the effectiveness and cost effectiveness of the identified service alternatives to acute care have been established, acute bed use cannot be classified as avoidable (Coast, 1996; Vetter, 2003). This is a powerful argument. Although the emerging evidence base does offer support for an expansion of services for intermediate care, important gaps in knowledge remain (O'Neill and Meade, 2001; Department of Health, 2002; Stevenson and Spencer, 2002; see also Chapter 8). Such concerns demonstrate the importance of monitoring and evaluating the impacts of schemes for intermediate care when they are introduced locally.

In addition, the limitations of existing tools to support the utilisation review process should also be recognised. This chapter has focused primarily on the use of the modified AEP. To reflect advances in medical practice, a number of the criteria contained in the original AEP were removed when it was adapted for use in the NHS (Bristow et al., 1997). This demonstrates that some of the criteria incorporated in screening instruments can become out of date, a concern raised by Vetter (2003). Hence, early in a utilisation review exercise, it is important to check that those professionals affected by a study agree that the criteria used by a screening instrument adequately define care that can be delivered only in an acute inpatient setting.

Finally, although the use of a screening tool such as the modified AEP increases the validity and reliability of the utilisation review process, the boundaries between the objective and subjective elements of the process should always be kept in mind. The testing of screening instruments has primarily focused on their ability to segregate appropriate and avoidable acute days of care. Less effort has been given to ways of assessing and improving inter-observer levels of agreement surrounding the causes of avoidable bed use and the actions and service initiatives that are required (Lorenzo et al., 1999). In other words, observers might agree that a day of care is avoidable but they might disagree about how this problem should be tackled. This is why the results of utilisation review studies offer only preliminary, but essential, guidance to support the development of schemes to reduce levels of avoidable bed use (McDonagh et al., 2000).

Summary

The NHS Plan promotes an expansion of services for intermediate care across the NHS and its adjacent agencies for supplying health and social care (Department of Health, 2000b). However, the relevance of intermediate care and the particular types of schemes promoted will vary from locality to locality. National policy directives therefore need to be interpreted locally to ensure that the 'right' services are set up for the 'right' people in the 'right' place (Audit Commission, 2000; Department of Health, 2001).

This chapter has shown how analysis based on routinely available performance indicators and utilisation review studies can provide essential information to support the planning of services for intermediate care. Performance indicator analysis helps to focus planning activity whilst utilisation review studies confirm the existence of avoidable bed use and help to clarify its causes. However, such analysis represents only the start of the planning task. Having confirmed the potential for an expansion of services for intermediate care, further work is needed to design the specific types of schemes required to meet the needs of potential users. Key design issues to be determined will include the appropriate settings for intermediate care (patients' homes, institutions etc.), and the scale and skill mix of services to be provided (for example, numbers and grades of nurses, social workers and therapists). Ways in which these complex issues can be tackled will be discussed in later chapters of this book.

References

Anderson, P., Meara, J., Broadhurst, S., Attwood, S., Timbrell, M., Gatherer, A. (1988) Use of hospital beds: a cohort study of admissions to a provincial teaching hospital. *British Medical Journal* **297**, 910–12.

Audit Commission (1997) *The Coming of Age: Improving Care Services for Older People.* London: Audit Commission.

Audit Commission (2000) *The Way to Go Home: Rehabilitation and Remedial Services for Older People.* London: Audit Commission.

Beech, R. (2003) Organisational barriers to access. In: Gulliford, M. and Morgan, M. (eds) *Access to Health Care.* London: Routledge, pp. 84–103.

Beech, R., Cropper, S. (2001) *An Analytical Framework for Supporting the Planning of Intermediate Care Services.* A Report Prepared on Behalf of the Research and Development Directorate West Midlands. Keele: Centre for Health Planning and Management, Keele University.

Bristow, A., Hudson, M., Beech, R. (1997) *Analysing Acute Inpatient Services: The Development and Application of Utilisation Review Tools.* Report prepared for the NHS Executive South East Thames. London: NHS Executive South East Thames.

Bristow, A., Hudson, M., Beech, R. (1998) Experiences of carrying out utilisation review in the NHS. *British Journal of Health Care Management* **4** (2), 74–7.

Clarke, G., Clarke, M. (1997) Spatial decision support systems for health care planning. In: Cropper, S. and Forte, P. (eds) *Enhancing Decision Making in the NHS: The Role of Decision Support Systems.* Buckingham: Open University Press.

Coast, J. (1996) Appropriateness versus efficiency: the economics of utilisation review. *Health Policy* **36**, 69–81.

Coast, J., Inglis, A., Frankel, S. (1996) Alternatives to hospital admission: what are they and who should decide? *British Medical Journal* **312**, 162–6.

Department of Health (2000a) *Shaping the Future NHS: Long Term Planning for Hospitals and Related Services. Consultation Document on the Findings of the National Beds Inquiry – Supporting Analysis.* London: Department of Health.

Department of Health (2000b) *The NHS Plan: A Plan for Investment, A Plan for Reform.* London: The Stationery Office.

Department of Health (2001) *Intermediate Care.* Health Service Circular/Local Authority Circular, HSC 2001/01, LAC (2001)1. London: Department of Health.

Department of Health (2002) *National Service Framework for Older People – Supporting Implementation. Intermediate Care: Moving Forward.* London: Department of Health.

Duffy, R., Bain, J., Neville, R., Staines, H. (1998) Relationship between route of referral for acute medical admissions, patient characteristics and appropriateness of admission. *Health Bulletin* **56** (6), 863–70.

Fellin, G., Apolone, G., Tampieri, A., Bevilacqua, L., Meregalli, G., Minella, C., Liberati, A. (1995) Appropriateness of hospital use: an overview of Italian studies. *International Journal for Quality in Health Care* **7** (3), 219–25.

Fenn, A., Horner, P., Travis, S., Prescott, G., Figgs, H., Bates, T. (2000) Inappropriate bed usage in a district general hospital. *Journal of Clinical Excellence* **1**, 221–7.

Gertman, P.M., Restuccia, J.D. (1981) The Appropriateness Evaluation Protocol: a technique for assessing unnecessary days of hospital care. *Medical Care* **19**, 855–71.

Jacobs, C.M., Lamprey, J. (1992) *The Isd-A Review System with Adult ISD Criteria*. Northampton: Interqual.

Lorenzo, S., Sunol, R. (1995) An overview of Spanish studies on appropriateness of hospital use. *International Journal for Quality in Health Care* **7** (3), 213–8.

Lorenzo, S., Beech, R., Lang, T., Santos-Eggimann, B. (1999) An experience of utilisation review in Europe: sequel to a BIOMED project. *International Journal for Quality in Health Care* **11** (1), 13–19.

McDonagh, M.S., Smith, D.H., Goddard, M. (2000) Measuring appropriate use of acute beds: a systematic review of methods and results. *Health Policy* **53**, 157–84.

National Audit Office (2000) *Inpatient Admissions and Bed Management in NHS Acute Hospitals*. Report by the Controller and Auditor General. London: The Stationery Office.

O'Neill, D., Meade, F. (2001) What evidence is there to demonstrate the effectiveness of health and social care interventions and services in reducing pressures on the acute hospital system? Service Innovations Background Research Rapid Reviews Report 4. Canterbury: University of Kent, Centre for Health Services Studies.

O'Neill, D., Pearson, M. (1995). Appropriateness of hospital use in the United Kingdom: a review of activity in the field. *International Journal of Quality in Health Care* **7** (3), 239–44.

Stevenson, J., Spencer, L. (2002) *Developing Intermediate Care: A Guide for Health and Social Services Professionals*. London: King's Fund.

Strumwasser, I., Paranjipe, N., Ronis, D., Share, D. et al. (1990) Reliability and validity of utilisation review criteria. *Medical Care* **28** (2), 95–111.

Vetter, N. (2003) Inappropriately delayed discharge from hospital: what do we know? *British Medical Journal* **326**, 927–8.

Chapter 3

Management and Planning of Services

Tom Bowen, Paul Forte and Chris Foote – The Balance of Care Group

Introduction

In the late 1990s the UK Government initiated a major and sustained increase in health service expenditure. This aimed to bring UK health expenditure up to the levels of other European Union states, in terms of the proportion of gross domestic product (GDP) used for such purposes (Department of Health, 2000a). Politically the commitment was driven by a wish to reduce the long waiting times for surgery that many patients experienced, and to improve access to services where delays were commonplace, such as Accident and Emergency departments.

An immediate practical implication was that acute hospitals needed to ensure that more beds were available as required to support increased levels of elective surgical activity. Many hospitals reported frequent cancellation of operations when inpatient beds were not available on the scheduled date of surgery. Bed occupancy was consistently very high for medical patients who often ended up placed in non-medical wards, squeezing the availability for surgical patients. To some degree the issue had been exacerbated by the reduction in hospital based rehabilitation during the 1990s, as hospital geriatricians increasingly focused their work on acute medicine, a trend encouraged by the practice of reimbursing hospitals on the basis of finished consultant episodes rather than bed days (Nocon and Baldwin, 1998).

The initial response was brought together in the report of the National Beds Inquiry (Department of Health, 2000b). This proposed some increase in general and acute beds, but indicated that the major development needed should be in intermediate care. This form of care aims to treat patients in settings other than mainstream primary and secondary care, through the introduction of new services and changes to patient care pathways. The principal objectives are to prevent acute hospital admission and to ensure early discharge when the acute phase of treatment is complete. Unlike conventional services, intermediate care is not designed around separate organisations or even a single budgetary resource, but is a collection of service elements, which may be managed by different agencies, including health, social services and the independent sector.

Although intermediate care has been described in the literature, and the various emerging models of care defined (Vaughan and Lathlean, 1999), the systems approach it requires is not a familiar one to many health service managers. Initial responses to the national initiative tended to focus on capacity changes, in particular the introduction of intermediate care beds in community hospitals, with the aim of providing rehabilitation services for patients recovering from an acute illness or trauma.

It quickly became apparent, however, that there were many other patients whose needs were not best met by continued stay in acute hospital beds. They did not require intermediate care, on the broad definitions above, but did clearly have continuing care needs. In many cases they would have been identified as requiring admission to a care home, but a place had not been arranged.

These issues reflect the way in which health services have been organised in the UK. There has been much comment on comparisons with other systems, most recently with Kaiser Permanente in California, which uses half the acute bed days for major conditions, a level of usage that is low by UK standards even when the US case mix is allowed for (Ham et al., 2003). However these systems have the additional provision and care practices in place that can make an integrated approach to care a viable option.

For managers to address these complexities requires a change in approach. Foote and Stanners (2002), looking at these issues from the viewpoint of redesigning care for older people, summarise this as requiring 'an ability to view things as systems and understand how systems behave'. This is not just about ensuring that resource requirements are soundly analysed but involves a recognition that the behaviour of people should be at the heart of any approach, not least because it is the choices made by clinicians and care professionals that determine whether any new investment delivers the intended benefits.

This chapter is concerned with the use of whole systems approaches to support managers and clinicians across the health economy to ensure that not only are suitable resources identified and provided to ensure most appropriate provision but, at the same time, to obtain consensus around – and practical implementation of – patient care pathways.

Developing a whole systems perspective

Our involvement in these issues has developed naturally from earlier work on the *Balance of Care* approach. This aims to provide a needs based approach to planning of future services, and has focused in particular on the complex and continuing care needs of older people (Forte and Bowen, 1997). The generic Balance of Care model is defined in terms of dependency groups within which people will have similar service requirements. For any given dependency group there may be a range of appropriate care options that can be specified; definitions of these will be subject to local circumstances and requirements. Depending on how people might be allocated across those options, there will be different

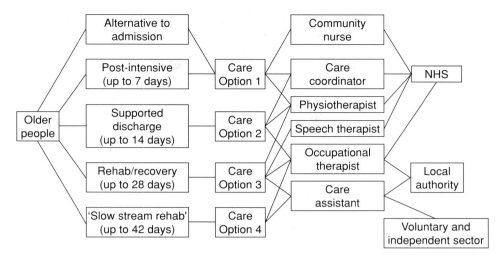

A simplified diagram of the Balance of Care model describing care options – combinations of services – to meet particular types of need for older people requiring 'intermediate care'. For example, people in the 'supported discharge' category might include arthritic patients recovering from a fall, while those classified as 'rehab/recovery' would include those recovering from a stroke.

Their medical and social characteristics can be defined in terms of assessment criteria that are used to determine care pathways (although at a much higher level of aggregation here, since we are concerned only with the resource requirements, rather than the detail of the care to be provided). Note that there may be more than one care option for any patient group.

These pathways, in turn, will require different mixes of skills-based services as well as bricks and mortar facilities – some of which may be provided by more than one agency in a locality.

Fig. 3.1   Simplified diagram of the Balance of Care model.

resource implications for volumes, costs and types of services to be provided – and different impacts on the agencies responsible for providing them. The Balance of Care model enables extensive – and fast – policy testing to see what these effects might be.

Figure 3.1 illustrates the structure of the planning issues, which the Balance of Care approach addresses. A client group – in this case older people – is classified into a series of dependency groups. For each dependency group a variety of appropriate care options can be specified and the implication for combination of resources on the supply side calculated and considered. As the focus of the approach is on helping to plan future requirements, it is possible to explore the potential resource implications of new models of care which people may want to introduce alongside existing care packages.

The structure of the modelling approach is described in Fig. 3.1, which for illustration includes some of the elements discussed above.

Fig. 3.1 is based on work undertaken to help identify the workforce implications of the NHS Plan (Department of Health, 2000a), in the context of limited understanding of how models of intermediate care might develop (Bowen and

Forte, 2000). This work, supported by a specially convened expert panel, provided initial estimates at a national level of future workforce requirements, but highlighted that:

- There was no established classification that would describe patients in terms of their suitability for alternatives to acute hospital care.
- Intermediate care could not always be differentiated from other forms of care that were delivered across organisational boundaries, especially if targeted at meeting continuing care needs.
- There was no readily available data that would help hospital management quantify the potential for change at a local level.

Subsequent projects undertaken for local health economies in various parts of the UK have addressed some of these shortfalls.

Of particular note in terms of establishing relevant and validated criteria for identifying patients for whom alternative care options may be possible is the Appropriateness Evaluation Protocol (AEP) instrument (Lang et al., 1999). This comprises two lists of criteria against which a patient is assessed from their case notes. One set of criteria relates to the patient's original admission into the current episode of acute care, the other relates to the patient's care requirements on the day of the survey itself. If a patient meets any single one of the criteria on either list (or on both of them) then their acute admission, their continued acute care, or both, are deemed 'appropriate' for the setting (it is usually preferable to state whether a patient falls 'within' or 'outside' AEP criteria). Note that it is possible for a patient to be admitted to an acute setting outside AEP criteria, but be within AEP criteria on the day of the survey, or vice versa. It is also possible for a patient to be within both sets of criteria, or be entirely outside both sets of criteria.

The AEP is a validated instrument that has been used successfully to provide criteria for evaluation of current practice. It was developed in the USA and has been adapted in the UK and Europe (Lang et al., 1999; see also Chapter 2). It has been validated and found to be a reliable tool (Goddard et al., 2000). It enables an analysis of the reasons for admission as well as those for continuing stay, identifying the underlying processes and any causes for delay. The data required can be found retrospectively in patients' casenotes. AEP focuses on issues relating to acute care and sets various criteria for judging the appropriateness of the care location, assuming alternative options were available. In the case study reported below and other similar exercises in the UK we have adopted the version of the AEP reported in Lang et al., 1999.

There are other instruments to identify the appropriateness of acute hospital care, for example the ISD (intensity, severity and discharge) instrument which looks in particular at the severity of illness, and is particularly targeted at identifying the threshold of admission and discharge (Lawrence et al., 1999). In general however we have found that the alternatives are more detailed than required for a strategic planning environment, and are more complex and resource intensive to use.

Methodology

To address the whole system issues in a context of incomplete data, the approach focused on the use of a point prevalence survey using the AEP, supported by a series of workshops to interpret the data and explore the implications for future service development and clinical practice. The main aim of the point prevalence survey is to gauge the extent to which the existing admissions and discharge system might contribute to patients being either unnecessarily admitted to hospital or delayed in their discharge from it when they are medically fit for discharge (or functionally stable). The survey is *not* an audit of existing clinical practice, but an attempt to understand whether, given 'perfect availability' of a range of alternative and supporting health and social services in other settings, there is (or could be) an alternative location for care for the patient either on the day of admission or on the day of the survey. It is assumed that such services would be available for all people who would be most likely to benefit from them. These would either avoid their admission to acute care altogether, or accelerate their discharge and recovery from it.

To supplement the 'snapshot' view, a longitudinal view of patients' progress is provided by the discharge outcomes, i.e. when and where the patient was discharged to. This follow-up allows some refinement of the patient analyses. For example, patients who returned home rapidly (say within a week) can be identified, for whom it may be assumed that appropriate services were available. These data are obtained by the extraction of administrative data from the local PAS (Patient Administration System) some weeks after the survey. This extract also provides information on the responsible PCT (Primary Care Trust), consultant and specialty.

Survey questionnaires are tailored to local requirements and set out to determine not just whether the patient's care met the AEP criteria both on admission and on the day of the survey, but also what alternatives might be possible if services were in place. All this requires a significant level of judgement on the part of the surveyors, who must be clinicians (whether medical, nursing or therapy) and undergo a short training course in advance of the survey. This level of involvement also has benefits in introducing frontline staff to whole systems issues that can facilitate subsequent changes in care practice.

Typically surveys include the following broad data items:

- *Patient details*: for confidentiality reasons personal details are restricted to age, general practitioner (GP) and location of residence.
- *Admitting circumstances*: the known source of referral; any known risk factors in the home circumstances of the patient; the recorded time of admission and the reason for it.
- *Appropriateness of admission*: whether, under ideal circumstances and a full range of alternative care provision available, an admission might have been deferred, or avoided altogether. If an admission is outside the AEP protocol, surveyors are asked to specify potential alternative care locations.

- *Continuing appropriateness of location of care*: given the presence of the patient in a hospital bed on the day of the survey, this question aimed to identify whether the patient still required care in that setting or, if not, what suitable alternatives existed.
- *Delays to hospital discharge*: where a patient was deemed medically or functionally fit for discharge, the final section of the survey asked for reasons why the patient was still occupying a hospital bed.

All adult medical and orthopaedic patients, who are the major groups for whom alternative care options may be available are included in the survey, plus other groups that are of concern or interest to local clinicians and managers. The survey itself is undertaken on a single day, thus the results are only as representative as the day itself. However, based on the experience of completing a number of surveys similar in scope to the case study described later (see for example Forte et al., 2003), there is a surprising similarity between hospitals in different areas. Clinicians have commented that the case mix across wards may also be relatively similar day to day, and some have predicted very accurately the proportions of their patients lying outside AEP criteria.

The AEP criteria will be a useful discriminator only if the hospital or ward being surveyed has an explicitly 'acute' purpose. Many district general hospitals over the years have developed specifically non-acute facilities such as rehabilitation wards, and community hospitals by definition provide only non-acute services. Looking across the whole system it would be helpful to have a similar discriminatory tool for non-acute facilities, though there is no validated instrument of the detail of the AEP. Donald et al. (2001) propose various useful criteria to examine the appropriate use of community hospital beds. A similar approach was adopted in the work reported here of identifying the reasons for admission (rehabilitation, sub-acute care, palliative care, respite etc.) and alternative care settings where identifiable.

It is important to make a distinction between different types of rehabilitation. Commentators such as Bowman and Easton (2000) and Foote and Stanners (2002) have identified three main types of rehabilitation:

- *Recuperative*: relatively 'low level' inputs of rehabilitation for patients convalescing from an illness or short acute care episode, typically requiring rehabilitation assistant skills only.
- *Restorative*: this requires more intensive and sophisticated rehabilitation skills and typically follows a more severe and prolonged acute episode or illness. The prognosis is that the patient will be re-trained to as close as possible a skill level that they had prior to the illness.
- *Reconstructive*: this is specialist rehabilitation, which typically involves the patient learning new skills or relearning old ones. Patients who have had a stroke or who are amputees would be typical examples of people requiring this level of rehabilitation.

The key to the success of the survey and subsequent analyses lies in the degree of participation of clinical and other care staff, and senior managers across the local health economy. Projects are typically arranged in three phases as illustrated by Fig. 3.2. The preparatory phase can take three months or more, and deliberately leaves time for clinicians and managers to become familiar with the methodology, to debate the issues to be addressed. The second, survey phase is designed to encompass as many as possible of these issues. The third phase aims to allow as many workshops and opportunistic meetings for stakeholders as resources allow. This allows the data to be reviewed and interpreted, and open discussion of the feasibility and extent of alternatives.

Case study

To illustrate the types of results encountered some summary data from an exercise which took place in October 2002 across the East Berkshire health community, involving an acute hospital operating across two hospital sites, two community hospitals, three Primary Care Trusts and related social services departments are presented here (Forte et al., 2002). It is worth mentioning that these results are broadly comparable to those obtained in five projects of similar size and scope over the past three years.

This exercise set out to survey all adult inpatients on the day, excluding maternity, paediatric and psychiatric patients, and all day cases. Total coverage of the target population was 96%, and altogether 598 adult inpatients in general and acute hospital beds across East Berkshire on the survey day. The majority of these were at the acute hospital sites (504, 84%) although this included 28 (4%) non-acute 'interim care' patients awaiting placement in a nursing or residential home. Excluding these, the total on acute hospital wards was 476 (80%). The remaining 94 (16%) patients were at two community hospitals providing non-acute care, principally rehabilitation: since the AEP would not be relevant for these patients an amended survey form to identify reasons for admission and continued stay was used.

Of all the patients surveyed, 77% were aged 65 years and over (see Fig. 3.3), including nearly all non-acute patients. Whilst it is commonly recognised that older people make greater use of hospital services, it is not always appreciated that the combined effect of higher admission rates and longer lengths of stay mean that bed usage in most UK hospitals is dominated by older people. Thus, alternatives to hospital care are often (though not exclusively) focusing on the complex service needs of older people.

Overall, 12% of acute admissions (55 out of 476) were identified as being outside the AEP criteria – that is, they might have been treated in another care setting rather than been admitted to acute care, assuming that these alternatives were readily available. Fig. 3.4 shows that this group is, again, dominated by older people, mostly those aged over 75. Most patients outside the AEP were admitted into medical specialties though there were some surgical patients, especially in the younger groups: five of these were being treated within AEP

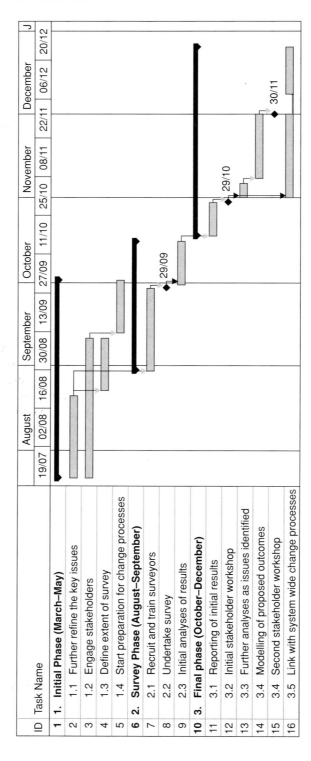

Fig. 3.2 Typical project plan in three phases.

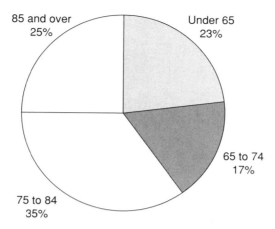

Fig. 3.3 All patients surveyed by age group (*n* = 598).

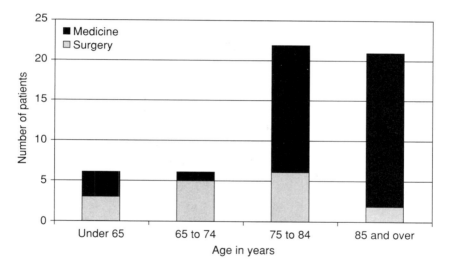

Fig. 3.4 Acute admissions outside AEP criteria by age and specialty group (*n* = 55).

criteria on the day of the survey, indicating that the admission might have been deferred but not avoided altogether.

The survey also asked what alternative locations for care to an acute admission might be appropriate for the 55 patients identified. Fig. 3.5 shows these for acute patients: the 'non-acute bed' option was favoured in over two-thirds of cases. This could mean a bed in a community hospital or in a nursing or residential home environment. EMH refers to Elderly Mental Health Services, which could be bed based or delivered through the patient's home or a day hospital setting.

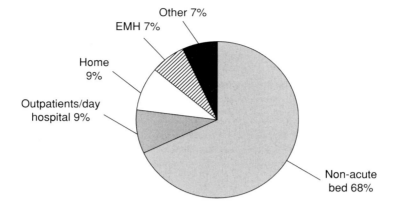

Fig. 3.5   Preferred alternatives to acute admission (*n* = 55).

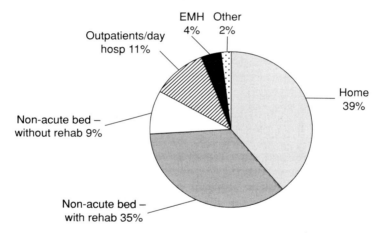

Fig. 3.6   Preferred alternatives for non-acute admissions (*n* = 46).

In the case of patients in non-acute settings, principally community hospitals or care homes with nursing or therapy input, for which the AEP instrument was not applicable, the professional judgement of the surveyors indicated that there were potential alternative settings for 46 out of 94 patients surveyed (Fig. 3.6). However, there was a wider range of alternatives for this group than for acute patients, and in 16 out of the 46 instances (35%) an alternative non-acute bed location was preferred. Sometimes these alternatives were referred to as 'intermediate care' reflecting a belief that the range of service in the current location was insufficient, but in other cases the choice may have reflected a preference for a location of care closer to the patient's own home.

Overall, 40% of all acute patients (189) were identified as not receiving care with AEP criteria on the day of the survey. While this may seem a very large

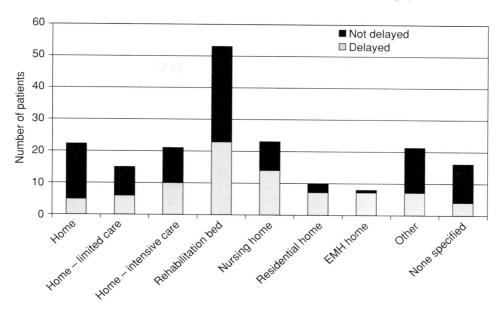

Fig. 3.7 Potential alternative locations for patients in acute hospitals (*n* = 189).

number, it is not inconsistent with all other surveys undertaken by the Balance of Care Group, and is also in line with comparative studies with other countries such as the Kaiser Permanente comparison (Ham et al., 2003). Some studies using AEP criteria include an override option, so that surveyors can indicate that for the treatment required an acute hospital stay was unavoidable. In this survey however such patients could be identified when no alternative location of care was specified, and no adjustment to the AEP was required: this applied to 16 of the 189 patients outside AEP criteria on the day. The 189 patients also identified also included 50 of the 55 patients whose admissions had been outside the AEP.

Fig. 3.7 shows that the 'rehabilitation bed' was the single largest alternative care type suggested. In part this is attributable to patients who require specialist rehabilitation, which is provided in an acute hospital setting but not included in the AEP protocol (e.g. recovery from road traffic accidents, severe strokes), perhaps up to 20 patients in all. However there are also significant numbers for whom home care would be possible, with varying intensity of domiciliary care. Only eight patients requiring EMH care were identified.

Fig. 3.7 also identifies patients for whom a delay to discharge had been noted. Of the patients also reporting delays, a higher proportion were waiting for care home places, but home based alternatives were recorded whether or not a delay had been identified. Similar counts of alternatives for non-acute patients were also derived.

The survey also collected a wealth of further data including admission reasons and routes, diagnostic details, and on the patient's location prior to hospital admission. Survey data are held on a relational database, and it is therefore easy to undertake multiple analyses, for example to see if there are any notable patterns in the time of admission, referral or admission route into the hospital. Understanding the patient's admission reasons is also significant: typically, patients with an indeterminate diagnosis and multiple risk factors (living alone, prone to falls or with confusion) are those who have the longest lengths of stay and are more likely to be recorded as being outside AEP criteria on the survey day (i.e. they may still require care of some description, but often not in an acute care setting).

A series of workshops were held: first with the surveyors themselves, then with key groups of clinicians and mangers with relevant responsibilities and interests. At the outset there was considerable reaction to the number of patients who could be discharged elsewhere, and to the indication that in a lot of cases these patients were delayed in various ways. Beyond this there was substantial debate about the extent to which those waiting for discharge were limited by system failings, such as the lack of availability or coordination of services, and the extent to which it was a simple matter of logistics – patients waiting for transport – or recuperation – the reasonable expectation that a few days recovery may be needed before risking a return home.

There is typically a wide range of issues raised by the survey results, some of which can be tackled in the immediate post-survey period (such as improving discharge planning processes), others requiring much longer term changes, for example investing in new forms of health care and services which will have a long-term impact on the need to admit to hospital.

The overall survey results are not out of line with experience from seven similar surveys undertaken by the Balance of Care Group (for example Forte et al., 2003), although the level of identified inappropriate acute admissions (12%) is on the low side (in other surveys this has ranged from 12 to 23%). This suggested that the existing admission system in East Berkshire is reasonably effective at preventing unnecessary admissions into the acute sector. However, a large proportion of patients not requiring admission to acute care, were still seen as needing a 'non-acute bed' of some description, which could be in an intermediate care facility, rehabilitation ward or care home setting.

For those patients who were directly admitted to a non-acute (or community) hospital but could have been treated in other settings there was a wide range of community based options, reflecting heterogeneity in the conditions and circumstances of the patients being admitted. This suggests that a range of alternative services needs to be developed in order to meet these demands. If such patients were cared for in community settings, this would release capacity at the community hospitals, and allow more routine use of non-acute beds for patients who present at Accident & Emergency requiring admission, but not necessarily acute care. Amongst the admission reasons to both acute and non-acute hospitals, falls were a major contributing factor. This implies that there is potential for placing greater emphasis on the development and resourcing of primary prevention strategies designed to prevent falls occurring in the first place.

The survey identified requirements for rehabilitation services in almost all parts of the system. This is a common requirement of patients no longer requiring acute hospital care, and it is not clear that existing acute wards are best placed to deliver such services. For many of these patients a rehabilitation bed was identified as a suitable alternative, and a proportion had already been identified as delayed and waiting for a bed in a community hospital. Earlier access to rehabilitation services could speed up return home, and various suggestions were made about the best approach to take, including the provision of a dedicated ward in the acute hospital itself.

Resolution of the overall approach to meeting rehabilitation needs would also go a long way towards defining the types of intermediate care provision that might be required. As noted earlier, there is a lack of clarity in the use of this term, and the survey forms deliberately avoided using it, since the form of provision would depend on the component elements (not least rehabilitation).

Generally there was a tendency to continue to see care alternatives in terms of bed based provision. In the case of community hospitals, the alternatives identified were mainly bed based, despite the range of community based alternatives to admission that surveyors identified. This may reflect the current lack of suitable community care services at the time of survey, so that staff continued to view alternatives in terms of what was readily available.

One of the additional data items collected in the survey was on the state of discharge planning procedures as evidenced from the notes, and a key finding was that there were large numbers of patients for whom no discharge plan had been initiated. This accelerated existing concerns that more could be done to address these needs and that this could be undertaken in the short term.

Discharge planning was a relatively poorly executed process at the acute sites (only 38% of the surveyed acute patients had plans in the notes) and, in many cases, these only appeared to begin once the patient had been declared medically fit for discharge. This has important consequences for the efficiency with which patient care is transferred and immediately introduces delay into the system. Furthermore, if social services are only involved at a late stage in this process, it invariably adds unavoidably to the delay as only then can they initiate some of their placement procedures. There appeared to be a lack of agreement between the different clinical professional groups and health and social care agencies as to who is ultimately responsible for overseeing the whole discharge planning process, and truly multidisciplinary working in this area is patchy. Many surveyors are already involved in consideration of improved procedures in the immediate aftermath of the survey itself.

Resulting from discussion and analyses five major recommendations were agreed and progressed by clinicians and managers working across the participating organisations:

- The provision of coordinated community based services to meet the needs of a proportion of the patients currently admitted to community hospitals, and to enable rapid discharge from acute beds when acute care and treatment is no longer required.

- Routine admission of patients without acute care needs from the Accident and Emergency or Medical Assessment Unit to the community hospitals.
- Development of one ward at a community hospital as an intermediate care resource.
- Review of the overall level and deployment of rehabilitation services across all locations.
- Major enhancement of discharge planning procedures.

Discussion

The case study above is not untypical of similar projects in terms of the range of the agenda covered at the local level. Certain 'common analyses' have recurred and progressed work into more complex areas, moving closer to quantifying the more detailed elements in the Balance of Care model described earlier in this chapter. While it is not possible to statistically test the variation between different survey results (owing primarily to differences in survey populations), nevertheless there is a consistency between them. Post survey follow-up with surveyors also indicates consistencies in their interpretation of patient case notes.

A major strength of all the projects lies in the provision, often for the first time, of an evidence base to begin to describe how the whole system is performing. This provides a shared focus for discussion between the various interested parties of existing problems with the operation of the system, and highlighted where changes to service design and availability, and to operational procedures, could make a difference.

In the above case study patients or older people were not directly involved themselves. However, in the context of a similar exercise elsewhere, the Balance of Care Group has experimented with a forum for older people: immediately this changed the emphasis of the solutions, with participants stressing the value they placed on 'convalescence' (not a term frequently used by care professionals these days, but related to the notion of 'recuperative rehabilitation' now used as standard in our surveys). Another key issue was proximity of services, and access to them: localisation wherever possible was valued.

It is important to recognise that these analyses are essentially retrospective, and this can create a tension for clinicians who necessarily are engaged in prospective decision making: faced with a patient with visible symptoms but unknown diagnosis a physician may quite rightly feel the need to admit, even if it transpires later that there was no acute condition. Similarly clinicians may judge that a patient who has progressed to a post-acute stage should stay in a few more days for monitoring, to ensure the condition has stabilised. Thus it is reasonable that patients outside AEP criteria should be cared for in acute hospitals. However our work aims to identify those for whom a more appropriate location of care might be recognised, should services be available.

Using the AEP protocol led to interesting interpretation over the use of intravenous therapy (IV) and whether it automatically defines a need for acute care.

In part this illustrates how acute care practice has changed since the AEP was first developed and, in that respect, is an issue for future deployment of the AEP itself. However, clinical practice can also dictate the extent to which IV therapy is employed with different clinicians choosing to use it or not in the same circumstances. The AEP is a relatively conservative instrument, but given the large numbers of patients still identified who might be suitable for alternative care options, such conservatism may help to generate consensus.

The case study also demonstrates a feature common in such projects, the potential for a 'cascade' of provision to occur: if community services are expanded for patients currently cared for in non-acute beds, potential additional capacity is released for patients in acute hospital who require a bed in a rehabilitative setting. However this implies that services in all locations change their practice to support these patient movements. The key element is to increase the number of 'slow stream' patients who are discharged earlier from an acute hospital setting, who may require several weeks or even months of therapy to return to independent living. New intermediate care services have often been introduced without clinical process change, and few benefits are apparent: a successful whole systems implementation requires that service capacity and clinical process are considered together, and that change occurs across all parts of the system.

Further research and development

Various issues are touched on above where further research would be desirable to strengthen the emerging methodologies outlined in this chapter. Of particular note:

- The potential to refine the AEP instrument, and to identify changing medical practice. This was noted for IV therapy, and it has been possible to check in subsequent surveys whether IV therapy was the only reason for admission. There may be other developing care practices, including those deploying specialist nursing, where acute hospital admission could be avoided.
- The AEP instrument is focused on normal inpatient beds and is not a good discriminator for intensive and high dependency care, nor for day case provision. In both instances most patients will fall within the AEP criteria, but the interest in resource planning terms is whether they might more appropriately be in other acute hospital settings (intensive care patients could sometimes be transferred to normal beds, day cases are sometimes called with an expectation that overnight stay will be necessary). Additional criteria are needed to provide such additional discrimination.
- In similar fashion there is a need to clarify the criteria for admission to community hospitals. There is currently little consistency in the way they are used, so there is a need for the introduction of commonly agreed, and validated, definitions of what types of service they aim to provide, in particular the different types of rehabilitation. The definitions given above, and now used

in a number of projects by the Balance of Care Group, provide some basis for this. There is the related possibility then of defining exactly what is intended – in terms of patient case mix and service delivery – when intermediate care arrangements are introduced.

- By taking snapshots of data at the time of admission and on the day of care, it is not readily apparent what might have been done at other stages in the patient's care pathway, for example what preventive measures could have been undertaken for particular risk groups of patients (prevention of falls in frail older people is a common example). However there is a wealth of data not commonly held on patient activity, hence one opportunity to use the survey and associated processes to start the redesign of preventive services, especially for identified chronic disease management.
- Similarly the wealth of data now held from a number of projects raises the possibility of some type of benchmarking exercise against health economies seen to have advanced levels of integrated services (not necessarily in the UK). Our exercises usually follow initiatives by progressive managements wanting to make rapid change in systems which are known to have deficiencies. Benchmarks could provide a practical view of the extent of change that can be readily demonstrated, both in terms of the types of patients and the service approach possible. For example, can intermediate care schemes be adapted to provide for 'slowstream' rehabilitation patients, whose immediate needs may require care over several months, and who are likely to need further integrated care packages thereafter?
- Finally there is, generally, a lack of quantified findings relating to the service elements to deliver integrated care across acute and community sectors. This reflects the information gap referenced when looking at national workforce requirements at the start of this chapter.

Summary

Substantial further service redesign, beyond the initiatives described above, are still needed in order to provide a fully quantified description of the care models needed to deliver innovative and integrated care appropriate to the 21st century. However, what has been described in this chapter is an approach and presents methodologies that can support the development of a shared vision for services. Bed usage surveys can provide evidence of the potential scale of change across the health economy and provide baseline data to enable complementary service developments to be specified and quantified through the use of the Balance of Care model.

References

Bowen, T., Forte, P. (2000) *Intermediate Care Services for Older People: Estimating Future Workforce Requirements*. Unpublished report to the Department of Health. London: Balance of Care Group.

Bowman, C., Easton, P. (2000) Rehabilitation in long-term care. *Reviews in Clinical Gerontology* **10**, 75–9.

Department of Health (2000a) *The NHS Plan: A Plan for Investment, A Plan for Reform.* Cm 4818-I. London: Department of Health.

Department of Health (2000b) *Shaping the Future NHS: Long Term Planning for Hospitals and Related Services.* Consultation document on the findings of the National Beds Inquiry. London: Department of Health.

Donald, I., Jay, T., Linsell, J., Foy, C. (2001) Defining the appropriate use of community hospital beds. *British Journal of General Practice* **51**, 95–100.

Foote, C., Stanners, C. (2002) *Integrating Care for Older People.* London: Jessica Kingsley.

Forte, P., Bowen, T. (1997) Improving the balance of elderly care services. In: Cropper, S. and Forte, P. (eds) *Enhancing Health Services Management.* Milton Keynes: Open University Press, pp. 71–85.

Forte, P., Bowen, T., Foote, C. (2002) *East Berkshire Inpatient Survey: Report of Findings.* Unpublished report by the Balance of Care Group. London: Balance of Care Group. Copy obtainable on application via www.balanceofcare.com.

Forte, P., Bowen, T., Foote, C. (2003) *Identifying Demand for Intermediate Care and Community Hospitals in Oxfordshire: Final Report.* www.oxfordshire.nhs.uk/ohse/balanceofcare.asp.

Goddard, M., McDonagh, M., Smith, D. (2000) Annex E: Avoidable use of beds and cost-effectiveness of care in alternative locations. In: *Shaping the Future NHS: Long Term Planning for Hospitals and Related Services. Consultation Document on the Findings of the National Beds Inquiry – Supporting Analysis.* London: Department of Health.

Ham, C., York, N., Sutch, S., Shaw, R. (2003) Hospital bed utilisation in the NHS, Kaiser Permanente, and the US Medicare programme: analysis of routine data. *British Medical Journal* **Nov. 327**, 1257.

Lang, T., Liberati, A., Tampieri, A., Fellin, G., Gosalves, M., Lorenzo, S., Pearson, M., Beech, R., Santos-Eggiman, B. (1999) A European version of the Appropriateness Evaluation Protocol. *International Journal of Technology Assessment in Health Care* **15**, 185–97.

Lawrence, D., Buxton, V., Solijak, M., Edwards, N., Illingworth, R. (1999) Emergency admissions: over the threshold. *Health Services Journal* **109** (5641), 26–8.

Nocon, A., Baldwin, S. (1998) *Trends in Rehabilitation Policy: A Review of the Literature.* London: King's Fund.

Vaughan, B., Lathlean, J. (1999) *Intermediate Care: A Directory of Developments.* London: King's Fund.

Chapter 4
Coordinating Intermediate Care
Wanda Russell

Introduction

At the start of the 21st century the UK Government produced a 10-year plan for investment in, and modernisation of, the National Health Service (Department of Health, 2000a). This plan, in part, reflected the public's concerns about the difficulties that they were facing in accessing hospital services for inpatient care. A national investigation into the demand for, and utilisation of, acute beds concluded that the difficulties in accessing acute inpatient care were also due to a shortage of service alternatives for preventing the acute admission of some patients and for facilitating the acute discharge of others (Department of Health, 2000b). Hence the implementation of the NHS Plan will result in both an increase in acute hospital capacity and the development of service alternatives for providing care that has traditionally been provided in acute hospital beds (Department of Health, 2000a). Such service alternatives go under the banner of services for intermediate care.

The principles that underlie intermediate care include: the targeting of mainly older people; the requirement of comprehensive assessments of potential users to ascertain appropriateness of services; a rehabilitative focus and/or preventive outcome; a limited timescale of intervention; a multi/interdisciplinary team of professionals providing intermediate care services in an integrated whole system approach (Department of Health, 2001).

The introduction of any new intermediate care service therefore introduces a range of uncertainties:

- Who is the service aiming to benefit?
- What will the service offer?
- Who will provide the service?
- Who will use the service?
- How will referrals be made, and who will make them?
- How will (appropriate) information flow between different care providers who may be involved in providing care at various stages during a client's journey through a care pathway?

- How will roles of care providers be delineated?
- How should effectiveness of the intermediate care service be measured and how should outcomes be identified?
- How should the service be evaluated?
- How should the public be involved in the evaluation and development of an intermediate care service, and who should take part in this involvement?

All of the above concerns link into issues relating to demand for the new service, its impacts on the quality of care, professional and lay attitudes to the service, effects on existing care models, the effectiveness of the service, and associated economic merits.

This chapter will explore a variety of aspects of the coordination of intermediate care by identifying a range of questions that should be posed both from the outset and on an ongoing basis during the delivery of an intermediate care service. Throughout the chapter, a case study is used to illustrate the issues covered. This case study illustrates the processes and issues involved in a recent implementation and evaluation of an intermediate care service in Hereford, namely a multidisciplinary Rapid Response Team (RRT) which aimed to facilitate earlier hospital discharge by providing home based care (Beech et al., 2004).

The intermediate care service

A wide variety of intermediate care services now exist having become established over recent years in response to a number of policy influences, for example the Community Care Act 1990, the National Bed Inquiry (Department of Health 2000b), the NHS Plan (Department of Health, 2000a), the *National Service Framework for Older People* (Department of Health, 2001) and the Community Care (Delayed Discharges etc.) Act 2003. Whilst intermediate care services share a range of common principles (as stated above), they are all nevertheless unique and often suffer from a mismatch of outcomes with respect to their initial aims. Many of these services develop within a 'trial and error' framework with administrative and operational issues taking precedence over evaluation owing to scarcity of resources. Several key issues thus need to be considered when a new service is planned and launched:

- The aims of a new intermediate care service, who provides the service and how, are all determined by the perceived need for the service.
- The intended clients.
- The aims of the service will determine the number and skill mix of the different health professionals who will become involved, e.g. both in a primary care setting and in the acute sector.
- Issues such as staffing, recruitment, training, roles, geographical boundaries, capacity etc. need to be identified and addressed.

The structure, processes and outcomes of the new service should be assessed by exploring a range of measures which together reflect the key issues above. This would involve a range of audit or evaluation activities which would be required:

- To identify the uncertainties which exist regarding the new service.
- To determine the methods which would need to be implemented to gather information to address the uncertainties.
- To inform future service development.

The process of audit or evaluation is necessary to provide evidence to demonstrate several important dimensions including the *relevance* of the new service (i.e. that it serves the needs of the intended users), the *effectiveness* of the service (that benefits are conferred to the users and providers of the service), the *acceptability* of the service (that expectations are met amongst both those receiving the service and those providing it) and *efficiency* (i.e. that the service has economic merit) (Norman and Redfern, 1995). Such an evaluation (or audit) would necessitate careful consideration with respect to the information that would need to be gathered as well as how data collection could best be implemented. These considerations would need to be underpinned by the availability of resources and therefore a balanced view that weighs up a pragmatic approach against the reliability of the evidence generated is required.

The service and the clients

When a new service is introduced, aspects of the service content and structure need to be defined. Key questions include:

- Who are the intended users of the service?
- What are the activities of care delivered by the service providers?
- What are the roles and skill mix of those providing care?
- What are the roles of the care providers with respect to the components of care provided by the service?
- What are the care needs of the clients?

Appropriate methods will need to be designed and implemented in order to provide answers to the above questions. In the case study of the Hereford based RRT an evaluation using a broad, descriptive approach was implemented to allow, amongst other objectives, an in-depth description of the new service to be produced. This descriptive model adopted a variety of complementary research techniques which included both audit and survey methods. Both primary and secondary sources of information were used and a mix of qualitative and quantitative techniques were applied to obtain numerical and descriptive data respectively from a variety of sources. Information was obtained from the RRT, stakeholders within both acute and primary care settings, patients and carers and hospital records. The multi-method design which was chosen reflects current guidance from the Medical Research Council (Campbell et al., 2000). More information about other components of the evaluation is given in appropriate sections throughout this chapter. In order to set the scene for the Hereford case study, Box 4.1 outlines the intervention provided by the intermediate care service established in the city of Hereford.

Processes and systems

In addition to concerns relating to the structure, content and delivery of care when a new service is introduced, there will also be a number of issues relating to the processes and systems which need to be in place and effectively monitored and developed to ensure quality of care, appropriateness of care and an optimal effectiveness of the service. Several factors which need to be considered in relation to the successful implementation of an intermediate care service include the ways in which referral criteria should be established and should operate (both in terms of 'referral from' and 'referral on') and the identification of other service providers linked into the intermediate care intervention.

The service therefore needs to gain awareness both pre- and post-launch, e.g. amongst those who refer to the service and those who accept referrals from the service. Referral criteria need to be set out and accessible as the clarity of referral criteria during assessments may be questionable and expectations may not match assessed need. Furthermore, potential clients need to be informed of the service, and thought needs to be given to the notions of 'choice' and alternatives. Problems may arise owing to the perception of intermediate care being free, which can influence referral behaviour and can introduce conflict between organisations, e.g. social services and NHS, with respect to funding. Guidelines need to be established to assist in identifying social compared with health inputs, with the decisions about such questions often being influenced by cost allocation. Such issues may overlap with client needs regarding the duration of care; for example, in the case of long-term intermediate care models such as those concerned with rehabilitation, interventions provided under a free NHS model will not require payment on the part of the client.

Information channels and mechanisms also need to be established and the types of questions which need to be asked include:

- Who needs to share information?
- What information needs to be exchanged?
- What mechanisms of information management exist or need to be put in place?
- What are the requirements with respect to the timeliness and the effectiveness of information exchange?

Box 4.1 Hereford's rapid response team: the service and the clients.

Background	In March 2001, Herefordshire Primary Care Trust launched a new multidisciplinary rapid response team (RRT) service to supply services for intermediate care for the population of the city of Hereford. The introduction of the RRT service was in part a response to a previous locally conducted study which had audited the use of beds in the Hereford Acute Trust (Sherlow, 2000). That study concluded that a substantial proportion of acute beds were occupied by patients who were suitable for discharge to home based intermediate care, a finding which was in keeping with those of studies reported in the National Beds Inquiry (Department of Health, 2000b). The introduction of the RRT was also in accordance with the current drive to expand services for intermediate care throughout the NHS. Furthermore the RRT service was set up because of plans to construct a new hospital with fewer beds to serve the local population.
Aims of the service	The overall aim of the RRT service was to provide a home based alternative to care currently provided in an acute hospital bed which was acceptable to patients and carers and which maintained standards of clinical care.
Who provided the service	The team consisted of a senior nurse coordinator, a senior social worker, four nurses, four generic workers and an administrator.
What the service covered	Activities of care included: intravenous therapy following an infection; baseline observations; catheter care; oxygen therapy; provision of equipment; wound care; personal care (washing and dressing); meals; help with housework.
Other service considerations	Prior to the launch of the service, individual team members attended appropriate training schedules with respect to their roles. The areas covered by the training schedule included catheter care, intravenous drug administration, cannulation, pain management, moving and handling, infection control, respiratory management and team building.
The clients	The service was offered to patients admitted into acute care at Hereford County Hospital and who lived within a five-mile geographical radius of the city. In order to qualify for early discharge and care at home from the RRT, ward staff would identify potential patients who matched the criteria for home based care under the RRT (e.g. this will have excluded patients with psychiatric problems or myocardial infarction cases). These patients were then referred for assessment by the RRT who would then, in agreement with the patient (and where relevant with their carer), arrange the patient's discharge to home.
Evaluation data, sources and methods of collection	A comprehensive set of data collection forms was developed by the evaluation team in close collaboration with the RRT to serve the joint purposes of routine data management for the RRT and data gathering for the evaluation. These forms included data regarding patients (such as socio-demographic data, clinical information, assessment and care information) which were captured from existing hospital records as well as being completed by RRT staff during assessments. Interviews with RRT staff and other health professionals in both the acute and community settings (e.g. hospital consultants, discharge liaison sisters, A&E admissions unit staff, hospital bed manager, physiotherapists, occupational therapists, general practitioners, district nurses and social workers) allowed information to be gathered at the launch of the new service and at follow-up time points. This information included opinions on the need for an RRT and perceptions of effectiveness of the new service. The latter dimension included an exploration of the potential impacts on other health care professionals (e.g. concerns about increased GP call-outs and role blurring between RRT staff and district nurses).

Information capture needs to be designed so as to be simple and quick to apply, for example during assessments. Accessibility of information is a key consideration and would typically include setting up mechanisms by which information about individual clients can be obtained from their general practitioners (GPs). Access to prescribing information, for example, can cause a 48-hour delay which could compromise the efficiency of an intermediate care intervention. In addition, the providers of an intermediate care service should ensure that steps are taken to conform to consistency in information technology (IT) hardware/software and adequate team skills in handling computer-based records.

Medical cover is another aspect which needs to be considered. Therefore, separate contracts are frequently set up between the intermediate care provider and the GPs on a patient basis. GP cover may be high in some models of intermediate care (such as hospital at home for chronic obstructive pulmonary disease cases) where patients may require substantial input owing to their frailty and complexity of needs. The provision of medical cover is becoming an increasingly important issue which needs sufficient thought during the design and implementation of intermediate care services. This is evidenced by the fact that some Primary Care Trusts (PCTs) have appointed salaried GPs specifically to work in intermediate care.

The roles of different care providers, such as referrers to an intermediate care service, those who provide intermediate care, and those who take on the clients' care needs after discharge from intermediate care need to be identified and any role blurring issues addressed. This includes consideration being given to the responsibility of care and costs. Box 4.2 uses the case of the RRT in Hereford to illustrate some of the issues surrounding the processes and systems in an intermediate care model.

Monitoring, public involvement and evaluation

An important aspect of setting up an intermediate care service is the identification of appropriate outcomes. These might include clinical outcomes, quality of care, professional acceptance, client satisfaction and economic dimensions.

Furthermore, the impacts of outcomes, for example increased workloads and positive or negative impacts in primary and acute sectors, need to be measured. Issues to be considered here include how outcomes should be measured, and how often, vis-à-vis the aims of the service. Clinical outcomes, for example, might be measured in terms of survival, quality of life or clinical improvement. However, the measurement of such outcomes might involve extending the period of data collection beyond the time span of intermediate care. Performance measures such as quality of care can include a wide range of parameters (e.g. satisfaction with the service, adequacy of information, issues around choice, client anxieties and concerns, and their understanding of the intervention *per se*) rated by both the individuals providing the care and the clients receiving care. Impacts may include resource use and costs as well as benefits such as those from training.

Box 4.2 Hereford's rapid response team: referral criteria, discharge criteria, information pathways, professional roles.

Promotion of the service	The RRT used a variety of methods to promote the new service, including promotional flyers, poster displays and seminar presentations. The information flyer about the RRT service was distributed to eligible patients in acute care.
Referral criteria	A list of criteria was drawn up by the RRT to assist hospital staff in the process of making referrals to the team. Although these criteria served the purpose of providing guidelines for the referral process, some patients were given additional consideration if their circumstances were such that the benefits of RRT care outweighed a possible mismatch with the recommended criteria. Similarly, a list of discharge criteria was drawn up and a protocol was established to ensure a smooth information exchange with follow-on care providers.
Mechanisms of care and patient management	Once successfully referred to the RRT and on completion of the RRT assessment in the acute setting, the team followed a sequence of procedures to ensure that the necessary activities of care and flows of information were adhered to for each patient. A flowchart of the protocol for patient referral and management was produced as part of the guidelines. A suite of data management forms was developed (for the joint purposes of internal information management within the RRT and for the evaluation of the service) to facilitate the capture of patient referral information, assessment data, activities of care including equipment supplied and medication given, and discharge information including outcomes and details of follow-on care where relevant.
Roles	An evaluation of the service (see below) showed that there were areas of concern with respect to roles and role blurring between the RRT staff and some of providers of follow-on care. District nurses in particular expressed concern over these issues, which included the provision of night and weekend cover. Both community care providers and local GPs also voiced anticipation of an increased work burden. In the case of the latter, these concerns were unfounded. Meetings between RRT staff and community nursing staff provided the opportunity to develop effective liaison strategies and allowed roles to be monitored and clarified on an ongoing basis.
Evaluation data, sources and methods of collection	A suite of data collection forms developed by the evaluation research team in collaboration with the RRT (see Box 4.1) also allowed data relating to the patient's care pathway to be collected. For example, a data form on 'transfer to the RRT' facilitated the capture of data on any investigations performed in acute care as well as outstanding investigations. Dates of transfer to the RRT were recorded for all patients, as were dates of discharge from the RRT, patient needs on discharge, details of any follow-on referrals, or information relating to re-admission to acute care where necessary. Interviews with RRT staff to collect perceptions of the new service, including referral issues and questions on information flows, were also carried out at the end-point of the evaluation study.

The question of whether to carry out an audit style approach may need to be considered. An audit can address one or more aspects of a service, for example by measuring overall quality of the service, by measuring quality issues directly relevant to a clinical specialty, or by specifically measuring the quality of care provision. There is a wide range of methods which may be used for the purposes of audit which may include surveys, peer review or case presentations. Research evaluations to assess new services often make use of audit methods. It is important to note that the purpose of conducting an audit is not only to measure quality or changes in practice, but also to bring about change and improvement in practice (Norman and Redfern, 1995).

Public involvement is also required to inform service development and to assess the quality of the service. Public forums, patient representatives and organisations such as the Patient Advocacy and Liaison Service ('PALS') can have an important role in obtaining the views of users and their carers. In the current culture of liability and complaints, issues such as patient consent, choice of care, and awareness and understanding of care models are of paramount importance amongst consumers and care providers. Consideration must therefore be given to appropriate ways of engaging the public (e.g. linking with PALS) and the use of evaluation tools such as satisfaction surveys and interviews. Responding to the views of the public is an important strategy in order to develop or reshape the service not just to meet the needs of intermediate care staff and care providers.

A formal evaluation of any new service is an invaluable process. Even evaluations conducted on a shoestring budget should aim at least to provide an in-depth description of the intervention or service being evaluated and an account of the context and environment in which the intervention is being delivered to facilitate a more informed judgement of the value of the intervention. A descriptive approach is therefore often relevant for developmental evaluations since key features of the intervention can be identified and the role of the new service can be assessed with respect to existing policies. This type of evaluation often includes measures of user satisfaction and also an economic dimension. The evaluation should aim to be conducted within a dynamic framework within which regular feedback sessions to an appointed steering group and stakeholders can inform the development of the intermediate care service.

Typical evaluation components might include:

- Quantifying the referral source, characteristics and care needs of users of the intermediate care service.
- Identifying the activities of care being provided in response to identified care needs.
- Monitoring the performance of the intermediate care staff using a range of performance indicators, for example: the response time and treatment duration of care; impacts of the service on acute bed use; the existence of adverse events in a given model of care (e.g. readmission rates, deaths during care and emergency calls to GPs).

- Assessing acceptability of the service amongst users and their carers.
- Determining acceptability to health and social care professionals in terms of the structure and outcomes of the new service (e.g. issues around role blurring, risk management etc.).
- Exploring the economic merits of the new and alternative models of care.
- Exposing existing gaps in the provision of intermediate care services which might be addressed by the service being further evaluated or other service developments.
- Clarifying the ways in which the nature of the service might need to change to better meet the care needs of existing or potential users.

Box 4.3 presents the outcomes and evaluation components of the RRT service in Hereford.

Box 4.3   Hereford's rapid response team: outcome measures and evaluation.

Outcome measures used	These included survival, hospital readmission and destination on discharge from the RRT (e.g. details of providers, if any, of follow-on care)
The evaluation	The role of the evaluation team embraced several key areas of activity: • To carry out an independent, unbiased evaluation of the RRT service • To collaborate with the project steering group for the purposes of the evaluation • To determine and use appropriate research methods to conduct the evaluation • To conduct appropriate analyses of the data collected • To identify the key findings emerging from the evaluation • To share the findings as they became identified with the steering group and stakeholders on an ongoing basis • To inform a range of audiences interested in the findings • To inform the development of the RRT service.
Evaluation methods and data sources	Data for the evaluation were obtained from the RRT using data collection forms, interviews and workshops. The perspectives covered were: • Patient profile • Activities of care • Process measures, e.g. duration of care, elapsed times between referral and discharge events, adverse markers and the impact of the RRT on acute bed use. Data for the evaluation were obtained from patients and carers by conducting a survey and interviews. The perspectives covered were: • Knowledge about the RRT • Issues concerning choice • Emotional concerns during RRT intervention • Service structure and delivery • Overall satisfaction. Data for the evaluation were obtained from other key stakeholders by conducting interviews and running workshops. The perspectives covered were:

- Professional roles
- RRT skill-mix
- Referral issues and processes
- Information flows
- Opinions on the need for an RRT
- Effectiveness of the RRT.

Other data collected for service development included a bed audit (Gertman and Restuccia, 1981; Bristow et al., 1997), interviews and workshops to address:
- Inappropriate or under-referrals to the RRT
- Scope for quicker referrals to the RRT
- Scope for other forms of intermediate care.

Sample key findings: the characteristics of service users	Patients accepted for the RRT service were elderly and the majority had both medical and social care needs at the time of referral. A one-year evaluation of the service showed that most referrals could also be grouped into five broad diagnostic categories, including respiratory conditions, heart/stroke, falls/other injuries, digestive system disorders and musculoskeletal/connective tissue disorders. The evaluation of the service also showed that having been accepted for RRT care, the majority of clients (74.2%) were transferred for care at home within one day of their assessment. Furthermore, 70.8% of clients who used the service in the first year received care lasting between one and seven days and 97.2% of clients received care of up to two weeks duration (Beech et al., 2004).

Summary

This chapter has addressed the key concerns which are typically encountered when a new intermediate care service is proposed and implemented. The key areas can be divided into issues surrounding the service framework (i.e. need for the service; aims, structure and content of the service; target population), the processes and systems which determine the efficiency of the service (i.e. referral mechanisms and information flows) and monitoring (including the choice of outcomes, public involvement, and performance measures and evaluation methods).

The wide variety of intermediate care services and the unique nature of these models of care suggest that each intermediate care service will have its own particular issues and uncertainties in terms of its coordination and implementation. None the less, the importance of investing time and resources to understand the diversity of potential impacts of a new intermediate care service, whether on care providers (both acute and in the community), or on users and their carers, cannot be underestimated. The case of Hereford's RRT provides a clear example of the range of issues which needed to be identified and addressed during an evaluation strategy in order to guide the development of the service.

References

Beech, R., Russell, W., Little, R., Sherlow-Jones, S. (2004) An evaluation of a multi-disciplinary team for intermediate care at home. *International Journal of Integrated Care* 4 October, 2004, http://www.ijic.org.

Bristow, A., Hudson, M., Beech, R. (1997) *Analysing Acute Inpatient Services: The Development and Application of Utilisation Review Tools.* Report prepared for the NHS Executive South East Thames. London: NHS Executive South East Thames.

Campbell, M., Fitzpatrick, R., Haines, A., Kinmonth, A.L. et al. (2000) Framework for design and evaluation of complex interventions to improve health. *British Medical Journal* **321**, 694–6.

Department of Health (2000a) *The NHS Plan: A Plan for Investment, A Plan for Reform.* London: The Stationery Office.

Department of Health (2000b) *Shaping the Future NHS: Long Term Planning for Hospitals and Related Services. Consultation Document on the Findings of the National Beds Inquiry.* Leeds: NHS Executive, Department of Health.

Department of Health (2001) *National Service Framework for Older People.* London: Department of Health.

Gertman, P.M., Restuccia, J.D. (1981) The Appropriateness Evaluation Protocol: a technique for assessing unnecessary days of hospital care. *Medical Care* **19**, 855–71.

Norman, I., Redfern, S. (1995) What is audit? In: Kogan, M. and Redfern, S. with Kober, A. et al. (eds) *Making Use of Clinical Audit: A Guide to Practice in the Health Professions.* Buckingham: Open University Press.

Sherlow, S. (2000) *A Strategy for Change.* Independent Study Dissertation: BSc(Hons) Field of Advanced Professional Studies. Worcester: University College Worcester.

Chapter 5
Service Development and Evaluation in Intermediate Care

Brenda Roe

Introduction

Intermediate care has been evolving since the early 1990s, with government policy since 2000 clearly recommending its continued development, evidenced by *The NHS Plan* (Department of Health, 2000a) and health and local authority circulars (Department of Health, 2001a). Standard Three in the *National Service Framework for Older People* (NSF) (Department of Health, 2001b) provides a rationale and specific recommendations for key interventions and milestones to be achieved between 2001 and 2004 aimed at providing integrated services to promote rcovery, prevent unnecessary hospital admission, facilitate discharge and maximise independent living by providing a range of care services at home or in local care settings, commonly termed 'step-up' and 'step-down' facilities (Department of Health, 2001b).

Recognition of insufficient investment in preventive and rehabilitation services resulting in unplanned hospital admissions of older people or their premature admission into long-term care (Audit Commission,1997), and the fact that the National Beds Inquiry (NBI) reported that significant numbers of older people were remaining in hospital beds (Department of Health, 2000b; McDonagh et al., 2000), provided the impetus for developing 'care closer to home' and investment in intermediate care (Department of Health, 2000a). This chapter builds on previous chapters by looking specifically at the development of intermediate care services and looking specifically at the development of intermediate care services and professionals, the evidence underpinning them and identifies some of the barriers and constraints to the development of services and professionals. The development of intermediate care and its evaluation as part of services provision is implicit within the government policy and guidance with clear milestones and targets (Department of Health, 2001a; 2001b).

Development of services and professionals

Use of evaluation to support service delivery and development

Intermediate care schemes commenced in the early 1990s with 'hospital at home' schemes being some of the first to be developed (Shepperd and Illiffe, 2000). Hospital at home is mainly intended to provide a level of nursing care for people with acute medical needs more than is usually provided by community services but not in a hospital setting. Since then new schemes have been added onto existing schemes without there being any systematic evaluation of their effectiveness. The drivers to this piecemeal approach and evolution tended to be winter pressures caused by increased admissions of patients to hospital and finances being made available to reduce them without any overall strategy.

Intermediate care is not a universally recognised term in health services in other countries. In the USA it is taken to mean ambulatory urgent medical care similar to 'walk in' or 'out of hours' general practice centres in the UK (see Tosteson et al., 1996). A more comparable term for intermediate care used in the USA would be 'sub-acute care'. A search of the Cochrane Library (2001, Issue 1) using the term 'intermediate care' located reviews and protocols covering mainly medical interventions and drug treatments rather than services or care, and provided further evidence that intermediate care is not a universally recognised term (Roe et al., 2003). Eight single studies were identified within the NHS Economic Evaluation Database and one systematic review (Shepperd and Illiffe, 2000). Two of the single studies were disease specific (O'Caithan, 1994; Rich et al., 1995) while the others were concerned with health care: patient management, screening and rehabilitation (Johansen, 1994; Styrborn, 1995; von Sternberg et al., 1997; Health Services Utilization and Research Commission, 1998; Stewart et al., 1998; Naylor et al., 1999). These studies looked only at single interventions and their economic evaluations were limited which meant their findings could not be generalised to other countries.

This lack of consensus of terminology was also recognised by Parker et al. (1999), who identified a plethora of terms and service models being used, such as intermediate care, hotel or hostel care, swing beds, nurse-led beds and hospital at home. As part of a national survey they mailed NHS Trusts that provided services for older people throughout England and Wales to establish the 'best place' of care following acute or during sub-acute illness (88% response rate, $n = 323$). At that time, before the NSF (Department of Health, 2001b), the largest provision remained with day hospitals and inpatient rehabilitation. Since 1997 there had been growth in the home care services (one-third) to facilitate early discharge and (two-thirds) to prevent hospital admission. By the time of the survey a quarter of the Trusts had discharge planning posts. There had been little development of GP beds in nursing homes or community hospitals. Few of the schemes had been evaluated in terms of outcomes or effectiveness although a minority of Trusts (25%) had undertaken evaluation of their home care services. Cost-effectiveness evaluations by an independent team had been undertaken by a very small minority of Trusts (5%), with the findings being mainly of use locally for operational services and development rather than being widely generalised.

Analysis of social, economic and demographic factors at Trust and regional levels to establish if they influence the development of older people's services following acute and sub-acute illness is warranted. This information is useful to identify local population needs and the development of intermediate care services (Roe et al., 2003; see also Chapter 3).

Shepperd and Illiffe (2000) in the Cochrane systematic review of hospital at home compared with inpatient care concluded there was insufficient data to assess the effects on patient outcomes or costs for the hospital at home schemes. They recommended future research to specify the types of service provided and the types of patients included. They concluded that formal economic evaluation measuring health outcomes and satisfaction of users and carers is warranted.

Parker et al. (2000) also conducted a systematic review of evaluation research looking at the costs, quality and effectiveness of acute, sub-acute, post-acute and rehabilitation of older people. Intermediate care schemes in the review included admission avoidance, nurse-led beds, early discharge, day hospitals and community rehabilitation. They found the evidence on costs and effectiveness of intermediate care was weak, but so too was that of traditional models of care. They did find that day hospitals and inpatient rehabilitation had economic disadvantage for the health service (Applegate et al., 1988; Young and Forster, 1991; Hedrick et al., 1993) while community rehabilitation provided a significant economic advantage (Young and Forster, 1991; Melin and Byrgen, 1992). Based on the evidence above, community or home care services which avoid unnecessary admission and facilitate early discharge appear to have an economic advantage and these form the basis of current policy on intermediate care (Department of Health, 2001a; 2001b). It is important to undertake evaluation and cost effectiveness studies to determine which types of patients and schemes are most suitable in terms of outcomes and effectiveness. Evaluation of intermediate care as part of service delivery and development is implicit within government guidance and policy and explicit in terms of commissioned research (Department of Health, 2001a; 2001b; Stevenson and Spencer, 2002).

Young (2002) acknowledges that whilst there is a paucity of research evidence to underpin intermediate care there is some evidence to support hospital at home as a genuine alternative to inpatient care and that it may be cost neutral. Day hospitals and community hospitals have roles to play in avoiding admission and after post-acute illness for older people. While comprehensive evidence is lacking, Young (2002) argues for a whole system approach that integrates the variety of intermediate care schemes currently available.

Whole system integrated services for intermediate care

Whole systems approaches are currently advocated as the basis for developing and integrating services for older people generally and not just specifically for intermediate care (Audit Commission, 2002; National Audit Office, 2002). The King's Fund, which was one of the earliest proponents of intermediate care, provides clear guidance for developing intermediate care for health and social services using a whole systems approach (Stevenson and Spencer, 2002). This is a comprehensive guide about putting policy into practice with ideas and suggestions about what needs to be considered and achieved. These include mapping of existing services; consulting with local organisations, providers, consumers and carers; analysing health and social data on demography and service use; Strengths, Weakness, Opportunities and Threats (SWOT) analysis; and management of change, to illustrate but a few. Suggestions include not only the development of services but also of people involved in commissioning and delivering intermediate care.

Policy on intermediate care has evolved since the late 1990s within health and social care and it has been singled out as an entity within its own right. It is implicit within current policy that older people's experiences of intermediate care should be routinely evaluated as part of service delivery. Cornes and Clough (2001) looked at older people's experiences of an intermediate care scheme and concluded that intermediate care treads a fine line between being compensatory for deficiencies in mainstream services and being an unwelcome addition to the mainstream system with extra bureaucracy and a barrier to seamless services. They argue that without comprehensive training and care management for interdisciplinary working, problems endemic in the mainstream system, such as inadequate assessment, can transfer to intermediate care. Cornes and Clough (2001) argue the importance of mapping the relationship of intermediate care to the whole continuum of care.

Using whole systems approaches to service development and delivery in intermediate care is key to providing efficient and effective services. It is this notion that intermediate care relates to the whole continuum of care including continuing care that provided the reasons for this book. National debate has not taken place as to where intermediate care and long-term care fit together in the continuum of care. Where does intermediate care end and continuing care begin? At present there is a notional cut-off of six weeks, which is what intermediate care is typically said to be able to provide (Department of Health, 2001a; 2001b).

Thinking in terms of the continuum of care fits with an integrated whole systems approach to service development, delivery and evaluation. The notion of intermediate care being considered as an 'add on' to mainstream services and systems means we are in danger of reinventing the wheel and not learning the lessons that have gone before – as is the case with the Elderly Persons Integrated Care System (EPICS) in South Buckinghamshire, England, which started in 1994 (Foote and Stanners, 2002). The focus of this whole system-integrated care initiative was not to separate out intermediate or continuing care but recognise that older people's needs and care will change over time, as part of a continuum ultimately culminating in the end of life. The EPICS project team has worked over the past decade to develop policies, services, people and systems that do not separate out whether care is intermediate, continuing or end of life, but that are sensitive to the needs of older people and their carers as they age over time. Foote and Stanners (2002) provide a detailed account of the project's journey and useful applied information on the management of change, development of services and systems, and how they undertook evaluation.

It is essential that intermediate care be considered as part of the whole system of health and social care and integrated within the continuum of care, so that as people age and their needs change over time appropriate, accessible, effective and efficient care and services can be provided.

Professionals as providers of intermediate care

There are a variety of multidisciplinary professionals involved with commissioning, developing and providing intermediate care. Intermediate care involves more than any one discipline (Steiner, 2001a) and requires cross-disciplinary working and comprehensive joint training in assessment and care management (see Chapters 6, 7 and 14). It is generally accepted that the success of intermediate care is dependent on the effective and successful working of interdisciplinary teams although continued recruitment and retention of nurses, therapists and health care assistants often on short-term contracts can pose a difficulty (Roe, 2001a; 2001b). There is evidence that team working can improve quality of care, staff satisfaction and well-being and the efficient use of resources (Stevenson and Spencer, 2002).

While not specific to intermediate care, studies of team working in mental health care, breast cancer care (Borrill and West, 2001) and stroke (Stroke Unit Trialists' Collaboration, 1997) provide valuable evidence that may be transferable. For example, teams that function effectively are more innovative and provide higher quality patient care; teams that work well together have lower stress levels; interdisciplinary working is associated with greater innovation in care; improved ways of delivering care are underpinned by teams having regular effective meetings, communication and integration processes. Clear leadership also contributes to these effective team processes, high quality care and innovation (Borrill and West, 2001). Kalra et al. (2000) and Parker (2002) found that key features of the best stroke units included:

- Interdisciplinary care that was coordinated.
- Involvement of family and carers.
- Staff that specialise in stroke rehabilitation.
- Education of staff, users and carers.

It has been suggested that these features are transferable to the effectiveness of rehabilitation in other situations, which also involve a number of distinctive and complementary disciplines where their roles and inputs need to be coordinated (Sinclair and Dickinson, 1998; Audit Commission, 2000). Of relevance to intermediate care is the fact that occupational therapy was found to significantly reduce handicap and disability in people with a stroke who were not admitted to hospital (Walker et al., 1999). Such improved functional abilities are associated with less need for institutional care and less dependence on health and social resources (Gladman et al., 1993; Walker et al., 1999). Also, physiotherapy at home has been found cost effective and able to improve instrumental activities of daily living compared with day hospital physiotherapy (Young and Forster, 1992). These examples are relevant to intermediate care where interdisciplinary team working is a key feature. Also of note is that the majority of people with a stroke (60%) are not admitted to hospital (Walker et al., 1999), and would be prime candidates for intermediate care.

Multidisciplinary and interdisciplinary team working are key characteristics of intermediate care. So too is the joint working and planning by health and social services in relation to commissioning, providing and developing intermediate care using shared or single budgets. Their close working with the voluntary sector and local authorities on falls prevention initiatives, Care and Repair schemes designed to provide practical help and alterations in the home, housing, and with care homes for 'step-up' and 'step-down' beds provides a variety of initiatives to help prevent people going into hospital and ensure that care is provided closer to home. This not only demonstrates interdisciplinary working in intermediate care but inter-agency working, which is essential for whole systems development (Jee et al., 1999; Audit Commission, 2002; Foote and Stanners, 2002; National Audit Office, 2002) and strategic alliances for public health promotion.

It is recommended that intermediate care be coordinated from a single base by a responsible individual in order to optimise operational management, referral and assessment processes (Department of Health, 2001a; 2001b). Having a single intermediate care coordinator and explicit referral criteria for operational services has been associated with high rates of referral and acceptance of people eligible for intermediate care (Roe 2001a; 2001b; Roe et al., 2003). It is generally recommended that another individual take a more strategic approach at a higher organisational level (Primary Care Trust or hospital trust) and at the strategic health authority level (Department of Health, 2001b; Stevenson and Spencer, 2002). At an operational level, intermediate care involves quite a number of staff and they too also need to be coordinated (see Chapter 4).

Clinical governance framework

Clinical governance is a requirement for maintaining and improving service quality in NHS organisations and provides a quality assurance framework so that intermediate care can deliver appropriate care (Department of Health, 1999). Young recommends that a named individual be responsible with the authority and accountability to lead the process, and that it is important that all intermediate care staff are involved and committed to clinical governance issues (Department of Health, 2002a, Appendix 6). Routine collection of information on patient outcomes, adverse events and service user feedback comprises the basic requirements of the clinical governance system. A suggested minimum clinical data set includes the following (Department of Health, 2002a, Appendix 6):

- Patient demographic data.
- Referral source, date and time.
- Intermediate care function (avoidance of admission, early discharge).
- Intermediate care response (rapid response team, transfer to community hospital, day hospital attendance).
- Patient outcomes (discharged to usual home address, new institutional care placement, death, emergency hospital admission).

This routinely collected information is available from the intermediate care coordinator and can be extracted from the single assessment process. Specific aims of intermediate care are providing appropriate person centred care involving robust assessment and integration of a full range of services (see also Chapter 4).

Assessment processes

Comprehensive assessment that leads to the development of care plans, particularly for older people, have been found to decrease mortality, improve physical function and improve living location (Stuck et al., 1993; Steiner, 2001b). The single assessment process (SAP) is recommended for intermediate care services (Department of Health, 2001a; 2001b; 2002b; 2002c) to avoid duplication and replication of effort and information. This is a requirement for efficiency and will form the basis of future electronic information technology (IT) systems for assessment and care planning. SAPs are being developed and evaluated locally without a national template having to be adhered to. This in itself could be seen as an inefficient duplication of effort although it does allow organisations to tailor their assessments to their current IT systems and configuration of services. The Department of Health has approved some assessment instruments, such as the Minimum Data Set for Home Care (Carpenter et al., 2003).

The SAP is to be undertaken by a single named individual to avoid duplication and replication of effort and over-assessment. This has resulted in members of the interdisciplinary teams reviewing their skills and competencies (see Chapters 6, 7 and 14), as part of their service organisation and delivery, and clinical practice. This has necessitated them identifying core competencies that all health and social care providers have in relation to assessment of health and social needs and transferable skills that can be shared across disciplines on assessment and rehabilitation. More specialist skills may be discipline specific, of note is the medical assessment required for some individuals. Medical assessment and input has been provided by contracts and additional payments to local general practitioners (Roe, 2001a; 2001b; Roe et al., 2003), salaried GPs with specialist interests or community geriatricians employed by NHS Primary Care Trusts.

Medical assessment and involvement have evolved according to local needs and arrangements. There is some national evidence that this seems to be well established (Martin et al., 2004), although some earlier local evidence found that medical assessment and involvement was not always clear or accessible (Roe, 2001a; 2001b; Roe et al., 2003). Although policy is clear that with intermediate care, where a person's condition or situation is not adequately explained, or a course of action to improve the situation is not clear, or the person is not improving, a GP should be involved in the first instance and, if necessary, a specialist medical assessment sought (Department of Health, 2002a).

Consumers and carers

Involving consumers and carers in the planning, development and evaluation of intermediate care comprises yet another element of interdisciplinary and inter-agency working and collaborations (see Chapters 15 and 16). So too is involvement with the voluntary sector, which provides specific comment and feedback on service integration and development as well as being providers of important initiatives such as falls prevention advice (e.g. Age Concern) and Care and Repair schemes (e.g. Care and Repair England). These latter schemes address the housing, health and care needs of older people that can prevent hospital admission and facilitate early discharge by providing essential home alterations such as keypads for carer access or handrails.

Barriers and constraints

A number of barriers and constraints in the delivery of intermediate care have been identified from local evaluations, which undoubtedly provide opportunities for service development and improvement. A number of different intermediate care schemes have evolved since the early 1990s and have been added on because of winter pressures and finance being available (Stevenson and Spencer, 2002; Roe et al., 2003). Consequently this has resulted sometimes in gaps and overlaps between the existing and recently developed schemes.

Of note have been schemes focusing on rehabilitation and recovery (R&R) and those of existing Community Rehabilitation Link Teams, which accept similar clients (Roe et al., 2003). This finding provided an opportunity to revisit inclusion criteria, care philosophies and short- and long-term goals of rehabilitation by the local intermediate care team to remove overlap and increase specificity.

Shortage of nursing home beds for 'step-up' or 'step-down' care has been a limitation in some areas. Equitable access to care home facilities has varied across Trusts serving large geographical and rural areas (Roe et al. 2003). Sometimes terminology was used, 'complex case' for example, without clear operational definitions of what was meant. Also, gaps in services were identified for meeting the needs of people who were immobile, heavily dependent, having dementia, or who required more technical nursing care requiring intravenous drug administration or 24-hour care.

Nurse prescribing for clients was also seen as an opportunity for development specific to intermediate care and merits further study (Roe, 2001b; Roe et al., 2003).

It is suggested that a lengthy process of development of intermediate care can be short-circuited by sharing examples of local good practice of which there are a number of published examples (Department of Health, 2002a; Foote and Stanners, 2002; Stevenson and Spencer, 2002). Dissemination of successful features makes pragmatic sense and based on Department of Health guidance (Department of Health, 2002a) these include:

- Having vision, drive and leadership.
- Senior level commitment.
- Shared objectives, clearly articulated and understood.
- Person centred care.
- Strategic and operational management and coordination.
- Clear appreciation of the potential and limitations of intermediate care.
- Confidence, trust and accepting risk.
- Clear professional accountability.
- Medical input with clear arrangements for assessment or referral.
- Shared financial arrangements between agencies.
- Pragmatism, problem solving and open-mindedness.
- Practicalities – single point of contact or access and shared base.

Range of schemes and services

As already stated a number of intermediate care schemes have evolved over the years, which comprise the intermediate care service. The purpose of this section is to provide an overview of these schemes. Information on their effectiveness and cost effectiveness is given in Chapters 8 and 9.

Hospital at home (HAH)

This was the first scheme to be developed and is now well established throughout the UK (Stevenson and Spencer, 2002; Young, 2002). Active treatment is provided by health and social care professionals in people's homes rather than in acute hospitals. HAH is aimed at facilitating early discharge and avoiding admission. It is aimed at people recovering from surgery or older people with a medical condition and can help to reduce hospital lengths of stay, where the views of carers are also taken into account. Admission avoidance may be less expensive than hospital care (Shepperd and Illiffe, 2002). HAH may not be suitable for people recovering from stroke, as there may be an increased mortality for people treated at the early stage of stroke at home (Parker, 2002).

Early supported discharge schemes

These are aimed at people needing to be cared for following acute care and a variety have evolved, for example Acute Medical Trauma, Rehabilitation and Recovery. They are aimed at people who have had falls or fractures and they have been found to reduce length of hospital stay for older people with hip fractures and increase their return to their previous living arrangements (Cameron et al., 2000). More older people remain in their own homes at 6–12 months following hospital admission rather than move into long-stay or institutional care without any increase in their mortality (Hyde et al., 2000). There have also been specific studies that have looked at early supported discharge for people with stroke and the use of rehabilitation. They have found early supported discharge to be cost effective (Beech et al., 1999), feasible and clinically effective, and that it resulted in considerable reduction in use of hospital beds (Rudd et al., 1997).

Rapid response

This provides a fast response to people's health and social care needs, usually within 2 to 24 hours. The idea is to prevent pressure on health and social care systems by providing rapid assessment and services to avoid hospital admission or facilitate early discharge. These schemes are relatively recent and arose following the National Beds Inquiry on delayed discharges (Department of Health, 2000b) and *The NHS Plan* (Department of Health, 2000a). According to local evaluations they do appear to be able to prevent hospital admissions and save on 'bed days' (Sanderson and Wright, 1999; Wilde et al., 2002; Beech et al., 2004).

Community rehabilitation teams (CRTs)

These tend to provide a comprehensive range of services, including equipment as well as therapy, not just specific to intermediate care. They provide living aids, bath aids, home based occupational therapy, exercise programmes for people with arthritis and falls prevention programmes. A national survey concluded that CRT is poorly defined, small in scale and fragmented, with teams having poor identities (Enderby and Wade, 2001) and overlapping with other services (Parker, 2002). Users of CRT prefer home based rehabilitation to hospital based (Sander, 2000) although no difference has been reported in outcomes or mortality (Parker et al., 2000). In order to maximise the effects of rehabilitation, CRTs are using enabling projects where therapists train care assistants to enable older people to regain their independence (Young, 2002).

Day hospitals and day care centres

These offer a range of services for whole or part day attendance, including multidisciplinary team assessment and treatment; specialist clinics for continence, falls prevention and Parkinson's disease; mental health assessment; rapid response; and therapy outreach by CRT (Stevenson and Spencer, 2002; Young, 2002). Day hospitals are used in a variety of ways, but poor coordination, inadequate transport and high running costs can result in them not being used to the full (Audit Commission, 2000). Day hospital appears to be as effective a service for older people as 'comprehensive elderly' inpatient care in terms of clinical outcomes (Forster et al., 1999; 2002; Young, 2002). It is also reported in an observational study that multidisciplinary assessments in the day hospital can take care of 63% of patients without the need for hospital admission (Black, 1997). Day centres, run by social services or the voluntary sector, also offer just as effective rehabilitation as day hospitals but cheaper. User satisfaction was not matched owing to the perceived stigma of day centres and perception of inferior treatment (Burch and Borland, 1999). Day centres do have a valuable contribution to make to intermediate care.

Community hospitals

These have a multipurpose role and provide a range of locally based inpatient and outpatient care, diagnostic services, rehabilitation, health promotion and day hospital care (Young, 2002). They may not be appropriate places for some forms of intermediate care or social rehabilitation (Audit Commission, 2000; Department of Health, 2002a) although they may well be appropriate for post-acute care of older people (Young, 2002).

Nurse-led units

Also known as nursing development units, these have been established for post-acute care. Patients tend to have longer lengths of stay on nurse-led units (Griffiths et al., 2000; 2001; Steiner et al., 2001), fewer medical reviews and less physiotherapy as their stay continues, with a focus on care rather than enabling and rehabilitation (Steiner, 2001).

Care homes

Care homes, which include nursing, residential and dual registered homes are used to provide 'step-up' or 'step-down' intermediate care. Partnerships between NHS Trusts, local authorities and the private sector have been encouraged (Department of Health, 2001a). Where the culture of the home focuses on enabling and independence rather than traditional care then rehabilitation of frail older people as part of intermediate care is possible (Ibbotson, 2001, cited in Stevenson and Spencer, 2002). A limitation is that access to therapies by care homes is difficult or absent (Stevenson and Spencer, 2002; Young, 2002). Physiotherapy is received by a small minority of people in nursing homes who pay for it themselves, while even fewer have occupational therapy (Barodawala et al., 2001). CRTs working with care home staff to focus on rehabilitation is warranted, so too is more work on the effectiveness of intermediate care in care homes.

Sheltered accommodation and assisted living

These may also have a part to play in intermediate care. Despite government recommendations for this (Department of Health, 2001a; 2002a) there has been very little work undertaken on sheltered accommodation and intermediate care (Stevenson and Spencer, 2002). Of the limited work that is available fourth-fifths of people unable to return to their own homes following acute illness regained independence and returned to their own home or remained in their new home. This scheme had high user satisfaction, reduced home care by five hours per week per person, and made financial savings for the local authority (Herbert, 2002). Information on continuing care in care homes, assisted living and retirement communities is covered in Chapters 11 and 12.

Equipment services

While not a specific scheme, these are essential to support intermediate care services and very important for older people in maintaining their activities of daily living and independence. They have a vital role in avoiding hospital admissions and facilitating early discharge (Audit Commission, 2002). There may be benefits for joint commissioning and finance of these services in order to optimise capacity and focus on meeting needs (Stevenson and Spencer, 2002).

Role of evaluation in service monitoring and development

It is recommended that evaluation of intermediate care services is implicit within their everyday provision (Department of Health, 2001a; 2001b). The information obtained can identify areas for future development and provide information on outcomes and effectiveness. Only a minority of intermediate care schemes developed in the 1990s had been subjected to any local evaluation and around 5% of NHS Trusts had completed evaluations of cost effectiveness of home care services by an independent team (Parker et al., 1999). Since the 2001 policy guidance on the evaluation of intermediate care, local evaluation of services has been undertaken but few studies by independent teams have been published (Foote and Stanners, 2002; Young, 2002; Roe et al., 2003; Beech et al., 2004).

Routine information can be collected locally on clinical data, patient outcomes, adverse events and user feedback as part of regular service monitoring and clinical governance assurance requirements (Department of Health, 2002a, Appendix 6). This information can be used to provide evidence of the services' appropriateness and effectiveness. Other useful techniques are undertaking SWOT analyses and facilitated workshops to identify strengths and gaps within services and the need for staff developments (Stevenson and Spencer, 2002; Roe et al., 2003). Evaluation can be used to benchmark existing services or the outcomes of new services. Dimensions to monitor include user satisfaction, care outcomes, processes, cost and resource use in order to establish effectiveness, with a variety of tools and measures such as quality of life, outcome tools, training programmes and length of stay (Foote and Stanners, 2002; Stevenson and Spencer, 2002). (See also Chapter 4.)

National evaluations, funded by the Department of Health and the Medical Research Council in England and Wales (2001–2004) have investigated the costs of intermediate care services for older people and the outcomes of different models and best practices (Gillian Parker, University of Leicester). A second project using a whole systems approach involving structure, process, outcomes and cost effectiveness has undertaken a national audit of intermediate care expenditure and a comparative case study (Gerald Wistow, University of Leeds). The third project has involved a multi-centre study of the effectiveness of community hospitals in providing intermediate care for older people (John Young, St Luke's Hospital, Bradford). These national evaluations will provide essential evidence for the future development of intermediate care services.

Summary

This chapter has looked at the role of evaluation in the development and monitoring of intermediate care. A wide variety of schemes have evolved and now comprise intermediate care services. Routine evaluation is essential not only for complying with clinical governance but also for providing evidence to measure success and effectiveness of current services and for developing future services. Interdisciplinary and inter-agency working are key to the commissioning and delivery of intermediate care. Whole systems approaches looking at structures, processes and outcomes of intermediate care services and how they integrate with other health and social services are essential. Intermediate care is part of the continuum of care.

References

Applegate, W.R., Akins, D., Beaver, T.B., et al. (1988) A randomised controlled trial of geriatric assessment and rehabilitation unit. *Journal of the American Geriatrics Society* **36**, 578.

Audit Commission (1997) *The Coming of Age: Improving Care Services for Older People*. London: Audit Commission.

Audit Commission (2000) *The Way to Go Home: Rehabilitation and Remedial Services for Older People*. London: Audit Commission.

Audit Commission (2002) *Integrated Services for Older People. Building a Whole System Approach in England*. London: Audit Commission.

Barodawala, S., Kesavan, S., Young, J. (2001) A survey of physiotherapy and occupational therapy provision in UK nursing homes. *Clinical Rehabilitation* **15**, 607–10.

Beech, R., Rudd, A.G., Tilling, K., Wolfe, C.D.A. (1999) Economic consequences of early inpatient discharge to community-based rehabilitation for stroke in an inner-London teaching hospital. *Stroke* **30**, 729–35.

Beech, R., Russell, W., Little, R., Sherlow, S. (2004) An evaluation of a multidisciplinary team for intermediate care at home. *International Journal of Integrated Care* **4**, October, 2004, http://www.ijic.org.

Black, D.A. (1997) Emergency day hospital assessments. *Clinical Rehabilitation* **11**, 344–6.

Borrill, C., West, M. (2001) *Developing Team Work in Health Care. A Guide for Managers.* Aston: ACHSOR.

Burch, S., Borland, C. (1999) A randomised controlled trial of day hospital and day centre therapy. *Clinical Rehabilitation* **13**, 105–12.

Cameron, I., Crotty, M., Currie, C., et al. (2000) Geriatric rehabilitation following fractures in older people: a systematic review. *Health Technology Assessment* **4**, 2.

Carpenter, I., Perry, M., Challis, D., Hope, K. (2003) Identification of registered nursing care of residents in UK nursing homes using the Minimum Data Set Resident Assessment Instrument (MDS/RAI) and resource utilisation groups version III (RUG-III). *Age and Ageing* **32**, 279–85.

Cochrane Library (2001) Issue 1. Oxford: Update Software.

Cornes, M.L., Clough, R. (2001) The continuum of care: older people's experiences of intermediate care. *Education and Ageing* **16** (2), 179–202.

Department of Health (1999) *Clinical Governance: Quality in the New NHS.* London: Department of Health.

Department of Health (2000a) *The NHS Plan: A Plan for Investment, A Plan for Reform.* London: The Stationery Office.

Department of Health (2000b) *Shaping the Future NHS: Long Term Planning for Hospitals and Related Services. Consultation Document on the Findings of the National Beds Inquiry – Supporting Analysis.* London: Department of Health.

Department of Health (2001a) *Intermediate Care.* Health Service Circular. Local Authority Circular. London: Department of Health.

Department of Health (2001b) *National Service Framework for Older People.* London: Department of Health.

Department of Health (2002a) *National Service Framework for Older People – Supporting Implementation. Intermediate Care: Moving Forward.* London: Department of Health, Appendix 6.

Department of Health (2002b) *The Single Assessment Process for Older People.* HSC 2002/ 01: LA 2002(1). London: Department of Health.

Department of Health (2002c) *The Single Assessment Process for Older People. Assessment Tools and Scales.* London: Department of Health.

Enderby, P., Wade, D. (2001) Community rehabilitation in the United Kingdom. *Clinical Rehabilitation* **15**, 577–81.

Foote, C., Stanners, C. (2002) *Integrating Care for Older People. New Care for Old – A Systems Approach.* London: Jessica Kingsley.

Forster, A., Langhorne, P., Young, J. (1999) Systematic review of day hospital care for elderly people. *British Medical Journal* **318**, 837–41.

Forster, A., Langhorne, P., Young, J., for the Day Hospital Group (2002) *Medical Day Hospital Care for the Elderly Versus Alternative Forms of Care* (Cochrane review). In: The Cochrane Library, Issue 3. Oxford: Update Software.

Gladman, J., Lincoln, N., Adams, S. (1993) Use of external ADL scale with stroke patients. *Age and Ageing* **22**, 419–24.

Griffiths, P., Wilson-Barnett, J., Richardson, G., Spilsbury, K., Miller, F., Harris, R. (2000) The effectiveness of intermediate care in a nursing-led in-patient unit. *International Journal of Nursing Studies* **37**, 153–61.

Griffiths, P., Harris, R., Richardson, G., Hallet, N., Heard, S., Wilson-Barnett, J. (2001) Substitution of a nursing-led inpatient unit for acute services: randomised controlled trial of outcomes and cost of nursing-led intermediate care. *Age and Ageing* **30**, 483–8.

Health Services Utilization and Research Commission (1998) *Hospital and Home Care Study*. Saskatoon: Health Services Utilization and Research Commission.

Hedrick, S.C., Rothman, M.L., Chapko, M., Ehreth, J., Diehr, P., Inui, T.S., Connis, R.T., Grover, P.L., Kelly, J.R. (1993) Summary and discussion of methods and results of adult day health care evaluation study. *Medical Care* **31** (9) (Suppl), SS94–103.

Herbert, G. (2002) *Tomlinson Court: A New Approach ro Rehabilitation in Sheltered Housing. Evaluation Report*. Leeds: Nuffield Institute of Health.

Herbert, G., Townsend, J., Ryan, J., Wright, D., Ferguson, B., Wistow, G. (2000) *Rehabilitation Pathways for Older People after Fractured Neck of Femur. A Study of the Impacts of Rehabilitation Services and Social Care Networks on the Aftercare of Older People with Rehabilitation Needs*. Leeds: Nuffield Institute for Health/York Health Economics Consortium.

Hyde, C.J., Robert, I.E., Sinclair, A.J. (2000) The effects of supporting discharge from hospital to home in older people. *Age and Ageing* **29** (3), 271–9.

Ibbotson, M. (2001) *Community Health Sheffield NHS Trust Community Rehabilitation Unit, Working in Partnership*. Presentation to King's Fund Workshop Nursing Homes and Intermediate Care. 20 March 2001. Manchester: University of Manchester.

Jee, M., Popay, J., Everitt, A., Eversley, J. (1999) *Evaluating Whole Systems Approach to Primary Health Care Development*. London: King's Fund.

Johansen, G. (1994) An economic appraisal of two strategies for geriatric screening. *Journal of Social Medicine* **22**, 293–8.

Kalra, L., Evans, A., Perez, I., Knapp, M., Donaldson, N., Swift, C. (2000) Alternative strategies for stroke care: a prospective randomised controlled trail. *Lancet* **356**, 894–9.

Martin, G.P., Peet, S.M., Hewitt, G.J., Parker, H. (2004) Diversity in intermediate care. *Health and Social Care in the Community* **12** (2), 150–54.

McDonagh, M.S., Smith, D.H., Goddard, M. (2000) Measuring appropriate use of acute beds: a systematic review of methods and results. *Health Policy* **53**, 157–84.

Melin, A.L., Byrgen, L.O. (1992) Efficacy of the rehabilitation of elderly primary health care patients after short-stay hospital treatment. *Medical Care* **30**, 1004–1015.

National Audit Office (2002) *Developing Effective Services for Older People*. London: National Audit Office.

Naylor, M.D., Brooten, D., Campbell, R., Jabobsen, R., Mezey, M.D., Pauly, M.V., Schwartz, J.S. (1999) Comprehensive discharge planning and home follow-up of hospitalised elders: a randomised clinical trial. *Journal of the American Medical Association* **281**, 613–20.

O'Caithan, A. (1994) Evaluation of a hospital at home scheme for early discharge planning and home follow-up of hospitalised elders: a randomised clinical trial. *Journal of Public Health Medicine* **16**, 205–210.

Parker, G. (2002) *What works and what doesn't work in intermediate care?* Presentation to King's Fund/BMA/Age Concern England Conference on Intermediate Care. 18 March 2002, London: BMA House.

Parker, G., Phelps, K., Shepperdson, B., Bhakta, P., Katbamna, S., Lovett, C. (1999) *Best Place of Care for Older People after Acute and During Sub-acute Illness: Report of a National Survey*. Leicester: University of Leicester, Nuffield Community Care Studies Unit.

Parker, G., Bhakta, P., Katbamna, S., Lovett, C., Pailsey, S., Parker, S., Phelps, K., Baker, R., Jagger, C., Lindesay, J., Shepperdson, B., Wilson, A. (2000) Best place of care for older people after acute and during sub-acute illness: a systematic review. *Journal of Health Services Research and Policy* **5**, 176–89.

Rich, M.W., Beckham, V., Wittenberg, C., Leven, C.L., Freedland, K.E., Camey, R.M.A. (1995) A multi-disciplinary intervention to prevent re-admission of elderly patients with congestive failure. *New England Journal of Medicine* **333**, 1190–95.

Roe, B. (2001a) *Evaluation of Intermediate Care Services: Pilot.* Keele: Centre for Geriatric Medicine, Keele University. (Unpublished report submitted to Cheshire Community Healthcare NHS Trust.)

Roe, B. (2001b) *Evaluation of Intermediate Care Services: Continuation.* Keele: Centre for Geriatric Medicine, Keele University. (Unpublished report submitted to Cheshire Community Healthcare NHS Trust.)

Roe, B., Daly, S., Shenton, G., Lochhead, Y. (2003) Development and evaluation of intermediate care. *Journal of Clinical Nursing* **12**, 341–50.

Rudd, A.G., Wolfe, C.D.A., Tilling, K., Beech, R. (1997) Randomised controlled trial to evaluate early discharge scheme for patients with stroke. *British Medical Journal* **315**, 1039–44.

Sander, R. (2000) *Evaluation of Portsmouth and South East Hampshire Community Rehabilitation Project.* Portsmouth: University of Portsmouth School of Health and Social Care.

Sanderson, D., Wright, D. (1999) *Final Evaluation of the CARATS Initiative in Rotherham.* York: York Health Economics Consortium, University of York.

Shepperd, S., Illiffe, S. (2000) *Hospital at Home Versus In-Patient Hospital Care* (Cochrane review). In: The Cochrane Library, Issue 4. Oxford: Update Software.

Shepperd, S., Illiffe, S. (2002) *Hospital at Home Versus In-Patient Hospital Care* (Cochrane review). In: The Cochrane Library, Issue 2. Oxford: Update Software.

Sinclair, A., Dickinson, E. (1998) *Effective Practice in Rehabilitation: the Evidence of Systematic Reviews.* London: King's Fund and Audit Commission.

Steiner, A. (2001a) Intermediate care: more than a 'nursing thing'. *Age and Ageing* **30**, 433–5.

Steiner, A. (2001b) Intermediate care: a good thing? *Age and Ageing* **30**, 30–39.

Steiner, A., Walsh, B., Pickering, R., Wiles, R., Ward, J., Broooking, J.I., Southampton NLU Evaluation Team (2001) Therapeutic nursing or unblocking beds: a randomised controlled trial of post-acute intermediate care unit. *British Medical Journal* **322**, 453–9.

Stevenson, J., Spencer, L. (2002) *Developing Intermediate Care. A Guide for Health and Social Services Professionals.* London: King's Fund.

Stewart, S., Pearson, S., Luke, C.G., Horowitz, J.D. (1998) Effects of home-based intervention on unplanned readmissions and out-of-hospital death. *Journal of the American Geriatrics Society* **46**, 174–80.

Stroke Unit Trialists' Collaboration, Langhorne, P. et al. (1997) Collaborative systematic review of the randomised trials organised inpatient (stroke unit) care after stroke. *British Medical Journal* **314**, 1151–9.

Stuck, A., Siu, A., Wieland, G., Adams, J., Rubenstein, L. (1993) Comprehensive geriatric assessment: a meta-analysis of controlled trials. *Lancet* **342**, 1032–6.

Styrborn, K. (1995) Early discharge planning for elderly patients in acute hospitals: an intervention study. *Journal of Social Medicine* **23**, 273–85.

Tosteson, A.N.A., Goldman, L., Udvarheyi, I.S., Lee, T.H. (1996) Cost-effectiveness of coronary care unit versus intermediate care unit for emergency department patients with chest pain. *Circulation* **94**, 143–50.

von Sternberg, T., Hepburn, K., Cibuzar, P., Convery, L., Dokken, B., Haefemeyer, J., Rettke, S., Ripley, J., Vosenau, V., Rothe, P., Shurle, D., Won-Savage, R. (1997) Post-hospital sub-acute care: an example of a managed care model. *Journal of the American Geriatrics Society* **45**, 87–91.

Walker, M.F., Gladman, J., Lincoln, N., et al. (1999) Occupational therapy for stroke patients not admitted to hospital: a randomised controlled trail. *Lancet* **354**, 278–80.

Wilde, K., Roe, B., Beech, R., Crome, P. (2002) *Evaluation of the Rapid Response Scheme Operating in North Staffordshire*. Keele: Keele Papers in Geriatric Medicine and Gerontology, Keele University.

Young, J. (2002) The evidence base for intermediate care. *Geriatric Medicine* **32** (10), 11–14.

Young, J.B., Forster, A. (1991) The Bradford community stroke trial: eight weeks results. *Critical Rehabilitation* **5**, 283–9.

Young, J.B., Forster, A. (1992) The Bradford community stroke trial: results at six months. *British Medical Journal* **304**, 108–109.

Chapter 6

Interdisciplinary Working in Intermediate Care: Generic Working or the Key to a Person Centred Approach?

Anne Marriott, Gaynor Reid, Kathy Jones, Rae de Villiers and Christine Kennedy

Introduction

'One man actually said to me, it was really good having just one person, tying things together. He had a sense that we were all coming together in the same place, doing, working towards the same goal, that we were connected to one another.' (Team member) (Reid et al., 2002, p. 67)

'Oh, yes . . . I got what I needed . . . Their coordination [made a difference] more than anything because what the care manager said was happening, it did. When you are on your own these things are vital, that you know who's coming and when.' (Client) (Reid et al., 2002, p. 58)

'I think the Rehabilitation Link Team does a vital job keeping older people in their own homes with the necessary support. The work efficiently crosses agencies preventing duplication and confusion and should be commended.' (Key stakeholder) (Reid et al., 2002, p. 57)

The above quotations are taken from the evaluation report on an interdisciplinary assessment and rehabilitation service in Cheshire. They illustrate some of the real benefits of interdisciplinary working such as effective coordination, clear communication and partnership working, with the person at the centre of the rehabilitation process. In East Cheshire interdisciplinary working has been defined as:

'a team of professionals from different disciplines (and possibly different organisations) who integrate their shared skills into a framework of core team skills. The team deliver a co-ordinated, person centred service by working across 'traditional' professional/organisational boundaries and targeting unique professional skills appropriately.' (Marriott and Wright, 2002, p. 38)

This new approach to rehabilitation began in 2000 when Cheshire County Council and health care providers established three interdisciplinary Rehabilitation Link Teams. Each team consisted of five to six rehabilitation coordinators and six rehabilitation assistants, with access to therapy practitioners and other specialist services. A team manager was appointed to each team and this position was available to a health or social work professional with management experience. The teams were part of a countywide project which was funded for two years through joint investment monies. In East Cheshire the Rehabilitation Link Team (RLT) became integrated within the intermediate care service in April 2002 with ongoing funding from East Cheshire Primary Care Trust and Cheshire County Council Social Services. As part of the intermediate care service, the RLT works alongside a Rapid Response Team and Discharge Liaison Team. Only the RLT operates as an interdisciplinary team. The overall emphasis of the RLT's work continues to be with older people who are experiencing general frailty and have complex needs, normally addressed by a series of different disciplines. The main aims of the team are:

- To promote independence in all aspects of daily life.
- To prevent or delay hospitalisation or entry to long-term care.
- To facilitate timely hospital discharge.

This chapter describes the implementation process and evaluation of the interdisciplinary rehabilitation team in East Cheshire. It explores the benefits and limitations of the interdisciplinary team approach based on the evaluation findings.

Background to the development of interdisciplinary working

Before the introduction of the new teams in Cheshire, national consultative exercises had indicated that older people wanted continuity within, and across, health and social services. Robinson and Turnock (1998) on behalf of the King's Fund, plus the Audit Commission (2000), the Department of Health (2001) and the Association of Directors of Social Services and Local Government Association (2003), had all produced documents that emphasised the importance of a partnership approach to intermediate care. In particular they emphasised the importance of each person's having only one rather than a collection of people taking responsibility for their overall care and that person being equipped to manage their particular concerns and needs.

National initiatives on rehabilitation, the single assessment process and person centred care all support a change in the delivery of rehabilitation to older people. It is therefore important to identify a way of working which puts the person at the centre of rehabilitation rather than setting up a system which allows a series of different uni-professional assessments to take place.

The care management model and process

Care management is defined as:

> 'a process of tailoring services to individual needs. Assessment is an integral part of care management, but it is only one of seven core tasks that make up the whole process.' (SSI/SOSWSG, 1991)

The application of care management was originally developed from the Griffiths Report (1988) and was initially referred to as case management. The process of care management was aimed at what would now be described as 'intermediate care', that is, to support people at home in order to avoid unnecessary admission to hospital or long-term care. The introduction of care management was also intended to put greater emphasis on the person and their carer(s). Care management was chosen as the model for developing interdisciplinary working because of the key features underpinning its use which include:

- Screening for priority individuals.
- Organising a full needs assessment.
- Consultation with the person and carers at all stages.
- Delivery of flexible and appropriate services.
- Clearly defined care planning with specified and agreed responsibilities for all those involved.
- Reviewing and updating of the care plan.
- Best value for money for a defined care plan.

The RLT applies the key features of care management to the rehabilitation setting with particular emphasis on achieving rehabilitation goals that are unique to each person's needs. The framework of care management holds the interdisciplinary process together and enables each team member to:

- Carry out an inter-disciplinary assessment.
- Define individual rehabilitation needs and goals.
- Plan and deliver rehabilitation programmes that integrate health and social services.
- Monitor and review the outcomes of intervention with service users.

This process has meant that health staff in the care manager role have had to learn the techniques of care management from their social work colleagues. Rather than undermine the social work role this has enhanced the respect of social work by health staff and revealed some of the mysteries of social care commissioning. Likewise the social worker has had to understand the relevance of nursing and therapy techniques and begin to integrate these into a new style of care management within the field of rehabilitation. In this way the breadth and the depth of the assessment has been enhanced.

Rehabilitation Link Team composition

The rehabilitation coordinator

The rehabilitation coordinators all have a professional qualification and experience as a nurse, physiotherapist, occupational therapist or social worker. The initial title for this role was care manager, but in East Cheshire the term 'rehabilitation coordinator' was adopted as this more accurately describes the team's work: rehabilitation rather than care, and coordination as opposed to an emphasis on the management process. The rehabilitation coordinator carries out a baseline assessment which covers all the domains of the overview assessment within the single assessment process. This team member also coordinates a rehabilitation programme that incorporates all aspects of a person's functioning: physical, psychological and social. Progress is reviewed at least every six weeks with individuals working on their rehabilitation goals for approximately three to four months.

Each rehabilitation coordinator uses the core team skills which exist across all professions involved in rehabilitation (e.g. communication, assessment and caseload management), plus learnt skills to an assistant level in a profession other than their own, and the skills and knowledge peculiar to their own profession, (see Fig. 6.1, Interdisciplinary team framework). This approach keeps the number of professional inputs to a minimum and helps to ensure that the rehabilitation programme focuses on an individual's particular needs. Fig. 6.2, Path of a single professional, provides an example of the development process of interdisciplinary working for a physiotherapist.

Practitioners and specialist services

The rehabilitation coordinators have access to physiotherapy and occupational therapy practitioners, a community psychiatric nurse and a general practitioner with a special interest in intermediate care. The skilled interdisciplinary worker is able to recognise the scope of their own practice and through discussion with colleagues make prompt and relevant referrals to practitioners. This is largely owing to a clear understanding of the unique skills of each professional (see Fig. 6.1) that are not shared across professions and can be delivered only by that professional. For example, the social worker is the lead professional for the management of abuse investigations, carer's assessment and family support; the physiotherapist has a key role in the knowledge and application of biomechanics and neuromuscular function, plus the application of relevant treatment modalities such as pain control or gait/balance re-education.

Sometimes, what is unique to a professional's input is the depth of knowledge and skill required. For example, it is expected that all rehabilitation coordinators can carry out a basic tissue viability assessment but any complex pressure care issues would need to be referred to either a community nurse or tissue viability nurse for further advice or care. The same procedure would be followed for a

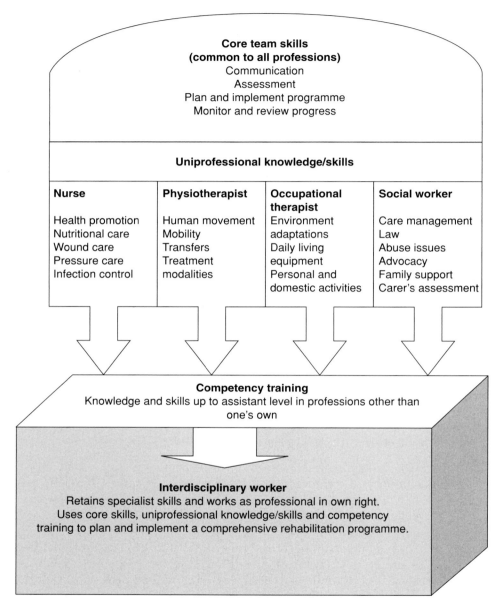

Fig. 6.1 Interdisciplinary team framework.

continence assessment. Likewise, the physiotherapy and occupational therapy practitioners have an active role in the rehabilitation programmes by providing detailed or specialised therapy assessment and treatment that are identified through discussion with the rehabilitation coordinator. Their input would be

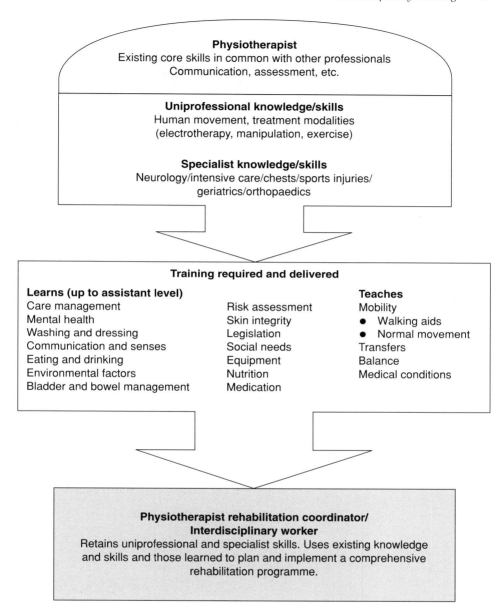

Fig. 6.2 Path of a single professional using physiotherapist as example.

reflected in the uni-professional areas identified in Fig. 6.1. They are also vital in training and supporting rehabilitation assistants when their input is appropriate.

In addition to therapy practitioners, the intervention of the community psychiatric nurse has ensured that a complete assessment is carried out of both a person's physical and mental health needs. This post has facilitated a rapid referral to psychiatric services where this is appropriate.

In 2003 the intermediate care service in East Cheshire benefited from the appointment of a part-time GP employed as a salaried GP by the Primary Care Trust (PCT). This post has enabled all intermediate care patients to have direct access to medical advice and diagnostic support should their condition deteriorate or they develop complex medical problems. The GP role focuses on providing medical input to individuals in an intermediate care bed. After discharge, the person's medical care is reinstated with their own local GP. Any medication changes, investigations and progress are communicated via a discharge summary letter to the registered GP.

All the above practioners and specialist services deliver a service across the range of intermediate care in East Cheshire: supported hospital discharges, rapid response care to both Accident and Emergency Department and the community, plus rehabilitation. All have an important role to play in supporting the development and maintenance of interdisciplinary working.

Rehabilitation assistants

The RLT benefits from access to dedicated rehabilitation assistants, employed within the home care service, who work closely with team members to support the person during their rehabilitation and provide regular opportunities for the person to practise day-to-day tasks such as dressing, walking and making a simple meal. The rehabilitation assistants have undergone a thorough training programme across health and social care that allows them to offer a range of social, nursing and therapy inputs under the supervision of the relevant professional. This has ensured an emphasis on the enablement approach and resulted in a reduction in home care input as the independence of the person improves. Care staff in social service residential centres also provide rehabilitation input to those who require a short period of rehabilitation in a residential setting.

Case study

The following case study is presented to illustrate the way in which interdisciplinary working is able to support a person's rehabilitation.

Mrs K was an elderly woman who had been admitted to hospital following a fall and chest infection. She was adamant that she wanted to return to live at home, but was currently unable to walk and was refusing rehabilitation within a hospital setting. Mrs K had a left-sided weakness from a previous stroke, and a history of extreme anxiety.

A rehabilitation coordinator, responsible for the overall care and rehabilitation programme for Mrs K, carried out a baseline assessment. This covered all aspects of Mrs K's needs, and established her rehabilitation goals which were:

- I want to return to live at home.
- I want to be able to walk short distances safely and confidently.
- I want to be able to use the toilet by myself.
- I want to be able to attend church.

She was willing to participate in a programme of rehabilitation in a residential community support centre.

Because of her long-standing mobility problems caused by extreme anxiety and physical weakness, a physiotherapist carried out a specialist assessment. A programme to practise transfers each day was developed for Mrs K, to be carried out under the supervision of trained rehabilitation assistants. This involved the repeated practice of transfers between bed, commode and chair. The layout of the room in the centre was arranged so that it was identical to her bedroom at home. This practice of transfers and walking helped Mrs K to establish a new pattern of movement and to overcome her debilitating anxiety. The rehabilitation coordinator, from a social work background, used her new interdisciplinary skills to carry out basic anxiety management work, and a home assessment.

Mrs K was involved in a gradual staged process towards discharge and when at home Mrs K received ongoing support from a comprehensive care package. The home care staff received training on how to enable Mrs K to move in the appropriate manner. Mrs K was pleased to have returned home, and that her needs had been understood. Using an interdisciplinary approach eliminated the need for multiple assessments and ensured that Mrs K and her goals remained the central focus of the rehabilitation programme.

The difference between multidisciplinary and interdisciplinary working

Interdisciplinary and multidisciplinary working are often used as mutually exchangeable terms; clinical experience demonstrates that they are different. Box 6.1 summarises some of the main differences of the various ways of team working. Multidisciplinary working has been defined as:

> 'a group of practitioners with different professional training (multidisciplinary), employed by more than one agency (multi-agency), who meet regularly to coordinate their work providing services to one or more clients in a defined area.' (Ovretveit, 1998, p. 9)

Traditionally this means that each discipline focuses on their own particular contribution and works in parallel with other disciplines. Very often communication takes place on an informal basis at the discretion of individual staff members and tasks outside the domain of one profession are not always channelled appropriately. In a multidisciplinary team that works well, the focus of communications

Box 6.1   Characteristics of multi- and interdisciplinary team working (Marriott and Wright, 2002). Published by kind permission of the Editor of *Community Care*.

Characteristics of multidisciplinary working	Characteristics of interdisciplinary working
• Reinforces boundaries between professionals • Generates multiple assessments and professionally orientated goals • Focuses on uni-professional skills • Allows only general sharing of information due to uni-professional focus • Perpetuates uni-professional models of training	• Emphasises the similarities across professional groups • Facilitates a single assessment approach and person centred goal setting • Acknowledges areas of shared skills • Promotes a shared understanding and viewpoint • Relies on shared training, mutual trust and respect

is usually on the coordination of individual contributions to care rather than integration. For example, the social worker will probably take responsibility for the social aspects of a person's care plan but does not have the authority to coordinate any health care aspects, which would be dealt with separately by the hospital medical staff or general practitioner, district nurses or therapists. Sometimes there is no real awareness of the depth of information and input being delivered by different agencies. The role of voluntary agencies in supporting older people at home may be underplayed or ignored.

Interdisciplinary working provides a more integrated and coordinated approach which overcomes some of the barriers of professional structures and organisations. It recognises the importance of each professional's philosophical perspective and unique skills but 'seeks to blur the professional boundaries and requires trust, tolerance, and a willingness to share responsibility' (Nolan, 1995).

This is not the same as generic working as it is rooted in the belief that every discipline's input is unique and is part of the whole picture for a particular person.

Although all rehabilitation coordinators are responsible for a single assessment as recommended by the *National Service Framework for Older People* (Department of Health, 2001), this is a baseline assessment and relevant professionals pursue any identified complex issues. As previously stated the social worker, therapist or nurse would learn the relevant knowledge and expertise to the level of an assistant in a profession other than their own. In this way interdisciplinary working is not aimed at creating a 'super-professional' working in a generic way. Instead the approach seeks to integrate the skills and knowledge that are common to all professions involved in rehabilitation and acknowledges the unique skills, expertise and knowledge of each profession. The rehabilitation coordinator is therefore equipped to identify a person's total needs and develop a comprehensive rehabilitation package.

Making it happen

Clearly interdisciplinary working cannot take place overnight. Much training is required to move staff away from the traditional and perhaps more comfortable ways of operating in a multidisciplinary setting. Chapter 7, 'Interdisciplinary training and development', explores in more detail the importance of inter-disciplinary training. Locally in East Cheshire the training for the RLT began on a countywide basis with all three teams and one to two training days allocated each month. This initially focused on working out what was meant by interdisciplinary working and defining what are core skills to all professionals and what is specific to each discipline (see Figs 6.1 and 6.2).

All professions share skills and knowledge related to the assessment process that involve effective communication and the ability to identify a person's needs and strengths. Likewise, all professionals have skills and knowledge related to the planning and implementation of the rehabilitation package, followed by the monitoring and reviewing of rehabilitation and finally the discharging of the person from the service. Within this overall framework of shared core skills, each professional has attained knowledge and skills in a wide area of rehabilitation practice to the level of an assistant. For this to work effectively all staff involved in the RLT have undergone training in a variety of competency areas described in Box 6.2.

A competency unit is described as an area of skill and knowledge that is related to the practice of rehabilitation and required to complete an interdisciplinary comprehensive assessment.

The competencies listed in Box 6.2 address all the key topics of our baseline assessment document and form the basis of each rehabilitation coordinator's continuing development programme. A series of workshops presented by the appropriate professional cover each of the competency units. Evidence for attainment of each competence includes observation by an appropriate professional, recording within the baseline assessment document and use of the 'think aloud' technique (Fonteyn et al., 1993) to determine the level of insight into the tasks carried out and their interrelationship. The competency framework has now been externally validated by University College Chester and team members have the opportunity to attain academic credits towards a first or Masters degree.

In addition to the structure of individual development plans, allocation and team meetings provide an ideal opportunity for staff to learn from each other and exchange ideas, views and knowledge with regard to all aspects of rehabilitation. This consolidates the learning, which has taken place on a formal basis and provides a realistic testing ground for different ways of working. In order to survive this degree of testing, individual staff members in our RLT have needed to demonstrate a resilience, self-confidence and personal integrity beyond all their previous experiences. Team support and a genuine tolerance for each other's learning needs have helped individuals through their own personal development. Together team members have learned to face the

Box 6.2   Competency units for the rehabilitation coordinator role.

Unit 1	**Bladder and bowel management** To be able to assess a client's bladder and bowel function and incorporate the findings into a rehabilitation plan.
Unit 2	**Care management** To be able to undertake all aspects of the care management process when working with individuals and work as an integral member of their interdisciplinary team.
Unit 3	**Risk assessment** To be able to undertake a risk assessment when working with individuals and incorporate the findings into the risk management and rehabilitation plans.
Unit 4	**Mental health** To be able to assess a client's mental health and incorporate the findings into a rehabilitation plan.
Unit 5	**Mobility and transfers** To be able to assess a client's mobility and transfers and incorporate the findings into a rehabilitation plan.
Unit 6	**Skin integrity** To be able to assess a client's skin integrity and incorporate the findings into a rehabilitation plan.
Unit 7	**Nutrition** To be able to assess a client's nutrition integrity and incorporate the findings into a rehabilitation plan.
Unit 8	**Washing and dressing** To be able to assess a client's washing and dressing ability and incorporate the findings into a rehabilitation plan.
Unit 9	**Medical conditions and medication** To be able to assess a client's medical conditions and medication and incorporate the findings into a rehabilitation plan.
Unit 10	**Eating and drinking** To be able to assess a client's eating and drinking and incorporate the findings into a rehabilitation plan.
Unit 11	**Legislation** To be aware of relevant legislation relating to clients and take appropriate action in accordance with appropriate policies and procedures.
Unit 12	**Social history and social needs** To be able to assess a client's social history and social needs and incorporate the findings into a rehabilitation plan.
Unit 13	**Environmental factors and equipment** To be able to assess environmental factors and equipment relating to a client and incorporate the findings into a rehabilitation plan.
Unit 14	**Communication and senses, including audiology, vision** To be able to assess a client's communication, senses, audiology and vision and incorporate the findings into a rehabilitation plan.

onslaught of criticism from established professional groups and teams which new ways of working inevitably bring. The team manager has needed to address these internal and external pressures whilst maintaining the energy and vision of the team members.

Evaluation of the service

Evaluation was seen as a core part of service delivery and a 21-month evaluation study (Reid et al., 2002) from July 2000 until March 2002 was commissioned. The evaluation had two main aims:

- To explore the way in which the care management model was implemented and translated to interdisciplinary working.
- To assess the extent to which the team achieved its aims.

An action research approach was used to give the team, the managers and the commissioners formative and summative results at different points during the evaluation. The evaluation took place across three teams in the county. A variety of methods were adopted to examine the different aspects of the team's functioning and effectiveness. Qualitative methods included open-ended interviews, observational work and focus groups. Quantitative methods included record review and standardised evaluation tools. The emerging findings were used to inform the decision making process and as a consequence contributed to the development of the service.

The effectiveness of the service for individuals was evaluated using validated outcomes measures (Modified Barthel Scale) (Shah et al., 1989), Hospital Anxiety and Depression Scale (Snaith and Zigmond, 1994) and EQ-5D (EuroQol Group, 1990) at the assessment, discharge and three-month follow-up. A health economic evaluation was undertaken to identify the cost-effectiveness of delivering rehabilitation in a new way. Surveys were also used to capture the perceptions of stakeholders.

The findings provided strong evidence of the effectiveness of the team's interdisciplinary approach:

- Individuals and carer(s) described very positive experiences of the way in which the team and the service met their needs.
- The achieved outcomes by individuals were very positive in relation to the areas measured by the validated tools (functional ability, levels of anxiety and depression, and overall health status) and improvements were maintained at least for three months post-discharge.
- The key stakeholders perceived the teams to have '*on average*' achieved their potential.

What works?

The evaluation identified the important role of team managers and team leaders in driving the change process forward and enabling the service to operate in its intended care management manner. The teams were prepared to challenge traditional ways of working, were supported as they worked through this, and encouraged to work creatively with the individual client as the main focus of attention.

Is it cost-effective?

The interdisciplinary approach of the RLT was evaluated as cost-effective:

- For those individuals who were likely to have been admitted to residential care or have been taken on by social services with an increased home care package.
- For those individuals who were likely to have been admitted to hospital or whose discharge from hospital was likely to have been delayed (had the RLT not been in place) and whose hospital stay had reached a break-even point.

The evaluation study has helped to inform the debate about the benefits and limitations of interdisciplinary working.

The benefits of interdisciplinary working in intermediate care

For the person

One of the main benefits of using an interdisciplinary approach is that it ensures that the person is at the centre of the rehabilitation process rather than for rehabilitation to be constructed around the input of individual professionals. This is made possible by the rehabilitation coordinator taking the lead role in delivering a baseline assessment in line with the overview assessment contained within the single assessment process. There are no serial assessments by different professionals and, as in the original quotation, the individual is clear about who is doing the coordination. By putting the focus on the individual rather than on different assessments, the individual is put in the driving seat of their own rehabilitation and road to independence. This is achieved by an individual setting their own goals and determining with the coordinator how they will get there. Several interview comments by clients in the evaluation report (Reid et al., 2002) confirm the client's appreciation of the coordination and real choices made available to them.

The person focused approach also changes the professional's ideas on risk assessment and management, by promoting a responsible and jointly agreed strategy to risk. This is linked with the evidence available on the relationship between risk management and the promotion of healthy ageing (Wistow et al., 2002). The individual is allowed to take control of their own independence and to decide what needs to change in order for them to live as independently and safely as possible. This is often a vital part of rehabilitation discussions if long-term care is to be avoided.

For team members

The focus of rehabilitation in intermediate care allows the process of interdisciplinary working to flourish because of the type of work being carried out and the possibilities for sharing skills. Most clients are medically stable and therefore the emphasis is on intensive therapy and balancing the issues of practical support and independent living. The need for acute nursing or medical intervention is usually limited and therefore the importance of a coordinated and relevant rehabilitation programme is high. For staff working in an interdisciplinary way, there are tremendous opportunities to learn new skills from team members and see the benefits of this translated to the people with whom they work. The rehabilitation coordinator is able to overview the whole process and follow this through to the end, often achieving remarkable outcomes for people previously destined for long-term or continuing care. The evaluation report (Reid et al., 2002) documents the rehabilitation coordinator's changing perception of their role from anxiety and tension to a deepening realisation of the benefits of their work. As their knowledge and skills grow the coordinator is therefore able to develop a deeper appreciation of each professional's role as well as affirmation of their own profession's worth. This is a far cry from the idea of generic working.

For the whole system of health and social care

A mature interdisciplinary approach encourages effective networking across all agencies and helps to break down the artificial boundaries across professions and organisations. Effective communication channels need to be established with the hospital, residential centres, primary care, housing department, specialist agencies and social services so that the individual receives a service which is as coordinated and seamless as possible.

The evaluation report (Reid et al., 2002) records the concerted and proactive efforts of team members to build effective links with key personnel in different organisations or departments. Where there are blocks in the system, interdisciplinary working will challenge this and actively look for solutions. Interdisciplinary working provides a way of reducing the number of serial assessments and inputs and a way of clarifying professional roles. It also values the contribution of assistants in working with the individual to fulfil their rehabilitation potential. As part of a whole system of health and social care, an interdisciplinary team therefore ensures that staff time is targeted appropriately, partnership working is promoted and people are promptly signposted to the service that will best meet their needs.

The limitations of interdisciplinary working

Within the RLT the individual views and abilities of rehabilitation coordinators have limited the extent to which role blurring can be actively pursued. Some rehabilitation coordinators find the responsibility of care management too stressful and are overwhelmed by the range of needs that have to be addressed. The evaluation study (Reid et al., 2002) used the evidence from focus group work with team members to examine the tension between the care management role and clinical status. Some rehabilitation coordinators reported concerns about maintaining their professional skills and self-esteem. They also emphasised the stress of being totally accountable for all aspects of a client's rehabilitation programme and were unable to perceive the development of new and different skills as a gain. By the end of the project phase this level of reported anxiety had lessened as rehabilitation coordinators described a growing confidence in their own competence and a strong belief in the validity of the interdisciplinary approach for the client. Some were unable to reconcile their professional concerns with the benefits of interdisciplinary working and left the team.

Within the wider system individuals and groups have not always been sympathetic to what interdisciplinary working is about and have failed to value the benefits. The evaluation study (Reid et al., 2002) records comments by team members such as 'being obstructive by not involving us', 'putting their own needs and services before client priorities' and 'testing us out' (Reid et al., 2002, p. 42). This is substantiated by some consistent comments in the two key stakeholder surveys that included that the approach was 'a waste of resources' (9% of respondents) and the acceptance criteria was too tight (33%).

A lack of belief in the team's purpose can sometimes jeopardise referrals to the team and make any handover to mainline services a complicated issue. Whilst some key stakeholders reported that they had stopped referring to the team because of its tight acceptance criteria, others mentioned that the achievement of positive results with clients was due to the clear referral criteria. An ongoing public relations exercise continues to be necessary for the team to maintain its profile and its relevance within the whole system of health and social care. The extent to which interdisciplinary working can be fully developed is therefore dependent on both the individual team members themselves and the support of the surrounding environment in which the team works.

Nevertheless, if interdisciplinary working has benefits, is it possible to generalise for all types of an intermediate care service? There are many aspects of interdisciplinary working that can be used to improve multidisciplinary working. For example, the opportunity to reduce the number of serial assessments must be seriously investigated across any intermediate care service as a whole. This will be supported by the implementation of the single assessment process (Department of Health, 2002).

All staff can benefit from having greater knowledge of another professional's role. All services need to be coordinated effectively. However, at the acute end of intermediate care such as hospital at home or rapid response, it is the specialist and in-depth skills of the nurse, general practitioner, social worker and therapist that are required. It is not helpful to dilute the role of the nurse who is required to identify and manage the sub-acute health care needs of a person so that they are safely cared for in the community rather than be admitted to hospital. It is none the less important that neither the nurse nor the social worker repeats a series of questions that an individual has already been asked. This is fundamental to the guidelines of the single assessment process. It is also important that any client who subsequently moves into a rehabilitation stage of their intermediate care is not asked the same questions and that there is clear communication between professionals. Intermediate care should at least operate as a seamless service regardless of its components.

Summary

The development of interdisciplinary working in East Cheshire has been a challenging but rewarding experience. During the most challenging times it has seemed that the fundamental beliefs in the professional's identity were being eroded. What has kept the team going was the vision of creating a better service for the people who need a rehabilitation service and their carers. The *National Service Framework for Older People* (Department of Health, 2001) has stressed the importance of each person having one rather than a whole collection of providers taking responsibility for their overall care. Interdisciplinary working promotes a coordinated approach to both assessment and the delivery of the rehabilitation package. Although there are limitations to its application across the range of intermediate care services, within the field of rehabilitation, there are clear benefits in using this approach. These benefits can be experienced by the individual at the centre of the rehabilitation process, the staff working in them and the whole system in which the process takes place.

Interdisciplinary working is not for the faint-hearted, but to grasp the challenges demanded of staff in the *National Service Framework for Older People* (Department of Health, 2001), both social and health care professionals must look beyond their professional title and work together in ways that challenge conventional lines of communication. The interdisciplinary approach allows staff to concentrate much more on the individual and their particular rehabilitation needs rather than on the input by any one or group of professionals. It is intrinsically linked to the implementation of a single assessment framework and the benefits are worth striving for.

Acknowledgements

The authors would like to thank the University of Salford, The Editor of *Community Care*, the Editor of the *British Medical Journal* and McGraw Hill Publishing for permission to use materials in this chapter.

References

Association of Directors of Social Services and Local Government Association (2003) *All Our Tomorrows: Inverting the Triangle of Care*. London: Association of Directors of Social Services.

Audit Commission (2000) *The Way to Go Home*. Oxford: Audit Commission Publications.

Department of Health (2001) *National Service Framework for Older People*. London: Department of Health.

Department of Health (2002) *Guidance on the Single Assessment Process for Older People*. Health Service Circular 2002/001: Local Authority Circular (2002)1. London: Department of Health.

EuroQol Group (1990) A new facility for the measurement of health-related quality of life. *Health Policy* **16**, 199–208.

Fonteyn, M.E., Kiupers, B., Grobe, S.J. (1993) A description of think aloud method and protocol analysis. *Qualitative Health Research* **3** (4), 430–41.

Griffiths, K. (1998) *Community Care: Agenda for Action* (Griffiths Report). London: HMSO.

Marriott, A., Wright, H. (2002) All for one. *Community Care* 16–22 May, 38–9.

Nolan, M. (1995) Towards an ethos of interdisciplinary practice. *British Medical Journal* **311**, 306.

Ovretveit, J. (1998) *Coordinating Community Care, Multi-disciplinary Teams and Care Management*. Buckingham: Open University Press.

Reid, G., Kneafsey, R., Hulme, C., Long, A. (2002) *Evaluation of an Assessment and Rehabilitation Service for Older People in South Cheshire*. Salford: University of Salford.

Robinson, J., Turnock, S. (1998) *Investing in Rehabilitation*. London: King's Fund.

Shah, S., Vanclay, F., Cooper, B. (1989) Improving the sensitivity of the Barthel Index for stroke rehabilitation. *Journal of Clinical Epidemiology* **42**, 703–709.

Snaith, R.P., Zigmond, A.S. (1994) *The Hospital Anxiety and Depression Scale*. Windsor: Nfer-Nelson.

Social Services Inspectorate/Scottish Office Social Work Services Group (SSI/SOSWSG) (1991) *Care Management and Assessment: Summary of Practice Guidance*. London: HMSO.

Wistow, G., Waddington, E., Lai, F.C. (2002) *Intermediate Care: Balancing the System*. Leeds: Nuffield Institute for Health, University of Leeds.

Chapter 7

Interdisciplinary Training and Development

Julie Howden

Introduction

The delivery of intermediate care requires interdisciplinary working across a number of agencies and professional groups. This chapter discusses how the development of interprofessional education and curriculum can enhance interdisciplinary working and provide a framework of core competencies for intermediate care teams. An illustration of an interdisciplinary training programme developed in South Staffordshire in 2001 presents the gains and benefits of such a programme in the development of intermediate care services. Wider discussion of the advantages of common learning programmes and consideration of learning styles and teaching strategies is also given.

Prior to the development of intermediate care services in 2000 a number of rehabilitative services already existed including day hospitals and specialist inpatient rehabilitation units, re-ablement services, local authority sheltered housing schemes and voluntary sector support schemes. All shared a common focus in the provision of client centred care designed to enable the individual to maintain maximum levels of independent living at home. In the past many of these services had been provided independently of each other with little or no collaboration, often struggling to meet the increasing demands made upon them due to the lack of dedicated investment (Audit Commission, 1997). In 2000 the National Beds Inquiry supported the findings of the Audit Commission suggesting that rehabilitative services showed wide geographic variations with the need for investment in order to meet the demands made upon them (Department of Health, 2000a).

Recent legislation supports the development of intermediate care services. *The NHS Plan* (Department of Health, 2000b) suggests that intermediate care has not been introduced to supersede existing rehabilitation provision but to complement it with the aim of developing integration between existing and new services. In 2001 health and social care commissioners were provided with a circular to be applied in the planning and development of new services (Department of Health, 2001c). The *National Service Framework for Older People* (Department of Health, 2001a) suggests that integrated commissioning for intermediate care will provide a 'seamless care pathway' across primary and secondary care, based on individual clients' needs. Inter-agency working between health services, social services, county councils and the independent and voluntary sector providers is crucial if a coordinated approach to care is to succeed in the future. This will avoid duplication of care through the introduction of shared protocols and procedures, integrated commissioning and a single assessment process allowing the patient to experience better continuity of care.

Inter-agency working can be facilitated through joint education and training across the different agencies and professional disciplines. Each individual profession contributes its own specialist skills to a care pathway, whilst a number of similar skills and knowledge are common to the whole team. Such skills and knowledge need to be developed into a joint curriculum for the provision of inter-agency/professional education in the future (Millar et al., 2001). The non-medical education and training consortia (NMET) provides funding for the education and training of health professionals other than doctors and dentists. Funding is distributed by contracts between higher educational institutes providing undergraduate and postgraduate courses. NMET is now working on the development of commissioning shared learning but there is little training available at present for existing services working in collaboration such as the developing intermediate care teams (Kesby, 2002). Although common areas within the curriculum can be identified across professional groups, common core programmes are limited in number and are the 'exception rather than the rule' (Lugon and Walker 1999).

The Department of Health (2003) has identified a number of success factors in the development of intermediate care provision over the past three years. Such factors include the ability of providers to see beyond their organisational boundaries and to have shared objectives in their purpose. Through collaborative learning it is possible to develop confidence and trust between professionals and organisations with clear lines of accountability for individual team members and a clear framework for intermediate care teams delivering services. There is continued recognition for the need of uni-professional training, but this should be more balanced with interprofessional training to meet the requirements of the changing workforce and the change in provision of health and social care services (Lugon and Walker, 1999).

There is a need for formalised training programmes to enhance the development of intermediate care provision at both undergraduate and postgraduate levels. Such training should be accessible to all health and social care workers within a variety of settings. Collaboration between higher educational institutes, the National Health Service, social services, and the voluntary and independent sectors is required to develop learning resources for all interested partners.

Joint working – the interdisciplinary approach and the multidisciplinary approach compared

The NHS Plan (Department of Health, 2000b) describes health and social services joining together to form a single organisation as part of the National Health

Service agenda for reform. In order for this to be successfully achieved health and social care providers should engage in joint working and training to achieve a more integrated approach to care. There is a need to move away from the multidisciplinary team approach towards the interdisciplinary team approach. In the past the multidisciplinary model has consisted of a number of professionals working in parallel towards their own discipline-related goals in the delivery of patient care. Although the team may all be working with the same patient they work within the boundaries of their own profession and the patient's role is often passive and minimal (Gorman, 1998).

The interdisciplinary model comprises a number of professionals working towards shared client centred goals. Team members cross professional boundaries according to the client's needs, working together in joint treatment sessions. The client's role is active and central to the process. The interdisciplinary approach supports the premise that all team members recognise and understand each other's skills and expertise but also that there are common core skills that all team members have. Interdisciplinary working nurtures a loss of role conflict and ambiguity as the team develops an appreciation of individual professional roles and competencies (Embling, 1995).

Through joint working and training, services are brought together to challenge the past delivery of care in order to promote a more client centred approach in the future. Intermediate care promotes the move towards collaborative working practice with an emphasis on an enabling philosophy empowering patients to do more for themselves, thus maximising their potential for independence (Department of Health, 2001a).

Inter-professional education and curriculum

As intermediate care teams have developed, commonalities in skills and knowledge have emerged across professional groups. There is often a role overlap between professions as described by Alsop and Vigars (1998) who suggest that occupational therapists and social workers could use shared learning, as could occupational therapists and physiotherapists. The British Geriatric Society (2003) also acknowledges that student doctors need to learn about a teamwork approach to patient care through inter-professional education. The undergraduate medical curriculum should involve medical students working alongside allied health and social care students. This would involve the pursuit of a separate qualification for each professional group but recognises common elements that could be taught across a number of professions together using collaborative teaching and learning strategies.

Over the past decade it has been suggested that 'therapeutic relationships' can develop between team members through shared learning (Jenkins and White, 1994; Ovreteit et al., 1997). Whilst there is a need for strict guidelines that govern the curriculum content for each professional group there is also a need for interdisciplinary training that will provide a framework of core competencies for intermediate care teams. Such teams are often inclusive of non-professionals and so it is important to provide core competencies that can be taught in modular format across all groups at different levels.

In 2001 the South Staffordshire Intermediate Care Training and Development Project carried out a training needs analysis of local staff providing intermediate care services in order to develop a suitable training programme to meet their needs (Howden, 2002). A number of interdisciplinary core topics were identified from the training needs analysis, which were developed into an intermediate care training catalogue. Courses were delivered to inter-agency staff providing intermediate care within South Staffordshire. Such topics included:

- *Person centred risk assessment*: developed to enhance the assessment skills of the practitioner regarding therapeutic risk taking, based upon a person centred approach that facilitates the sharing of information between team members and other agencies. The course outcomes were to raise awareness of risk assessment and risk management, to consider therapeutic risk taking when promoting independence, and to develop skills in risk assessment in order to avert a crisis.
- *The theory and practice of rehabilitation*: made up of two different training sessions: 'Promoting Independence through Activities of Daily Living' and 'Purposeful Activities in Promoting Independence'. The course outcomes of the first session were to explore the theoretical and practical aspects of rehabilitation in daily life and the principles of client centred goal planning. The course outcomes for the second session gave an understanding of the therapeutic value of activity and how activities can be broken down and used to achieve independence through rehabilitation.
- *Communication awareness*: developed to allow students to gain an insight into the importance of developing effective communication skills in order to work in a person centred approach. The course outcomes were to explore the importance of communication in the delivery of person centred care and the barriers to effective communication, considering ways of engaging with individuals who challenge the conventional way of engaging in communication.
- *Mental health awareness*: developed as two courses, one to raise 'Awareness of Mental Health' difficulties relating to dementia and depression, and the second considering 'Medication in Mental Health'. The course outcomes were to raise awareness of person centred approaches in the rehabilitation of individuals with mental health difficulties. The emphasis was on care of the client within the intermediate care settings. The second course was designed to raise awareness of current medication management of mental health clients and to explore issues of consent to treatment and the consideration of complementary therapies.
- *Basic conditions awareness*: developed to standardise the common foundation knowledge of staff concerning the basic physical and mental health conditions relevant to the team's caseload so that early recognition of signs and symptoms may help prevent deterioration of the patient, and in turn avoid hospital admission.

- *Models of intermediate care services*: developed to consider the principles and models of intermediate care services and how they can benefit the patient. The course outcomes were to increase knowledge of the political drivers of intermediate care and the different intermediate care models with exploration of their application in practice.

The above modules were taught across inter-agency groups at appropriate levels to suit the learning group's needs. A number of clinical skills were also taught to nurses and health care assistants to enhance their professional practice including venepuncture, catheterisation, percutaneous endoscopic gastrostomy (PEG) feeds and the administration of subcutaneous fluids. In the future such training has the potential to be developed in line with the National Qualifications Framework for academic study at both undergraduate and postgraduate levels. For example, the learning outcome statements at undergraduate or certificate level would be based upon the acquisition of knowledge and understanding introducing some enquiry and problem solving applicable to the student's level of learning. At postgraduate or Masters level, learning outcomes would be based on a greater depth of learning including analysis, application and reflection of new knowledge (Wilts, 2002).

For health and social care assistants the present National Vocational Qualification (NVQ) in Care (Level 3) could be used with specific intermediate care endorsements added as the NVQ is based upon a competence based model of learning outcomes. The endorsements could be written under the same course headings as above designed at a level appropriate for health care assistants (Reep, 1995). Such training available to intermediate care teams allows assistants to be taught in an interdisciplinary way providing modules of common knowledge and skills that can be used across the different professions within the team.

Common learning programmes

The Scholfield Report (1996) suggests that all health care professionals can learn 'core team competencies' allowing for more 'generic working' so enhancing collaborative practice. Some, such as Millar et al. (2001), advocate inter-professional learning at undergraduate level, whereas others, such as Barr (2000), suggest postregistration learning is more effective in promoting collaborative working as practitioners are more able to reflect on their past experiences to enhance their professional expertise.

In 2001 the Department of Health published the paper *Investment and Reform for NHS Staff – Taking Forward the NHS Plan* (Department of Health, 2001b). The paper recommends 'common learning programmes for all health professionals, based on core skills'. Such skills can be taught at foundation level to a range of health and social care students enabling them to move on to their chosen field of expertise following successful completion of the foundation course. This will encourage more flexible entry routes into a wide range of health and social care professions such as physiotherapy, occupational therapy, nursing, medicine, psychiatry and social work. It also allows easier routes for students to transfer between programmes giving greater opportunities for career pathways in the future. The paper gives examples of inter-agency programmes such as the Common Foundation Programme (CFP) teaching nursing, physiotherapy, biomedical sciences and social work students together provided by St George's Hospital Faculty of Health and Social Care Sciences in London. Workforce development confederations and universities must now consider opportunities for interdisciplinary programmes with all future commissioning.

Intermediate care lends itself to common learning programmes where training provision should be based upon the principle of preparing the practitioner to enable the client to achieve maximum levels of independence and autonomy in day-to-day living. Curricula development for intermediate care should start with a set of learning outcomes that need to be achieved for each level of study. Intermediate care training should include modules from NVQ Level 3 to certificate, degree and Masters level for all disciplines. Allowing Accreditation of Prior Experiential Learning (APEL) will widen the access to learning for all students moving away from theory based courses to more work based learning practice.

Learning styles

It is important that the teaching of intermediate care involves the interdisciplinary team training alongside each other. Teaching should be varied to suit a wide range of learning styles and abilities. Adult learning is known as 'andragogy' and should be problem centred rather than content orientated as adults learn best experientially and when the topic is of immediate value (Knowles, 1984).

Adult learners have their own individual learning styles and so it is important that curriculum development takes into account a wide range of learning activities to suit all student needs. Honey and Mumford (1992) and Kolb (1976) suggest four different learning styles adopted by adults. Some may prefer an 'activist' style where learning occurs through brainstorming problems, through role-play exercises, by competitive teamwork and by tackling new experiences and learning from them. The activist learner does not learn well from being passive – listening to lectures, reading a book or through writing.

The 'reflector' style learner prefers to stand back from events, listen, observe and then think about what has occurred in order to learn from the experience. They do not learn well from role-play situations or when they have to take action without all the necessary information to do so. They tend to listen and take a passive role during discussions receiving all the information available before making a decision or judgement.

The 'theorist' style learner prefers to question assumptions and methodologies. They like to read or listen to others giving lectures, learning well from discussions and question and answer sessions. They do not learn well from situations emphasising emotions and feelings or from open ended problems, as they prefer to think problems through in a step-by-step logical way.

The 'pragmatist' style learner is practical, using simulation or demonstration with coaching or feedback to learn new skills. They are able to formulate action plans to solve problems and learn least from lectures or theoretical situations.

Intermediate care covers a range of inter-professional knowledge and skills that can be taught in a variety of ways to suit all learners putting equal emphasis on experience and academic ability. Shared learning involves a common structure of knowledge and skills that can be taught across the inter-disciplinary team using a range of teaching and learning strategies.

Teaching strategies

Health and social care training in the past has followed a traditional 'talk and chalk' style of teaching where the learners are passive recipients of information presented through lectures and tutor-led seminars. Such teaching strategies do not suit all learning styles as they fail to encourage problem solving or allow practical integration of the knowledge being taught. It is now recognised that students learn best when information is presented to them in a teaching style most congruent to the individual's preferred learning style (Schmidt et al., 1991). Intermediate care training needs to be taught in a way that suits different learning styles and allows practitioners to apply their knowledge and skills to a variety of unique cases.

Problem Based Learning (PBL) originated from Canada in the 1960s and is an educational approach that encourages students to become 'self-directed learners' (Engel, 1992). It is a teaching style particularly suited to practice based professionals, as students work together in small groups on real case studies selected to encourage critical thinking, problem solving and team working. The teacher acts as a prompt and guide to the students providing them with feedback as they progress through a problem and students are responsible for identifying their own learning needs.

The Problem Based Learning approach begins with a problem being presented to the students that acts as a 'trigger' for learning. This may take the form of a written case study or perhaps a video or role-play of a patient's situation. Students work both as a group to identify what needs to be done to solve the problems, and also individually to explore relevant knowledge to bring back to the group. This may be by literature review, critical appraisal or by seeking the opinion of specialists and peers. The group meet together to discuss and debate the information gathered before applying their new knowledge to practice. Group discussion is a useful teaching strategy to develop reasoning skills and team building in the workplace (Romiszowski, 1993).

The problem solving may then be presented back to the teacher via a report, seminar or role-play usually taking the form of a patient goal plan or case conference. The teacher evaluates the students' abilities to identify their own learning needs applied to the given problem, their analysis of information and the application of their learning to practice. The final stage of the process involves students reflecting on what they have learned and how they will then apply this to practice (Sadlo et al., 1994; Savin-Baden, 1998).

Problem Based Learning is a teaching style that fits well into the theory of adult learning (andragogy) where instruction should be task orientated and self-directed allowing learners to discover things for themselves (Knowles, 1984). Beyond the traditional lecture format and problem based learning approach other suitable teaching styles may include: demonstration of a skill, individual study, multimedia work, project work or simulation of a real life situation. An important consideration when planning a teaching package is to ensure it includes a wide range of teaching strategies to suit the different learning styles (Romiszowski, 1993).

Gains and benefits

Inter-professional education is now being developed within health and social care courses. At present there is little evidence to suggest the efficacy of inter-agency training as many courses are still in their infancy. As they are developed, further evaluation of inter-agency programmes is required to ascertain the gains and benefits of joint learning (Lugon and Walker, 1999).

An independent evaluation of the South Staffordshire Intermediate Care Training and Development Project was carried out at the completion of the project in 2002. This provided some evidence for the gains and benefits of inter-agency learning (Jinks and Linell, 2002). The project evaluation had two strands. These included examination of the intermediate care training teams' perspectives of the project's development and effectiveness, and investigations into the effectiveness of the training offered. The latter strand was carried out by a telephone survey of participants of the intermediate care training courses. 'The key objectives of the training were to raise awareness of intermediate care for staff and to teach a range of skills required in order to integrate intermediate care philosophy into practice' (Jinks and Linell, 2002, p. 12). Results showed that 75% of staff interviewed believed the course objectives had been achieved. Respondents were also asked if an increased awareness of inter-agency working had occurred as a result of inter-agency training. Respondents believed that joint training did serve to promote mutual respect and understanding of each other's roles and increased recognition of the clinical expertise of each team member. As staff became more aware of each other's roles this served to avoid role duplication or professional protectionism that can be evident in multidisciplinary based working.

The Intermediate Care Training and Development Project provides evidence of how joint training can serve to integrate services and enhance the skills of individuals working within inter-agency teams. Lathleen and Le May (2002) suggest that inter-agency training allows professionals to learn from each other, sharing their knowledge and skills and becoming more reflective in their practice, leading to more positive outcomes in patient care. As common learning programmes develop, greater exploration of students' perspectives on shared learning in relation to influences on provision of services is required.

With new knowledge and skills, professionals have greater opportunity for self-development as advanced practitioner roles emerge. Through the recognition of Accreditation of Prior Learning and Experience there is also the possibility for professionals to study for dual qualification providing more flexible career pathways in the future. Professionals with a dual qualification in both occupational therapy and physiotherapy or occupational therapy and social work could serve to lessen the recruitment and retention problems within health and social care as individuals become able to extend their role in the future (Department of Health, 2000c.)

For the patient, benefits include a 'seamless pathway' of care between hospital and the community as providers work with shared protocols and procedures. Duplication of assessment from many different professionals can be avoided through the application of a collaborative single assessment process. Through intermediate care the patient is encouraged to state his or her own perceived priorities for care promoting a client centred approach. An appreciation of the uniqueness of each patient allows him or her to achieve their optimum levels of independence, as professionals work together in the best interests of the patient (Department of Health, 2001a).

User involvement in the development of the curriculum for intermediate care training is also a consideration for the future, identifying the patients' views through patient satisfaction questionnaire or interview. Much can be learnt from engaging users in the planning and implementation of training.

Summary

While there are both champions and critics of intermediate care, all should applaud its guiding principles of person centred care, whole system working and the promotion of health and active living (Department of Health, 2003). Through interdisciplinary training staff can learn how to work within a single assessment process and provide the physical, mental and social dimensions of treatment required for person centred care. Interdisciplinary training staff can learn how to break down organisational barriers and professional boundaries from an enhanced understanding of each other's roles and through shared responsibilities for patient care. With shared learning staff develop greater skills and knowledge from each other and from reflecting together as a team.

Intermediate care supports patient empowerment, appreciating the uniqueness of every individual and their need to engage in purposeful activity and maintain social roles. Through interdisciplinary training intermediate care teams share a common philosophy for promoting maximum levels of independence for all patients, facilitating them to achieve their full potential in active healthy living.

Acknowledgements

To the South Staffordshire Intermediate Care Training and Development Team for their hard work and commitment in developing a local intermediate care training catalogue and in their delivery of training between 2001 and 2002: including Julie Jones, Project Administrator, Heather Brundrett (RMN), Lucy Pursehouse (RMN), Julie Myatt (RN), Trudi Wheeler (RN) and Alison Overton (OT).

To Professor Annette Jinks and Sue Linnell as authors and researchers of the final evaluation of the Intermediate Care Training and Development Project conducted at the Centre for Health Policy and Practice at Staffordshire University.

To Staffordshire University School of Health (now Faculty of Health and Social Sciences) for their accommodation and hospitality to the project team.

To the Stafford and Shropshire Education Consortia (now Shropshire and Staffordshire Development Directorate) for funding the project.

To all members of the project steering group made up of representatives across the health and social care organisations of South Staffordshire for their support and direction to the project team.

References

Alsop, A., Vigars, C. (1998) Sharing learning, joint training or dual qualification in occupational therapy and social work: a feasibility study. *British Journal of Occupational Therapy* **61** (4), 146–52.

Audit Commission (1997) *The Coming of Age: Improving Care Services for Older People*. London: Audit Commission.

Barr, H. (2000) *Interprofessional Education: 1997–2000. A Review*. London: United Kingdom Central Council for Nursing, Midwifery and Health Visiting.

British Geriatric Society (2003) *Core Content of Undergraduate Curriculum in Elderly Care Medicine*. www.bgs.org.uk/compendium/compf2.htm (accessed 9/08/03).

Department of Health (2000a) *Shaping the Future NHS: Long Term Planning for Hospitals and Related Services*. London: Department of Health.

Department of Health (2000b) *The NHS Plan: A Plan for Investment, A Plan for Reform*. London: Department of Health.

Department of Health (2000c) *A Health Service of all the Talents: Developing the NHS Workforce. Consultation Document on the Review of Workforce Planning*. London: Department of Health.

Department of Health (2001a) *National Service Framework for Older People*. London: Department of Health.

Department of Health (2001b) *Investment and Reform for NHS Staff – Taking Forward the NHS Plan*. London: Department of Health, pp. 37–41.

Department of Health (2001c) *Intermediate Care*. Health Service Circular/Local Authority Circular, HSC 2001/01, LAC (2001)1. London: Department of Health.

Department of Health (2003) *Intermediate Care: Moving Forward*. London: Department of Health.

Embling, S. (1995) Exploring multidisciplinary teamwork. *British Journal of Therapy and Rehabilitation* **2** (3), 142–5.

Engel, C.E. (1992) Problem Based Learning. *British Journal of Hospital Medicine* **48** (6), 325–9.

Gorman, P. (1998) *Managing Multidisciplinary Teams in the NHS*. London: Kogan Page.

Honey, P., Mumford, A. (1992) *The Manual of Learning Styles*. Cited in: *Learning Styles of UK Higher Education Students – Four Studies of the Reliability and Replicability of the Learning Styles Questionnaire*. www.uwe.ac.uk/bbs/trr/Issues3/Is3-1_4.htm (accessed 8/02/04).

Howden, J. (2002) The South Staffordshire Intermediate Care Training and Development Project. *British Journal of Occupational Therapy* **65** (3), 138–40.

Jenkins Curtis, G., White, J. (1994) Action Learning, a tool to improve interprofessional collaboration and promote change. Counsellors, general practioners and the primary care team. *Journal of Interprofessional Care* **8** (3), 265–73.

Jinks, A., Linell, S. (2002) *Charting the Processes and Outcomes of the South Staffordshire Intermediate Care Training and Development Project*. Stafford: Stafford Centre for Health and Policy and Practice, Staffordshire University.

Kesby, S.G. (2002) Nursing care and collaborative practice. *Journal of Clinical Nursing* **11**, 357–66.

Knowles, M. (1984) *Andragogy in Action*. San Francisco: Jossey-Bass.

Kolb, D.A. (1976) *Learning Styles Inventory: Technical Manual*. Boston, MA: McBer and Company.

Lathleen, J., Le May, A. (2002) Communities of practice: an opportunity for interagency working. *Journal of Clinical Nursing* **11**, 394–8.

Lugon, M., Walker, J.S. (1999) *Clinical Governance – Making it Happen*. London: Royal Society of Medicine Press, pp. 131–43.

Millar, C., Freeman, M., Ross, N. (2001) *Interprofessional Practice in Health and Social Care: Challenging the Shared Learning Agenda*. London: Edward Arnold.

Ovreteit, J., Mathias, P., Thompson, T. (1997) *Inter-professional Working for Health and Social Care*. London: Macmillan.

Reep, J. (1995) An evaluation of the design and implementation of an NVQ in an occupational therapy service. *British Journal of Occupational Therapy* **58** (4), 163–70.

Romiszowski, A.J. (1993) *Designing Instructional Systems. Decision Making in Course Planning and Curriculum Design. Copernicus Team (1996)* www.pit.ktu.It/HP/coper/kiev.new/cit/ap_ch3/les31a.htm (accessed 8/02/04).

Sadlo, G., Warren-Piper, D., Agnew, P. (1994) Problem based learning in the development of an occupational therapy curriculum. Part 1: The process of problem based learning. *British Journal of Occupational Therapy* **57** (2), 49–54.

Savin-Baden, M. (1998) Problem based learning. Part 3: Making sense of and managing disjunction. *British Journal of Occupational Therapy* **61** (1), 13–16.

Schmidt, H.G., Neufeld, V.R., Nuoma, Z.M., Ogunbode, T. (1991) Network of community orientated educational institutes for the health sciences. *Academic Medicine* **66** (5), 259–63.

Scholfield, M. (1996) The future healthcare workforce: the steering report. Health Services Management Unit, University of Manchester, UK. Cited in: Scholes., J., Vaughan, B. (2002) Cross boundary working: implications for the multiprofessional team. *Journal of Clinical Nursing* **11**, 399–408.

Wilts, N. (2002) *Staffordshire University Award Outcomes. Interpreting the National Qualifications Framework*. National Qualifications Framework Working Group (last updated April 2002) (unpublished). Stafford: Staffordshire University.

Chapter 8
Evidence on the Effectiveness of Intermediate Care

Roger Beech

Introduction

The current policy of expanding services for intermediate care began towards the end of the 1990s and was a response to the problems that patients were experiencing in accessing services for emergency acute inpatient care, particularly during winter months. Professionals were encouraged to develop 'whole systems' responses for addressing problems that were occurring within acute hospitals (NHS Executive, 1998; Social Services Inspectorate/NHS Executive, 2000): in other words, to consider ways of diverting care away from acute settings towards non-acute settings. The findings of the National Beds Inquiry further endorsed this growth in services for intermediate care (Department of Health, 2000a) and as a result the expansion of these services was a key element of the UK Government's NHS Plan (Department of Health, 2000b) and the *National Service Framework for Older People* (Department of Health, 2001).

Intermediate care services have been defined as those 'designed to prevent avoidable admissions to acute care settings, and to facilitate the transition from hospital to home and from medical dependence to functional independence' (Department of Health, 2000c, p. 13). The types of scheme promoted in the NHS Plan include: multidisciplinary rapid response teams for preventing avoidable acute admission by providing care in patients' homes; for those patients who do require hospital admission, the use of 'step-down' beds in non-acute institutions or integrated home care teams to facilitate their timely acute hospital discharge; intensive rehabilitation services to help patients regain their independence more quickly; and one-stop clinics to improve patient access to services for health and social care (Department of Health, 2000b).

Available scientific evidence at that time did offer some support to justify an increased role for such services. For example, it had been demonstrated that amongst older people at least 20% of bed use could probably be avoided by expanding the supply of service options beyond the acute setting (McDonagh et al., 2000). In addition, findings were available of studies which had evaluated schemes which transferred elements of patient care away from the acute hospital to non-acute or community based settings. For example, studies had demonstrated that, by using community based rehabilitation teams, it was possible to reduce acute bed use whilst maintaining clinical outcomes for patients with stroke and with chronic obstructive pulmonary disease (Rudd et al., 1997; Beech et al., 1999; Davies et al., 2000). However, prevailing wisdom at that time was that more evidence on the effectiveness of schemes for providing intermediate care was needed (Hensher et al., 1999; Goddard et al., 2000; Lambert and Arblaster, 2000; Luff et al., 2000; Parker et al., 2000).

Key issues that need to be investigated when evaluating the merits of schemes for intermediate care reflect, in part, the overall aims of such schemes. Hence, there is a need to identify what impact services for intermediate care have on levels of 'avoidable' acute bed use. In addition it is important to assess whether or not these services are capable of maintaining clinical outcomes and that they are acceptable to both service users and health and social care professionals. Finally, it is important to assess how schemes for intermediate care affect the costs and cost-effectiveness of services for health and social care. In relation to each of these areas of investigation, the following section of this chapter summarises and updates the research evidence that was used to inform the current policy to expand services for intermediate care. For the purposes of this review, intermediate care schemes have been grouped into the categories adopted by Stevenson and Spencer in their guide for developing intermediate care: hospital at home; early supported discharge schemes; rapid response schemes; community rehabilitation teams; residential intermediate care; and day rehabilitation (Stevenson and Spencer, 2002; see also Chapter 5). However, in classifying services for intermediate care in this way it is accepted that there is potential overlap between the nature of schemes and that services grouped under the same label may perform quite different roles and functions.

This review of current evidence about the merits of schemes will reveal that key gaps in current knowledge remain. To a large extent, these gaps reflect the difficulties that are encountered when attempts are made to evaluate schemes for delivering intermediate care. Hence the subsequent section of the chapter includes a discussion of these methodological challenges and of the ways in which they might be addressed. The concluding section of the chapter summarises the key areas where more research is needed to inform the ongoing development of services for intermediate care.

Current evidence about the merits of schemes to deliver intermediate care

Hospital at home schemes

These schemes aim to offer a home based alternative for the supply of health care that would traditionally have been delivered in an acute inpatient setting (Shepperd and Iliffe, 2004). The role of hospital at home schemes is to prevent avoidable acute admissions and/or facilitate timely acute discharge (Stevenson and Spencer, 2002). Shepperd and Iliffe (2004) undertook a systematic review of randomised controlled trials which had compared the merits of hospital at home schemes and traditional acute hospital care. The results of this review indicated that hospital at home schemes are capable of reducing levels of avoidable bed use by shortening patient acute stay. However, Shepperd and Iliffe noted that the overall duration of patient care increased when comparisons included the period of care in a patient's home. Sheppard and Iliffe were unable to offer firm conclusions about whether or not hospital at home schemes can reduce acute bed use by avoiding, as well as shortening, spells of acute inpatient care. A previous systematic review by Lambert and Arblaster (2000) also found insufficient evidence about whether or not hospital at home schemes can reduce levels of avoidable admission. However, Shepperd and Iliffe's conclusion that hospital avoidance schemes may reduce health care costs does, in turn, imply that they found that they may also reduce rates of avoidable acute admission.

Shepperd and Iliffe's review of studies where hospital at home schemes had been used to care for elderly patients who had either undergone acute elective procedures or had a mixture of medical conditions found that, relative to inpatient acute care, these schemes had a neutral impact on patient health outcomes. Studies reviewed where hospital at home schemes had been used for stroke care reached differing conclusions: one trial concluded that hospital at home improved patient independence but another that it led to reduced levels of communication and psychosocial well-being three months after the onset of stroke (but not at six months post-stroke).

In terms of patient acceptability, Shepperd and Iliffe concluded that published findings indicated that patients were more satisfied with hospital at home care than they were with hospital care. For example, as part of a randomised controlled trial, Wilson et al. (2002) used a patient questionnaire and semi-structured interviews to explore the patient acceptability of a hospital at home admission avoidance scheme. The questionnaire survey revealed higher levels of satisfaction amongst patients who had been randomised to hospital at home care rather than hospital care, differences in satisfaction levels that were statistically significant in all but one of the domains covered. The semi-structured interviews revealed that patients felt that being at home facilitated their recovery and led to better communication between care professionals and themselves. The review of the literature by Shepperd and Iliffe also indicated that the informal carers of patients (for example, spouses and relatives) preferred hospital care to care at home. This conclusion is again in keeping with the study by Wilson et al. (2002): carers thought that any increased demands on their role as carers were offset by them no longer having to undertake hospital visits.

As indicated above, Shepperd and Iliffe argued that hospital at home admission avoidance schemes may reduce the overall costs of health care. However, they also concluded that schemes which aim to facilitate acute discharge should not be viewed as a less costly alternative. This is because the cost 'savings' from reduced hospital stay may be offset by the extra costs of home based care and the fact that the patient's overall duration of care is increased. Following a review of available evidence, Young (2002) concluded that hospital at home schemes probably have a neutral impact on costs.

Early supported discharge schemes

Schemes within this classification aim to facilitate patient discharge from acute care by providing care in patients' homes (Stevenson and Spencer, 2002). Hence, there are potential overlaps between schemes grouped here and those classified as hospital at home schemes. Any distinction seems to surround the types of care provided. Shepperd and Iliffe (2004) stated that hospital at home schemes provide 'active treatment by health care professionals' whereas early supported discharge schemes may draw on the skills of a broader range of professionals from other disciplines and agencies. For example, in addition to therapists, one example of an early discharge team for stroke care included a person to carry out structural modifications to patients' homes (Rudd et al., 1997). Interestingly, in his review for the Department of Health, Young (2002) did not attempt to separate early discharge and hospital at home schemes.

Following a review of available literature, Goddard et al. (2000) concluded that early discharge schemes can bring about reductions in acute lengths of stay. For example, the introduction of a community based rehabilitation team for stroke care led to a significant reduction in acute lengths of stay (Rudd et al., 1997). Early discharge schemes have also been shown to reduce the lengths of acute stay of patients admitted for hip fractures (Cameron et al., 2000). In addition, it has been found that such schemes can reduce patient admissions to long-term care (Hyde et al., 2000).

Moreover, published research demonstrates that patient health outcomes can be maintained when care is delivered within an early discharge scheme (Goddard et al., 2000; Parker et al., 2000). Finally, the reviews undertaken by Goddard et al. (2000) and Parker et al. (2000) both concluded that early discharge schemes may reduce the overall costs of health care, even after allowing for any additional costs incurred by non-health care agencies and by informal carers. For example, a cost analysis of the early discharge scheme for stroke referred to above concluded that it led to net reductions in the overall costs of health and social care per patient (Beech et al., 1999).

Rapid response schemes

Such schemes allow patients rapid access to services for health and social care with the aim of reducing acute bed use by avoiding acute admission or by facilitating acute discharge (Stevenson and Spencer, 2002). However, although all intermediate care schemes are time limited, the duration of care from a rapid response scheme is much less than than offered by other types of scheme for providing intermediate care. For example, a rapid response team for facilitating acute discharge in Hereford had five days as a target duration of patient care: actual average duration of care per patient was 5.6 days (Beech et al., 2004). Similarly, a community health and social care treatment team established in Rotherham aimed to prevent acute admission and facilitate acute discharge by offering care for up to 72 hours (Sanderson and Wright, 1999).

The literature review conducted by Stevenson and Spencer (2002) did not present the results of any randomised controlled trials which had compared rapid response schemes with traditional hospital care. This means that it is not possible to reach definitive conclusions about the merits of this form of inter-mediate care. In the absence of trials, only evidence generated by descriptive studies is available. Such studies solely describe the impacts of a service but do not indicate whether or not it is better, the same as, or worse than the previous approach to delivering care. For example, an evaluation of Hereford's rapid response team described the characteristics of service users, the types of care that they received, the duration of this care, and the acceptability of the service to professionals and service users (Beech et al., 2004). In terms of the latter, both professionals and service users had positive attitudes towards the rapid response service. A descriptive evaluation of Rotherham's community assessment treat-ment team also revealed that professionals and service users had positive atti-tudes towards this service (Sanderson and Wright, 1999).

Community rehabilitation teams

Such teams aim to change the setting in which rehabilitation is provided and, in particular, move it away from the hospital setting (Stevenson and Spencer, 2002). However, in keeping with some of the schemes discussed previously, attempts to review the merits of community rehabilitation can prove problematic because of difficulties in distinguishing community rehabilitation from other approaches to delivering intermediate care (Stevenson and Spencer, 2002; Young, 2002). Indeed Young (2002) argued that community rehabilitation should be seen as a component of other schemes for delivering intermediate care rather than a scheme in its own right.

In his review of the literature, Young (2002) was able to identify only one trial of community based rehabilitation and, as a result, was unable to reach definit-ive conclusions about the merits of this form of intermediate care. However, he noted that trials which had studied specific elements of community rehabilita-tion (for example, the supply of living aids, exercise programmes and occupa-tional therapy) had generated some support for such a transfer in care. The studies that he reviewed also offered support for the development of aspects of community based rehabilitation for stroke care and, in particular, an increase in community based occupational therapy. A more recent systematic review by Ward et al. (2004) attempted to compare the merits of providing rehabilitation for older people in care homes, hospitals and patients' own homes. They were unable to identify any studies which met their inclusion criteria so, like Young (2002), they concluded that it was not possible to reach firm conclusions about the merits of this form of intermediate care.

Residential intermediate care

The schemes discussed below aim to reduce levels of avoidable acute bed use by providing intermediate care in non-acute institutions. They are targeted at individuals who need a level of support above that which can be delivered in a patient's home.

Delivering intermediate care in community hospitals

In his review of the literature, Young (2002) was unable to find sufficient evidence to draw any conclusion about the ways in which care in this setting affects patient health outcomes and the cost-effectiveness of services. He argued that the development of trials to supply this information is a research priority given that community hospitals are widely used for post-acute care. Concerns have also been raised that some individuals admitted to community hospitals may have care needs that could be met by other approaches to delivering care (Audit Commission, 2000). This concern reflects the potential overlaps between the nature of schemes for intermediate care. It also indicates the need for trials which compare the merits of alternative ways of delivering intermediate care (Coast et al., 2000): traditionally the merits of acute hospital care and individual schemes for delivering intermediate care have been compared. This issue will be discussed further later in this chapter.

Delivering intermediate care in nurse-led units

In a systematic review of the literature, Griffiths et al. (2004) compared traditional hospital care and nurse-led units in terms of their success in supporting the recovery of patients and their move from hospital to home. The evidence reviewed indicates that although there are no statistically significant differences in the inpatient mortality generated by the two models of care, there is a suggestion that mortality rates might be higher in nurse-led units.

The evidence also indicates that patient functional status at discharge is better following care in a nurse-led unit and that a lower proportion of patients are discharged to institutional settings. However, Griffiths et al. argued that these improved outcomes at point of hospital discharge might be linked to the fact that care in a nurse-led unit can lead to increases in hospital stay, increases that are approaching statistical significance. As a result, nurse-led units can also increase the overall costs of patient care in UK settings (Steiner et al., 2001; Griffiths et al., 2004).

Wiles et al. (2003) used qualitative interviews to obtain the opinions of patients about care in a nurse-led unit. They found that care in the unit was acceptable to the majority of patients. However, there was less consensus amongst users about the role and purpose of the unit: most but not all patients thought that the unit supported their convalescence and rehabilitation from hospital to home. Wiles et al. argued that this may have been due to the fact that, in addition to being a setting for the delivery of intermediate care, the nurse-led unit was also being used as a 'holding area' for patients requiring long-term care. As a result, Wiles et al. argued that it is important to agree appropriate criteria for the referral of patients to nurse-led units.

Delivering intermediate care in nursing homes

A lack of randomised controlled trials meant that Young (2002) was unable to reach any conclusions about the adequacy of nursing homes as a setting for intermediate care. In the absence of such trials he argued that the findings of studies of nurse-led units might be applied to nursing homes. He also noted that nursing home residents have, in the past, had inadequate access to services for rehabilitation, a situation that will need to be addressed if the supply and philosophy of intermediate care in nursing homes is to expand. Within any attempts to improve patient access to services for intermediate care, it might be best to view nursing homes as the setting for other schemes for intermediate care. This is because, in many cases, a nursing home has become a resident's 'own home'.

Delivering intermediate care in sheltered housing

Department of Health guidance to support the development of services for intermediate care noted that changes to a person's home environment might have a vital role in achieving some of the key aims of services for intermediate care – preventing acute hospital admission and facilitating acute hospital discharge (Department of Health, 2002). For example, in a study referred to earlier in this chapter, a person to carry out structural modifications to a patient's home was included as a member of an early discharge team for stroke care (Rudd et al., 1997).

In the same spirit, the Department of Health (2002) argue that there might be potential to expand the use of sheltered housing as a setting for intermediate care. The review by Stevenson and Spencer (2002) did not identify any trials which had assessed the merits of this setting for intermediate care. However, they did present the results of a study by Herbert (2002) which found that: after a period of care in sheltered housing, almost 80% of service users returned to their 'own home'; users had positive attitudes to this form of care; and that it reduced the overall costs of health and social care.

Delivering intermediate care in residential rehabilitation units

As indicated above in the discussion of community rehabilitation schemes, following a systematic review of the literature, Ward et al. (2004) were unable to draw any conclusions about the relative merits of traditional hospital based rehabilitation, home based rehabilitation and that based in residential units. In the absence of findings from trials, Stevenson and Spencer (2002) presented the results of a study by Trappes-Lomax et al. (2002) which compared the merits of home based rehabilitation and rehabilitation in a residential unit for patients discharged from a community hospital. That study found that the two alternative settings for rehabilitation achieved similar health outcomes at similar overall cost, although the balance of spending on health and social care differed between the two.

Intermediate care in day hospitals and centres

Day hospitals

A systematic review of the literature by Forster et al. (2004) concluded that rehabilitation programmes and services delivered in day hospitals are capable of achieving equivalent clinical outcomes to those based on a traditional model of inpatient and outpatient geriatric care. Young (2002), one of the authors of that review, has suggested that the quality of care delivered in day hospitals may, however, be increasing because, for example, of an expansion in the range of rehabilitation services provided. Forster et al. also concluded that the use of day hospital care may help to reduce patient demands for acute beds. In his review for the Department of Health, Young (2002) also argued that past reductions in the number of day hospital places due to industrial disputes have been associated with a rise in hospital admissions.

On a more cautionary note, the review by Forster et al. (2004) and a report by the Audit Commission (2000) warned that day hospital care may be more costly than alternative care options. The Audit Commission report also indicated that transport arrangements may mean that users have difficulty accessing services in day hospitals and that these services may be inadequately coordinated.

Day centres

Day centres have emerged as an alternative setting for the delivery of intermediate care (Stevenson and Spencer, 2002). In a randomised controlled trial, Burch and Borland (1999) compared the merits of rehabilitation programmes delivered in day hospitals and in day centres. They found that the two alternative settings for care achieved similar clinical outcomes but that the costs of care were lower in day centres. However, the perception of patients was that the quality of care was higher in day hospitals.

Methodological challenges in generating evidence about intermediate care schemes

The previous review of the evidence base of the effectiveness of intermediate care services has revealed that important gaps in knowledge remain. Following systematic reviews of the literature, for a number of schemes and/or service impact areas (e.g. impact on patient acceptability, costs etc.), authors were unable

to reach definitive conclusions about the relative merits of traditional and intermediate care scheme approaches to delivering patient care. Such gaps in knowledge mean that, according to a recent editorial in the *British Medical Journal*, there
is still a view that 'little scientific evidence exists on the benefits of intermediate
care' (Melis et al., 2004).

One of the reasons for this apparent lack of evidence surrounds the difficulties of using 'scientific' methods to evaluate schemes for delivering intermediate
care. The innovative nature of intermediate care schemes means that they
take time to stabilise in terms of, for example, their patient mix and working
arrangements. During this period it is inappropriate to evaluate their impacts
using randomised controlled trials. The Medical Research Council recognises
this problem and suggests a phased approach to evaluating the types of interventions that fall under the umbrella of intermediate care (Medical Research
Council, 2000; Campbell et al., 2000). The suggested phases of evaluation, in
chronological order, are:

- Defining the intermediate care intervention, its purpose, and the key areas
  of uncertainty surrounding its impacts.
- Monitoring the initial performance of the intervention in terms of, for
  example, the client group and their use of services.
- Designing the main experimental study, including the appropriate control
  situation, and relevant measures of cost and outcome.
- Conducting the main experimental study.
- For successful interventions, monitoring their ongoing effects.

During the first two phases of the evaluation framework, descriptive evaluation designs can be used to generate information to refine the nature of the
intermediate care scheme and to identify any ways in which it might need to be
adapted so that, for example, it more appropriately meets the care needs of its
users. Such a descriptive design was used to evaluate the Rapid Response Team
for intermediate care established in Hereford (Beech et al., 2004; see also Chapter
4). Once the nature of the service has been confirmed, the next two phases of the
evaluation framework focus on its formal evaluation using 'scientific' methods.
In practice, however, it might prove difficult to introduce 'scientific' approaches at
this stage of the evaluation process. This is because local support for the intermediate care scheme may have been generated during the period of stabilisation
so a comparison of traditional (old) and new ways of delivering care may be
seen as unacceptable.

Assuming that it is possible to undertake a randomised controlled trial, the
Medical Research Council Framework indicates the importance of identifying the appropriate comparative situation. Traditionally, care delivered within a
scheme for intermediate care has been compared with care delivered in an acute
hospital setting. As services for intermediate care become more established,
the relevance of using the acute hospital as the comparative situation may
reduce and it may be more appropriate to use alternative schemes for inter-

mediate care as the comparison (Coast et al., 2000). To some extent this requirement reflects the current difficulties of categorising intermediate care schemes in terms of, for example, their roles and the types of care need that they meet (Stevenson and Spencer, 2002). For example, a report by the Audit Commission (2000) raised concerns that patients referred to intermediate care schemes in community hospitals had care needs that could be met by other types of intermediate care scheme. In such a situation a relevant question for evaluation is, 'For an individual with given care needs, which type of intermediate care scheme is best?'

The difficulties in defining and categorising intermediate care schemes create more general difficulties in generating an evidence base: schemes that have similar 'labels' might have quite different roles and functions (Stevenson and Spencer, 2002). For example, earlier in this chapter the difficulties in trying to distinguish hospital at home and early discharge schemes were highlighted. Melis et al. (2004) suggest a new classification of intermediate care schemes based upon the types of care that they aim to provide. As the review of current evidence demonstrated, current classification systems tend to define schemes according to the setting in which care is delivered: for example, hospital at home, residential care in nursing homes. The setting in which care is provided may have an impact on patient health outcomes, but probably of greater importance is the precise nature of the care. Hence, a classification system that also incorporates care needs met would facilitate a more patient centred approach to analysing the impacts of schemes for intermediate care.

Finally, information on the merits of intermediate care schemes in terms of their costs and cost effectiveness continues to be an important gap in knowledge. As they address this gap in knowledge, Coast et al. (2000) emphasise that it will be important for researchers to indicate the basis for any cost comparisons. For example, they argue that different conclusions about the relative cost effectiveness of a scheme are likely to be reached if it is seen as a means of addressing an increase in overall demands for health care (comparator, the costs of meeting this demand by increasing the number of hospital beds) rather than a means of meeting existing demands for care by using existing resources in an alternative manner (comparator, savings generated by reductions in hospital beds because patients have been diverted to intermediate care). The first of these scenarios reflects the situation faced by the authors of the National Beds Inquiry (Department of Health, 2000a). They argued that an expansion of services for intermediate care was probably the most feasible way of meeting the expected increase in demands for health care that will be generated by the ageing of the population.

Summary

This chapter has discussed the existing evidence base of effectiveness to support the current policy of expanding the supply of services for intermediate care. For each of the various schemes for intermediate care, this review has focused on:

their potential impacts on levels of avoidable acute bed use and patient clinical outcomes; their acceptability to service users and health and social care professionals; their impacts on the costs and cost effectiveness of care. The current consensus seems to be that more evidence about the merits of schemes for intermediate care is needed (Young, 2002; Melis et al., 2004). Most 'scientific' evidence is available for hospital at home and early discharge schemes. This evidence indicates that these schemes can maintain clinical outcomes and reduce patient acute stay at lower or equivalent health care costs. The extent to which hospital at home schemes can reduce levels of avoidable acute admission is less clear. In addition, patients and carers appear to have positive attitudes towards hospital at home schemes. 'Scientific' evidence in relation to the merits of other schemes for intermediate care is generally lacking.

However, there are difficulties in using scientifically robust methods to evaluate the merits of schemes for delivering intermediate care and researchers will need to address these difficulties in their efforts to increase the evidence base. Alongside these efforts more work is needed to identify improved ways of categorising schemes for intermediate care that place more emphasis on the care needs of the patient and the nature of care provided and less emphasis on the setting in which care is delivered. Such a shift would mean that the results of evaluations facilitate a more patient centred approach to the selection and implementation of intermediate care schemes. In addition, given that the policy to expand services for intermediate care resulted from whole system concerns about the delivery of care, it will be important to evaluate schemes in terms of their impacts within a complete network of services for providing health and social care.

References

Audit Commission (2000) *The Way to Go Home: Rehabilitation and Remedial Services for Older People*. London: Audit Commission.

Beech, R., Rudd, A.G., Tilling, K., Wolfe, C.D.A. (1999) Economic consequences of early inpatient discharge to community based rehabilitation for stroke in an inner-London teaching hospital. *Stroke* **30** (4), 729–35.

Beech, R., Russell, W., Little, R., Sherlow-Jones, S. (2004) An evaluation of a multidisciplinary team for intermediate care at home. *International Journal of Integrated Care* 4 October, 2004, http://www.ijic.org.

Burch, S., Borland, C. (1999) A randomised controlled trial of day hospital and day centre therapy. *Clinical Rehabilitation* **13**, 105–12.

Cameron, I., Crotty, M., Currie, C., Finnegan, T., Gillespie, W., Handoll, H., Kurrle, S., Madhok, R., Murray, G., Quinn, K., Torgerson, D. (2000) Geriatric rehabilitation following fractures in older people: a systematic review. Southampton. *Health Technology Assessment* **4**, 2.

Campbell, M., Fitzpatrick, R., Kinmouth, A.L., Sandercock, P., Spiegelhalter, D., Tyrer, P. (2000) Framework for the design and evaluation of complex interventions to improve health. *British Medical Journal* **321**, 694–6.

Coast, J., Hensher, M., Mulligan, J.A., Shepperd, S., Jones, J., et al. (2000) Conceptual and practical difficulties with the economic evaluation of health services developments. *Journal of Health Services Research and Policy* **5** (1), 42–8.

Davies, L., Wilkinson, M., Bonner, S., Calverley, P.M.A., Angus, R.M., et al. (2000) 'Hospital at home' versus hospital care in patients with exacerbations of chronic obstructive pulmonary disease: prospective randomised controlled trial. *British Medical Journal* **321**, 1265–8.

Department of Health (2000a) *Shaping the Future NHS: Long Term Planning for Hospitals and Related Services. Consultation Document on the Findings of the National Beds Inquiry.* London: Department of Health.

Department of Health (2000b) *The NHS Plan: A Plan for Investment, A Plan for Reform.* London: Department of Health.

Department of Health (2000c) *Shaping the Future NHS: Long Term Planning for Hospitals and Related Services. Consultation Document on the Findings of the National Beds Inquiry – Supporting Analysis.* London: Department of Health.

Department of Health (2001) *National Service Framework for Older People.* London: Department of Health.

Department of Health (2002) *National Service Framework for Older People – Supporting Implementation. Intermediate Care: Moving Forward.* London: Department of Health.

Forster, A., Young, J., Langhorne, P., for the Day Hospital Group (2004) *Medical Day Hospital Care for the Elderly Versus Alternative Forms of Care* (Cochrane Review). In: The Cochrane Library, Issue 4. Chichester, UK: John Wiley.

Goddard, M., McDonagh, M., Smith, D. (2000) Avoidable use of beds and cost-effectiveness of care in alternative locations. In: *Shaping the Future NHS: Long Term Planning for Hospitals and Related Services. Consultation Document on the Findings of the National Beds Inquiry – Supporting Analysis (Annex E).* London: Department of Health.

Griffiths, P.D., Edwards, M.H., Forbes, A., Harris, R.L., Ritchie, G., et al. (2004) *Effectiveness of Intermediate Care in Nursing-Led Units* (Cochrane Review). In: The Cochrane Library, Issue 4. Chichester, UK: John Wiley.

Hensher, M., Fullop, N., Coast, J., Jeffreys, E. (1999) Better out than in? Alternatives to acute hospital care. *British Medical Journal* **319**, 1127–30.

Herbert, G. (2002) *Tomlinson Court: A New Approach to Rehabilitation in Sheltered Housing. Evaluation Report.* Leeds: Nuffield Institute of Health.

Hyde, C.J., Robert, I.E., Sinclair, A. (2000) The effects of supporting discharge from hospital to home in older people. *Age and Ageing* **29**, 271–9.

Lambert, M., Arblaster, L. (2000) Factors associated with acute use of beds by older people: a systematic review of the literature. In: Department of Health (2000c) *Shaping the Future NHS: Long Term Planning for Hospitals and Related Services. Consultation Document on the Findings of the National Beds Inquiry – Supporting Analysis (Annex G).* London: Department of Health.

Luff, D., Nicholl, J., O'Cathain, J., Munro, J., Paisley, S., et al. (2000) Patient preferences. In: Department of Health (2000c) *Shaping the Future NHS: Long Term Planning for Hospitals and Related Services. Consultation Document on the Findings of the National Beds Inquiry – Supporting Analysis (Annex F).* London: Department of Health.

McDonagh, M.S., Smith, D.H., Goddard, M. (2000) Measuring appropriate use of acute beds: a systematic review of methods and results. *Health Policy* **53**, 157–84.

Medical Research Council (2000) *A Framework for the Development and Evaluation of RCTs for Complex Interventions to Improve Health.* www.mrc.ac.uk.

Melis, R.J.F., Rikkert, M.G.M.O., Parker, S.G., van Eijken, M.I.J. (2004) What is intermediate care? An international consensus on what constitutes intermediate care is needed. *British Medical Journal* **329**, 360–61.

NHS Executive (1998) *Second Report of the Emergency Services Action Team (ESAT)*. Leeds: NHS Executive (available on Department of Health website).

Parker, G., Bhakta, P., Katbamna, S., Lovett, C., et al. (2000) Best place of care for older people after acute and during sub acute illness: a systematic review. *Journal of Health Services Research and Policy* **5** (3), 176–89.

Rudd, A.G., Wolfe, C.D.A., Tilling, K., Beech, R. (1997) Randomised controlled trial to evaluate early discharge scheme for patients with stroke. *British Medical Journal* **315**, 1039–44.

Sanderson, D., Wright, D. (1999) *Final Evaluation of the CARATS Initiatives in Rotherham*. York: York Health Economics Consortium, University of York.

Shepperd, S., Illife, S. (2004) *Hospital at Home Versus In-patient Hospital Care* (Cochrane Review). In: The Cochrane Library, Issue 4. Chichester, UK: John Wiley.

Social Services Inspectorate/NHS Executive (2000) *Millennium Executive Team Report on Winter 1999/2000*. Available on Department of Health website.

Steiner, A., Walsh, B., Pickering, R., Wiles, R., Ward, J., Brooking, J., et al. (2001) Therapeutic nursing or unblocking beds? A randomised controlled trial of a post-acute intermediate care unit. *British Medical Journal* **322**, 453–60.

Stevenson, J., Spencer, L. (2002) *Developing Intermediate Care: A Guide for Health and Social Services Professionals*. London: King's Fund.

Trappes-Lomax, T., Ellis, A., Fox, M., Rohini, T., Stead, J., Sweeney, K., et al. (2002) *The User Voice: a Qualitative Study of User Views about 'What Worked and What Could Have Worked Better' at a Joint Health/Social Care Short-term Residential Rehabilitation Unit for Older People*. Exeter: University of Exeter.

Ward, D., Severs, M., Dean, T., Brooks, N. (2004) *Care Home Versus Hospital and Own Home Environments for Rehabilitation of Older People* (Cochrane Review). In: The Cochrane Library, Issue 4. Chichester, UK: John Wiley.

Wiles, R., Postle, K., Steiner, A., Walsh, B., on behalf of the Southampton NLU Evaluation Team (2003) Nurse-led intermediate care: patients' perceptions. *International Journal of Nursing Studies* **40** (1), 61–71.

Wilson, A., Wynn, A., Parker, H. (2002) Patient and carer satisfaction with 'Hospital at Home': quantitative and qualitative results from a randomised controlled trial. *British Journal of General Practice* **52**, 9–13.

Young, J. (2002) Review of research evidence. In: Department of Health (2002) *National Service Framework for Older People – Supporting Implementation. Intermediate Care: Moving Forward*. London: Department of Health.

Chapter 9

Economic Evaluation of Intermediate Care

Richard Little

Introduction

This chapter explores some of the economic issues raised by intermediate care. Chapter 5 identifies that there are several different models or schemes covered by the term 'intermediate care'. Key issues surrounding the introduction of any of these models include: its appropriate design, its comparative costs and benefits, and which different agencies need to be involved in delivering the service. This chapter briefly reviews the main aims of intermediate care schemes and some of the key assumptions surrounding their development. This is followed by a discussion of some basic economic concepts and of their relevance for intermediate care. Next, a review of published economic evidence is presented, the approaches used and the challenges faced. Given the current shortage of evidence, later sections of the chapter explore the main economic questions that arise from deciding to implement an intermediate care initiative.

Some key issues behind intermediate care

During the 1990s concerns were raised about the appropriate use of acute beds and the strain upon emergency services, which manifested as winter pressures. In the 20 years to 1997/8, general and acute ordinary admissions rose by 1.8% per annum while at the same time the number of acute beds fell by 47 000 and elderly beds by 26 000 (Vaughan and Lathlean, 1999). The NHS responded by reducing the average length of stay; falling from 9.3 to 5 days for acute specialties, and 66.1 to 18.6 days for the elderly (Vaughan and Lathlean, 1999). Chapter 1 identifies a decade of government policy responses.

Table 9.1 shows the percentage of the population aged 65 and over for 1981 and ten yearly to 2031. It shows that the elderly population is set to grow by almost 6 million, constituting almost a quarter of the population in 30 years, compared with a growth of fewer than one million in the past 20 years when the NHS found itself under pressure. The exceptional growth of gross domestic product allocated to the NHS is highly unlikely to continue beyond 2008. Therefore,

Table 9.1 Number and percentage of United Kingdom total population aged 65 or more, 1981–2031.

Year	Percentage of total	Number
1981	15.0	8 475 700
1991	15.8	9 059 100
2001	15.9	9 340 999
2011	17.2	10 507 814
2021	20.1	12 736 633
2031	23.5	15 266 545

Sources: Mid 1981 Population Estimate Based on 1981 Census (ONS); Mid 1991 Population Estimate Revised in the light of 2001 Census (ONS); 2001 Census (ONS); Government Actuary Department 2002 Based Population Projections.

intermediate care needs to plan not just for the present, but for a very different situation in 20 years. What is efficient now may not be so efficient as the population ages rapidly. Schemes need to be prepared to respond to these changes.

The policy advocating intermediate care assumes that treating patients in other settings will relieve pressures upon acute beds. Some in the NHS have also assumed that it is cheaper (e.g. NHS Executive Anglia and Oxford, 1997). Similar arguments were used for community care in the 1980s, yet the NHS discovered that such arguments were not always correct. Local NHS organisations often find themselves implementing intermediate care schemes because of policy pressure and a local belief that it will be cheaper, rather than based on evidence. This could lead to an inefficient position. This is the reason why evidence from evaluations is important, and in particular why economics should form part of evaluation.

Relevant health economics theories and concepts

Intermediate care schemes are advocated to reduce pressures on acute beds by either avoiding inappropriate admissions or by reducing the length of stay, or by both. It is assumed that patients cared for in alternative settings achieve at least the same health outcomes and are treated, some assume, at a lower resource input.

Economics rests on the principles that scarce resources are always exceeded by the wants of human beings. Choices have to be made; this entails priorities. Doing more of A means doing less of B, subject to constrained resources. This leads to the important concept of *opportunity cost*. In the example of the options of A and B, the opportunity cost of doing more of A are the benefits which have been foregone by sacrificing some of B. Elderly patients eligible for intermediate care could continue to be treated in acute hospitals. However, the opportunity cost of such a policy is that those patients who need acute care have reduced access to acute beds.

All possible options should be considered and ranked. Many see the choice as being between the selected intermediate scheme and acute care. However, this perspective is too narrow, as alternative options for delivering intermediate care may exist. For example, relevant options might be acute hospital care and intermediate care either delivered in a community hospital or the patients' homes. If all options achieved the same benefits, the one using the least resources would be seen as the best, enabling the saved resources to be used to treat other patients. The opportunity cost of something is therefore the foregone benefit of the *next best alternative*.

This leads to the concept of efficiency, which seeks to maximise the benefits from the available resources. Efficiency entails two concepts. Technical efficiency focuses on production at least cost, subject to the required quality. For example, within a rapid response team in an intermediate care scheme technical efficiency requires setting up the team so that the mix of staff, health facilities and consumables is at least cost, subject to achieving a given quality level of treatment and care required for a specific group of patients. This demonstrates that economic evaluations need information about both costs and benefits (see Drummond et al., 1997, and Chapter 5).

Often decisions are based not on whether or not to introduce a new service, but on whether to expand or contract an existing one. This entails additional or marginal costs and benefits. The margin is central to decisions. Marginal decisions entail identifying the costs and benefits of expanding (or contracting) something. For example, it is now policy to offer the elderly the influenza vaccination each winter. A marginal decision might entail considering whether to expand the vaccination programme to the carers of the elderly. Some carers would undoubtedly already qualify for the vaccination as they themselves were elderly, but others would be younger.

Often decisions entail comparing two (or more) technologies to treat the same condition. In this case the term incremental (difference) is used (see Drummond et al., 1997, p. 62). An evaluation of an intermediate care project which compared a hospital at home scheme with inpatient care for the same mix of patients would look at the incremental differences in costs and benefits of the two modes of care. Evaluations of intermediate care differ from health technologies such as drugs, because what is of interest is the mode of service delivery, which is more complicated than providing a given health technology (Coast et al., 2000).

The second concept of efficiency is allocative efficiency. This focuses upon the appropriate allocation of resources between different groups, for example the appropriate balance of resources for the elderly (which will include intermediate care) compared with that for children. Technical efficiency questions often entail allocative questions (Donaldson et al., 2002). For example, should a new treatment to treat chronic obstructive pulmonary disease (COPD) at home, proven to be effective but costing more, become available, it could only be implemented if additional resources could be identified from somewhere else. Others might not now be treated.

Existing economic evidence

Several researchers have published evaluations of intermediate care or literature surveys which included costs and benefits. Most of the comparisons have been between early discharge hospital at home and routine acute inpatient care for a specific diagnostic mix of elderly patients.

The evidence in the first half of the 1990s was contradictory. An evaluation of a varied case mix of patients in Peterborough suggested that early discharge hospital at home was cost effective (Knowelden et al., 1991). Scott (1996) undertook a survey of the literature published between 1990 and 1996 (with aspects pertinent to intermediate care) and found no evidence to support the claim that substituting services from secondary to primary care saved resources.

The second half of the 1990s saw a number of studies published which bolstered confidence upon clinical outcomes, but less so upon costs. They also raised some important questions. An evaluation of a randomised controlled trial (RCT) of stroke patients receiving conventional care compared with those discharged early with specialist clinical rehabilitation found both modes equally clinically effective at one year (Rudd et al., 1997). Shepperd et al. (1998a) compared hospital at home with routine inpatient care for patients requiring hip replacements, knee replacements, hysterectomies, elderly medicine and COPD; no major differences in outcomes at three months follow-up were found. Hospital at home was questioned as possibly inappropriate for knee replacements. This raises the issue of identifying appropriate patients. Hospital at home did not reduce total health care costs for the conditions studied. Indeed, costs were higher for COPD and hysterectomy patients. There was some evidence of cost shifting to primary care for elderly medical and COPD patients (Shepperd et al., 1998b). This underlines the importance of analysing diagnostic groups separately in any evaluation.

Richards et al. (1998) evaluated an early discharge hospital at home scheme compared with routine acute hospital care in Bristol. Patients were mainly emergency orthopaedic with fractures, a few were elective hip or knee replacements, and a category of 'other' included conditions such as chest infections and falls without fractures. No significant differences in outcomes was found at one and at three months, except that hospital at home patients perceived higher levels of involvement. The hospital at home costs were lower than those of routine care: this was true for both the NHS and social services viewpoint, and that of the patients (Coast et al., 1998). Jones et al. (1999) evaluated a hospital at home scheme in Leicester: costs were similar or lower to acute inpatient care and were sustained at three months.

A systematic literature review of interventions to improve health and social care access after discharge from hospital identified 15 RCTs, mainly from the USA (Richards and Coast, 2003). Schemes that both assessed need and facilitated or implemented the care plan were more successful, as measured in the short term. Levels of morbidity and diagnostic groups were important factors in generalisability. Work previously undertaken by the author with the NHS indicates that mechanisms to facilitate a form of care management are critical when different providers work together in the interests of clients or patients.

Existing health economics evaluations have revealed that intermediate care does not always save resources and that service design and client groups require careful consideration. If we return to the basic questions outlined in the introduction, it is clear that there remains a shortage of evidence about the economic merits of intermediate care. Most published studies compare intermediate care schemes with acute care, focusing upon technical efficiency. Not enough is known about the alternatives in terms of appropriate design, costs, benefits, upon whom these fall, and the involvement of different agencies. Turning theory into practice is not straightforward. The challenges are largely methodological, but these need to be addressed in the best way possible, if the evidence base is to be developed. It is to this that we now turn.

The role of evaluation: knowledge needed

One of the reasons why economic knowledge is not as plentiful as it might be is that the NHS has been encouraged, in spite of limited evidence, to adopt intermediate care as a solution to the regular winter beds crisis. Early discharge and hospital at home schemes are adopted as solutions in waiting, despite the lack of local evidence. Health economists have also focused more on the challenges of undertaking RCTs to evaluate new drugs, with fewer researchers looking at intermediate care. The paper by Coast et al. (2000) contains thoughtful reflections of some health economists who have looked at this area. Key issues that need to be addressed when designing economic evaluations of intermediate care schemes are discussed below.

Reasons investment in intermediate care is being considered

The objectives need to be unpacked to determine the precise questions. Two crucial questions are:

- What group of patients is the scheme intended for?
- What will happen to the 'liberated beds'?

In relation to the first question, the scheme might be targeted at a distinct group, for example those with hip replacements, strokes, COPD or a mix of these. The levels of morbidity that are deemed appropriate for the scheme also need to be clarified.

In relation to the second question, if the intention is to close beds and redeploy staff, resources may be saved at some future point, should the intermediate care scheme achieve sufficient thresholds in terms of its scale and impact (Coast et al., 2000). The nature of these thresholds and the feasibility of their being achieved needs to be determined: for example, whether beds could be closed if half a ward were liberated; whether a full ward could be closed if replaced by a scheme. If so, resources might be released to offset the intermediate care scheme. In this case the scheme is *substituting* the current provision. If the scheme uses fewer resources, some resources may be released, but release may be delayed. Double running costs may be needed for a time. Some costs are fixed and take time to be released, for example buildings and land. Others can be released sooner, but will still take time (i.e. they are semi-fixed), for example staff who may need to be trained in additional skills and redeployed. Some will be easily released (i.e. variable), for example consumables such as bed linen. Decisions might become difficult if the scheme cost the same as routine acute inpatient care, or were deemed to provide more appropriate care at greater cost.

If the objective is not to abolish beds but to use them for other patients, three things will follow:

(1)   The intermediate care scheme will be in addition to the existing provision. In economic terms, it will *complement* the current provision.
(2)   It will be important to ensure that freed up beds are now used by more 'appropriate' patients.
(3)   Whether or not the patients who occupy the freed up beds require less, the same or more resources will need to be assessed. If less or the same, only the intermediate care scheme will incur a need for additional resources. However, if the patients now using the freed up beds require a greater resource input, both the intermediate care scheme and the new inpatients will require additional resources. In all scenarios the question will be about allocation: where the additional resources will come from and who will incur the opportunity cost.

The NHS also has an equity objective, which is interested in the distribution of health care and health benefits. It has come to prominence recently in the discussion of health inequalities. If equity is an objective of the intermediate care scheme, the distribution of costs and benefits across different groups of interest will need to be part of an audit or evaluation.

In summary, it is critical that decision makers are explicit about the objective and resulting questions raised by the scheme: whether additional resources will be required and where they will be obtained.

Appropriate comparators

Evaluations tend to compare, for a particular range of ages and diagnostic conditions, a specific intermediate care scheme with inpatient acute care. This is a starting point. Coast et al. (2000) ask whether other intermediate care schemes should be included as options. Once intermediate care is accepted, all options, including those within intermediate care, need to be evaluated. It is important to consider all the feasible options if the most efficient option is to be determined. See Mooney et al. (1986) and Posnett and Street (1996) for a discussion on the implications of this.

It is also important to reconsider all the options when a scheme is being expanded to a new area. For example, a hospital at home scheme with a dedicated team of nursing and general care staff may be efficient in an urban situation. The same may not be true if it is expanded to a rural community: travel times will increase, raising staff costs and reducing staff time in direct care. It may be that some form of community hospital or nursing home may be more appropriate. Alternatively, it may be more efficient if staff already visiting patients take on additional care responsibilities (maybe by increasing their range of skills and numbers) rather than having dedicated staff. Because a scheme works efficiently in one setting does not mean it can be simply transposed to another one.

Costs included in the evaluation

As indicated earlier, economic analyses require information on both the costs and the benefits of the options being considered. In order to determine costs, all the resources that are consumed in the production of care for each of the options of interest need to be identified, the quantities used measured and unit costs (prices) attached. (See Chapter 4 in Drummond et al., 1997, for a technical discussion of costs.) Intermediate care throws up both common and more specific issues.

The viewpoint taken determines what costs are included. Intermediate care often involves several agencies. From the economics perspective, it is what resources are critical for a service that matter, irrespective of who provides them. Thus, if a scheme requires inputs from both acute and community Trusts, social services and primary care, ignoring one or more of these inputs would mean that the evaluation identifies resources for only a partial and incomplete service. For example, if a social worker forms part of a hospital at home team, from an NHS accounts perspective the social worker incurs no cost as they are paid by the local authority (either directly or through the NHS). From an economic point of view, however, if the social worker is an integral part of the hospital at home team they are a resource input and must be costed.

It is often the case in intermediate care that some items will be paid for by different parts of the NHS or local authorities depending on where the patient receives them. For example, hospital patients have their drugs issued and paid for by the acute Trust, whereas patients cared for in their homes are likely to have their drugs paid for from the primary care drug budget. The NHS may provide some equipment, while the local authority social services department may provide others. The identification and collection of resource items is therefore more challenging when evaluating intermediate care schemes because it is the modality of care which is being changed and crossing different NHS and non-NHS agencies.

There are also dangers in perceiving a resource input as a free good. A facility provided by a Trust for delivering services may not appear in the budget line of those providing the care and consequently be viewed as free. For example, a scheme that requests patients who live at home to be assessed at care facilities located near to where they live in order to plan care will be convenient to patients, but will also entail the use of more facilities. They are necessary resources irrespective of whether they are shown in the scheme's budget line. If they did not exist, the facilities would have to be rented or bought. This reflects their value.

A related issue is that of cost shifting. The intermediate care scheme may not draw upon certain resources directly, but lead to a change in their use. For example, a concern sometimes expressed by GPs is that their workload may increase as a consequence. There may also be an effect on patients and carers. If a patient is cared for in hospital, their carers would visit them and hospital staff would provide all care. When patients are cared for at home, however, the duties of the carer are likely to increase. The patient or carers may have to pay for items or equipment because of where they are received. Intermediate care schemes need to be sensitive to changes that affect the wider society. Many carers of the elderly are themselves elderly, the next group of carers are the patients' grown-up children, more often than not daughters. The past thirty years or so has seen a dramatic increase in women participating in full time employment. These carers balance work, home, social life and care, which may lead to choosing lower wages and/or working hours. These issues need monitoring. A useful discussion upon valuing informal care can be found in the chapter by Brouwer in Drummond and McGuire (2001).

Hence, the task of identifying all relevant cost areas for inclusion in an economic evaluation is not straightforward. However, the following resource areas are most likely to be relevant when evaluating intermediate care schemes.

Set-up and administrative costs

A new service will entail set-up costs. Services delivering care to patients in their homes are likely to make greater use of post and telephone communication and support staff.

Buildings

All buildings, rooms and other facilities need to be identified, measured and valued, irrespective of who provides them.

Overhead charges

Buildings incur overhead charges for common functions such as cleaning, maintenance, administration, power and so forth, including non-NHS organisations (see Drummond et al., 1997, Chapter 4).

Staff

Staff by type, grade and time spent on main activities need to be identified. Wage or salary rates, including employer costs of national insurance and pensions, should be applied to value the different groups of staff. The mix of staff and time spent between care and travelling is likely to vary between urban and rural schemes.

Other resource areas

Other resources to capture may include various items of equipment and drugs and who provides and funds these. In addition, it is likely that both patients and carers will be in receipt of various benefits payments. Current guidance recommends that benefits paid to patients and carers be included in estimates of benefits from schemes along with changes in quality of life, satisfaction etc. (Gold et al., 1996).

Some resource inputs may be common in all the options. For example, it is possible that potential patients for a scheme to avoid admissions for a particular condition may be assessed in the same place irrespective of which mode of care delivery is used. While these costs are the same for the options, they will form part of the total cost.

Finally, if applicable, an estimate should be made of the costs of those patients who now use beds freed by the intermediate care scheme.

Sources of relevant cost information

The sources for costing the resources affected by intermediate care schemes will include NHS and local authority finance departments. Purchased items can be valued at their market prices; drug costs are obtainable in the *British National Formulary* (biannual). The Personal Social Services Research Unit at Kent University produces a useful annual document with estimates of unit costs for health and social care (Netten and Curtis, 2003).

Two related issues stem from the sources used for costs. First, the policy of payment by results will increasingly mean that trusts are paid for inpatient acute care based upon a tariff constructed from the average reference cost for each Health Resource Group (HRGs are the UK equivalent of diagnosis related groups), adjusted for specific local factors (Department of Health, 2002). Second, the costs of patient care delivered by new intermediate care services are likely to be constructed locally from separately identified resource inputs with unit costs applied. Consider a situation where the inpatient costs used in an evaluation are based upon the national tariff while those of a hospital at home scheme, for example, are locally determined. Table 9.2 shows the possibilities.

True hospital costs could be above, equal to or below those based on the tariff. If the hospital at home cost is (b) it will appear cheaper than the tariff (e) but the costs of the hospital at home scheme relative to actual costs will remain unclear:

Table 9.2 Costs relative to tariff used in local commissioning of services.

True costs relative to tariff	Inpatients	Hospital at home
Above	a	a
Equal	e	e
Below	b	b

they could be below, equal to or above actual costs. Hence, a false impression of the costs of inpatient care and intermediate care could result. In addition, if tariff costs are used, it might be difficult to match HRG patient categories with the categories of inpatients eligible for the new intermediate care scheme.

The second issue to be aware of when estimating savings in the costs of acute care is that the use of average costs may distort true resource savings, such as, where an intermediate care scheme reduces inpatient acute stay from eight to five days. Will an average inpatient cost accurately estimate the cost saving of this reduction? Drummond et al. (1997) point out that an inpatient stay incurs a hotel cost that is the same for each day, and a treatment cost which is incurred in the first few days of the stay. The average cost is constructed from these two elements. The cost of the first few days is above the average, whereas that of subsequent days, consisting wholly (or mainly) of the hotel cost, will be below the average daily cost. Applying the average cost to estimate the cost saving for the last few days will overestimate the actual saving. A scheme that prevented admissions would avoid both the inpatient treatment and hotel costs.

Benefits to consider

Information about benefits is critical to put alongside costs. The role of the information depends upon the evaluation question. The interest may be in which modality of care to provide for one or more diagnostic groups: technical efficiency. Alternatively, interest may be in identifying how much resource to allocate to specific patient groups.

What do we mean by benefits? An acute hospital may be interested in shorter lengths of stay or fewer patients admitted. The hospital is interested in using its facilities more appropriately: the efficient production of health care. This is a very important question in its own right, but belongs to the service design and its costs. The objective of the NHS in providing health care to patients is to maintain or improve individuals' health. It is the impact upon an individual's health in terms of quality and quantity of life that is the benefit. There may be other benefits linked to the process of care. There may also be benefits to carers and relatives.

Early evaluations of intermediate care were driven by clinical concerns of effectiveness and safety for specific diagnostic groups. They tended to use measures specific to the disease of interest, for example stroke (Rudd et al., 1997) or COPD (Cotton et al., 2000; Davies et al., 2000; Swarska et al., 2000). Specific measures enable comparisons within the disease of interest but not with other diseases. Sometimes more generic measures were used, for example Rudd (1997) included the Nottingham Health Profile, Shepperd et al. (1998a) looked at several diagnostic groups and used the Short Form 36 (SF–36).

Appendix 9.1 provides references for more information upon generic measures. In addition to the Nottingham Health Profile and the SF–36, the role of Quality Adjusted Life Years (QALYs) as a measure of health benefit is also discussed. QALYs have been developed over the past twenty years or so to enable comparisons to be made across and between different disease states. Quality and quantity of life are summarised as a single figure, which can be expressed as a cost per QALY ratio for each option. Several QALY measures have been developed but the one most widely used in the UK is the EQ5D (Brooks, 1996).

Intermediate care, however, can include multi-faceted benefits with both health and non-health attributes. Benefits may include factors additional to health status, such as the provision of clear and meaningful information, the respect and sensitivity shown by professionals, the location of care, and access to regular contact with known carers (family). These cannot all be measured by clinical measures, health profiles or indeed EQ5D.

Satisfaction surveys are sometimes used alongside other measures in intermediate care. Scott (1996) argued that satisfaction surveys do not measure the strength of importance of schemes to individuals and suggested that the tools of Willingness To Pay and Conjoint Analysis might be helpful with this. To use these tools inputs from specialist researchers are required. They do not appear to have been tested in intermediate care to date, and certainly appear worth using in a well-designed piece of research.

The reality of many intermediate care schemes, that are implemented by the NHS and not evaluated, is that none of the benefit issues are addressed. This means that whether or not the schemes are more or less efficient than what they replace is completely unknown. It is probable that as intermediate care schemes develop, there will be more confidence to expand them to either patients with greater morbidity in diagnostic groups currently covered or to new diagnostic groups. The issues raised by this discussion of benefits will remain.

When costs and benefits should be measured

Intermediate care is time limited but is not the end of the patient journey. It is important to reflect upon the appropriate time-frame to analyse costs and benefits when comparing an intermediate care scheme with a comparator. For example, if a hospital at home scheme is compared with routine inpatient care, an early cut-off could lead to spurious results. Patients receiving routine inpatient care will be discharged to district nursing and other health professional care. They may receive social care from social services, or from private or voluntary organisations for which they may have to pay. Patients receiving intermediate care are likely to have social care earlier. Too short a cut-off could miss the health and social care with the cost consequences to the inpatient group.

Benefits are also likely to accrue at different points of care. A challenge faced by any evaluation is the time-scale available, a time period that may only represent one part of the patient journey. One possible approach might be to measure outcomes on an ongoing basis; this would raise issues of attributing causal inference. Both costs and benefits are affected by the choice of cut-off.

In addition, the Treasury requires costs and benefits to be discounted at 3.5% per annum up to 30 years (HM Treasury, 2003). These are the discount rates, which should be applied to intermediate care schemes if costs and benefits are collected for more than 12 months.

How to allow for uncertainty surrounding the results of an evaluation

Uncertainty stems from the evidence base and for intermediate care this is limited. Statistical techniques developed to address uncertainty in health economics costs and benefits are described by Briggs (2001). One approach is to model data and explore the impact of different assumptions in a sensitivity analysis. Campbell et al. (2001) compared the costs of a hospital at home scheme with inpatient care in a discrete event simulation model for elderly medical and orthopaedic patients. Modelling to explore different assumptions and uncertainties in the data might strengthen some evaluations of intermediate care schemes.

Potential ways forward

Programme budgeting and marginal analysis

There is an economic tool that addresses prioritisation of resource allocation across different investment options, which may be of help for intermediate care. The tool is programme budgeting and marginal analysis (PBMA) (Mitton and Donaldson, 2001) and it may have merit where decisions straddle different sectors: primary, acute, community hospitals, rapid response teams, hospital at home teams, nursing homes and local authority social service departments, to name the main ones. It would enable a health care commissioner to investigate the merits of alternative schemes for intermediate care, an evaluation requirement that some have raised (Coast et al., 2000). The tool also offers a framework to investigate resource investment options across different sectors and options and could be used to help the NHS and local authorities to work together. The tool does not appear to have been tested in the field of intermediate care to date.

Care management

Another approach, which may help the management of care across different agencies is that of care management. This is supported by the findings from the systematic literature review undertaken by Richards and Coast (2003). Curiously, it resonates with developments that have occurred in social care over the past twenty years or so: for example see Davies (1992). Care management is a model that appears to have considerable potential in intermediate care to manage patients in an efficient manner. This entails a lead professional monitoring the implementation of the care package with a multidisciplinary team. It is possible for the lead professional to be drawn from the NHS when health is the main issue, or social services when social care issues are more important. Efficiency is not simply determined by building the findings of an evaluation into a system and then standing back: mechanisms within the system to navigate it to improving efficiency as it develops are critical. Interestingly, the NHS has models of multi-agency working which sometimes use a form of care management in community psychiatric care from which intermediate care may benefit.

Summary

This chapter has argued that the demographic and health technology changes facing the NHS make implementing efficient intermediate care schemes critical. It is impracticable to expect every scheme to have an RCT design prior to full implementation. However, it is equally impracticable to implement intermediate care across the NHS without sufficient information upon costs and benefits.

Surveying the existing evidence is critical, although schemes may not be transplantable root and branch. Identifying what factors are the same and what are different is a first step.

Schemes implemented without a full evaluation, which includes appropriate comparators, means the estimation of benefits will be very limited and that of costs partial, depending on what is available from local finance departments. Building some evaluation in from the start will enable NHS decision makers to steer the schemes appropriately.

Identifying the key cost drivers and monitoring these, together with collecting information about benefits, such as the EQ5D, is feasible. It is important to keep an eye on the potential impact of cost shifting across providing agencies, be they NHS primary care or social service departments, and especially to patients and their carers. Hospitals with actual costs below the tariff may have a revenue incentive to treat patients as inpatients, especially if intermediate care schemes mean patients will incur payments at below the inpatient rate, or even receive care from another trust.

Previous work at Keele University has found examples of scope to shorten patient lengths of stay by speeding up the time to report test results and timetable consultant ward rounds. This points to the fact that hospitals may find ways to increase their efficiency alongside intermediate care initiatives.

While technical efficiency questions have dominated evaluations to date, allocative efficiency is also critical. If a scheme entails more resources, where they come from and who loses must be considered.

Commissioning and funding studies to fill gaps in knowledge is important if intermediate care is to move in an appropriate direction to address the challenges posed by an ageing population and provide evidence to inform upon policy development.

Appendix 9.1

Nottingham Health Profile

Further information upon the Nottingham Health Profile can be found in Hunt et al. (1985) and limited information for non-members on the websites http:// www.qolid.org/public/NHP.html and http://www.atsqol.org/nott.asp#ats1.

Short Form 36 (SF–36)

Further information can be found on the SF–36 website http://www.sf–36.org/.

Some have suggested that the SF–36 may be less applicable to the over 65s (Brazier et al., 1992), which may be an issue to consider in intermediate care given that most of the patients are elderly. Shorter forms are available such as the SF12 and SF8. The SF–36 and its shorter forms have been subject to continual development.

Both the Nottingham Health Profile and SF–36 (and its variants) are limited from an economic point of view as to the extent they measure individual preferences; the dimensions cannot be summarised as a single measure so they cannot be compared directly with the costs; and the instruments are not calibrated so that they can combine quality of life with quantity of life (Drummond et al., 1997, p. 130). There has been work recently exploring converting SF–36 information for use in quality and quantity measures (Brazier et al., 1998; 2002), however, this work is still under development and requires more testing.

Quality Adjusted Life Years (QALYs)

Quality Adjusted Life Years (QALYs) have been developed over the past twenty years or so to enable comparisons to be made across and between different disease states. Several QALY measures have been developed, but the one most widely used in the UK is the EQ5D (Brooks, 1996). The EQ5D has been designed to be simple and quick to answer; there is one main sheet with five questions, each having three possible answers. These are used by the EQ5D to construct a five-dimensional health state classification system with each of five dimensions having three statements representing degrees of perceived severity. Patient perceptions are elicited through close-ended questions. The five dimensions are:

- Mobility,
- Self-care,

- Usual activities,
- Pain/discomfort,
- Anxiety/depression.

Each dimension has three levels: no problem, some problems, and major problems. The combination of three levels in five dimensions produces 243 possible health states, to which have been added 'unconscious' and 'dead' which produces a total of 245. These are converted to scores using health state values, derived from European population surveys, which include the general UK population using a time trade-off method (Dolan et al., 1995). The health state values generate a single index value for health status, in which full health is assigned a value of 1 and death a value of 0; states deemed worse than death can be assigned negative values. These are then combined with expected length of life. If a health state is valued at 0.6 and the length of life is 10 years, the calculated QALY equivalent is $10 \times 0.6 = 6$ QALYs. The EQ5D also includes a Visual Analogue Scale with endpoints of 100 for best imaginable health and 0 for worst imaginable health state. The EQ5D has been extensively used alongside other measures in both clinical trials and epidemiological evaluations of health status. The study by Richards et al. (1998) used several outcome measures, including the EQ5D. The main advantage of the EQ5D in economic evaluations is that health benefits are summarised in a single number that can be compared with costs. Health benefits accruing across different conditions may be compared. This enables technical efficiency questions to be addressed for different diagnostic groups and can inform some allocative questions if the sole benefit of interest is changes in health *per se*. The disadvantage is that the single score does not enable movement in separate dimensions to be identified, which may be of specific interest. This is the reason why it is often used together with other outcome measures. There would appear to be great scope for the EQ5D to be used more often in intermediate care. Further information on the tool is available at the EQ5D website http://www.euroqol.org/.

References

Brazier, J.E., Harper, R., Jones, N.M.B., O'Cathain, A., Thomas, J.K., Westlake, L. (1992) Validating the SF–36 health survey questionnaire: new outcome measures for primary care. *British Medical Journal* **305**, 160–64.

Brazier, J., Usherwood, T., Harper, R., Thomas, K. (1998) Deriving a preference-based single index from the UK SF–36 health survey. *Journal of Clinical Epidemiology* **51**, 1115–28.

Brazier, J., Roberts, J., Deverill, M. (2002) The estimation of a preference-based measure of health from the SF–36. *Journal of Health Economics* **21**, 271–92.

Briggs, A.H. (2001) Handling uncertainty in economic evaluation and presenting the results. In: Drummond, M.F. and McGuire, A. (eds) (2001) *Economic Evaluation in Health Care – Merging Theory with Practice*. Oxford: Oxford University Press.

British National Formulary (biannual). London: British Medical Association and The Royal Pharmaceutical Society of Great Britain.

Brooks, R., The EuroQol Group (1996) EuroQol: the current state of play. *Health Policy* **37**, 53–72.

Campbell, H., Karnon, J., Dowie, R. (2001) Cost analysis of a hospital-at-home initiative using discrete event simulation. *Journal of Health Services Research and Policy* **6** (1), 14–22.

Coast, J., Richards, S., Peters, T.J., Gunnell, D.J., Darlow, M.A., Pounsford, J. (1998) Hospital at home or with acute hospital care? A cost minimisation analysis. *British Medical Journal* **316**, 1802–806.

Coast, J., Hensher, M., Mulligan, J.A., Shepperd, S., Jones, J. (2000) Conceptual and practical difficulties with the economic evaluation of health services developments. *Journal of Health Services Research and Policy* **5** (1), 42–8.

Cotton, M.M., Bucknall, C.E., Dagg, K.D., Johnson, M.K., Macgregor, G., Stewart, C., Stevenson, R.D. (2000) Early discharge for patients with exacerbations of chronic obstructive pulmonary disease: a randomised controlled trial. *Thorax* **55**, 902–906.

Davies, B. (1992) *Care Management, Equity and Efficiency, the International Experience*. Canterbury: Personal Social Services Research Unit, University of Kent.

Davies, L., Wilkinson, M., Bonner, S., Calverley, P.M.A., Angus, R.M. (2000) 'Hospital at home' versus hospital care in patients with exacerbations of chronic obstructive pulmonary disease: a prospective randomised controlled trial. *British Medical Journal* **321**, 1265–8.

Department of Health (2002) *Reforming NHS Financial Flows: Introducing Payment by Results*. London: Department of Health.

Dolan, P., Gudex, C., Kind, P., Williams, A. (1995) *A Social Tariff for Euroqol: Results from a UK General Population Survey*. Discussion Paper 138. York: University of York, Centre for Health Economics.

Donaldson, C., Currie, G., Mitton, C. (2002) Cost-effectiveness analysis in health care: contraindications. *British Medical Journal* **325**, 891–4.

Drummond, M.F., O'Brien, B., Stoddart, G.L., Torrance, G.W. (1997) *Methods for the Economic Evaluation of Health Care Programmes*, 2nd ed. Oxford: Oxford University Press.

Drummond, M.F., McGuire, A. (eds) (2001) *Economic Evaluation in Health Care – Merging Theory with Practice*. Oxford: Oxford University Press.

Gold, M.R., Siegel, J.E., Russell, L.B., Weinstein, C. (1996) *Cost-Effectiveness in Health and Medicine*. Oxford: Oxford University Press.

HM Treasury (2003) *Appraisal and Evaluation in Central Government* (The Green Book). London: HM Treasury.

Hunt, S.M., McEwen, J., McKenna, S.P. (1985) Measuring health status: a new tool for clinicians and epidemiologists. *Journal of the Royal College of General Practice*, **35**, 185–88.

Jones, J., Wilson, A., Parker, H., Wynn, A., Jagger, C., Spiers, N., Parker, G. (1999) Economic evaluation of hospital at home care with hospital care: cost minimisation analysis of data from randomised controlled trial. *British Medical Journal* **319**, 1547–50.

Knowelden, J., Westlake, L., Wright, K.G., Clarke, S.J. (1991) Peterborough hospital at home: an evaluation. *Journal of Public Health Medicine* **13**, 182–8.

Mitton, C., Donaldson, C. (2001) Twenty-five years of programme budgeting and marginal analysis in the health sector, 1974–1999. *Journal of Health Services Research and Policy* **6** (4), 239–48.

Mooney, G.H., Russell, E.M., Weir, R.D. (1986) *Choices for Health Care: A Practical Introduction* (2nd edition). London: Macmillan.

Netten, A., Curtis, L. (2003) *Unit Costs of Health and Social Care 2003*. Canterbury: Personal Social Services Research Unit, University of Kent.

NHS Executive Anglia and Oxford (1997) *Opportunities in Intermediate Care. Summary Report from the Anglia and Oxford Intermediate Care Project.* Oxford: NHS Executive.

Posnett, J., Street, A. (1996) Programme budgeting and marginal analysis: an approach to priority setting in need of refinement. *Journal of Health Services Research and Policy* **1** (3), 147–53.

Richards, S., Coast, J., Gunnell, D.J., Peters, T.J., Pounsford, J., Darlow, M.A. (1998) Randomised controlled trial comparing effectiveness and acceptability of an early discharge, hospital at home scheme with acute hospital care. *British Medical Journal* **316**, 1796–801.

Richards, S., Coast, J. (2003) Interventions to improve access to health and social care after discharge from hospital: a systematic review. *Journal of Health Services Research and Policy* **8** (3), 171–9.

Rudd, A., Wolfe, C., Tilling, K., Beech, R. (1997) A randomised controlled trial to evaluate early discharge scheme for patients with stroke. *British Medical Journal* **315**, 1039–44.

Scott, A. (1996) Primary or secondary care? What can economics contribute to evaluating the interface? *Journal of Public Health Medicine* **18**, 19–26.

Shepperd, S., Harwood, D., Jenkinson, C., Gray, A., Vessey, M., Morgan, P. (1998a) Randomised controlled trial comparing hospital at home care with inpatient hospital care. I: Three month follow up of health outcomes. *British Medical Journal* **316**, 1786–91.

Shepperd, S., Harwood, D., Jenkinson, C., Gray Vessey, M., Morgan, P. (1998b) Randomised controlled trial comparing hospital at home care with inpatient hospital care. II: A cost minimisation analysis. *British Medical Journal* **316**, 1791–6.

Swarska, E., Cohen, G., Swarski, K.M., Lamb, C., Bushell, D., Parker, S., MacNee, W. (2000) Randomised controlled trial of supported discharge in patients with exacerbations of chronic obstructive pulmonary disease. *Thorax* **55**, 907–12.

Vaughan, B., Lathlean, J. (1999) *Intermediate Care: Models in Practice.* London: King's Fund.

Part 2
Continuing Care

Chapter 10

Continuing Care: Policy and Context

David Challis and Ann Netten

Introduction

The term 'continuing care' in the UK has often, if erroneously, been associated narrowly with the definition of what amounts to residual responsibilities of the NHS for the provision of care for particularly vulnerable individuals (Department of Health, 1995). This confusion has been made the subject of guidance in policy (Department of Health, 2001a) which discriminates continuing care in general from 'continuing NHS health care', 'continuing health and social care' and 'intermediate care'. 'Continuing care' is defined therein thus:

> 'Continuing care (or long-term care) is a general term that describes the care which people need over an extended period of time, as the result of disability, accident or illness to address both physical and mental health needs. It may require services from the NHS and/or social care. It can be provided in a range of settings, from an NHS hospital, to a nursing home or residential home, and people's own homes.' (para. 5)

For the purpose of this chapter reference is made to the provision of what is called in the policy documents of many countries 'long-term care', or continuing care in its broadest sense. This refers to the provision of this mode of support (irrespective of the administrative division of responsibilities in the United Kingdom) which has evolved since the 1940s. Following the 1948 National Assistance Act the accommodation provided by former workhouses was divided into Part III accommodation, the responsibility of the local authority sector, and infirmaries, the responsibility of the then infant NHS (Means and Smith, 1998). From this can be seen the administrative separation of the provision of long-term care into the health and social care sectors, which markedly changed its balance during the 1970s and 1980s with the reduction of long-stay hospital beds for older people, the growth in provision of beds in care homes and the development of community based care.

It has been suggested that there was an excessive focus on residential care in the 1948 National Assistance Act (Townsend, 1964), perhaps inevitably given the need to address the needs of those then in institutional settings, with a lack of focus upon the development of community based services. None the less, this lack of emphasis was partially offset in the 1946 NHS Act, which empowered local authorities to establish district nursing and home help services (Means and Smith, 1998).

While policy objectives place increasing emphasis on improving functioning, preventing decline and maximising independence, and indeed there is epidemiological evidence that becoming disabled in old age is not an irreversible event (Manton, 1988), inevitably there will be a need for continuing care for a substantial number of people. There are debates as to whether the growth in numbers of older people will be associated with what has been termed compression of morbidity (Fries, 1980), although US estimates indicate that active life expectancy may be greater than expected (Manton and Land, 2000). None the less, for many older people the last years of their lives will be characterised by long-term impairment. Sauvaget and colleagues (2001), using data from Leicestershire, suggest that estimates of healthy life expectancy for very old people – over the age of 85 years – indicate that few years will be spent without restriction in performing activities of daily living, although less than one-third of remaining life would be with cognitive impairment.

This chapter produces a summary of the developing policy and service arena of continuing care, defined in its widest sense as above, thereby setting the subsequent chapters in context. The chapter is divided into four parts: first a summary of policy from the 1940s to the 1990s; second, a summary of changes occurring as a result of the community care reforms of the early 1990s; and third, a discussion of a number of facets of the modernisation of social care from the late 1990s. Finally, reference is made to the variations in national and local context and the future funding needs of long-term care.

Past policy and history

Long-term commitment to community based care

As long ago as 1946 the National Health Service Act empowered local authorities to provide home nursing and home help services, but the development of long-term care services after this and the passing of the 1948 National Assistance Act has been viewed as a failure to address the development of community based care (Townsend, 1964; 1981; Parker, 1965). There was no marked growth in services to reflect a policy shift towards support of vulnerable people at home (Means and Smith, 1998) and home care was frequently targeted to those living alone and lacking family support (Shanas et al., 1968; Hunt, 1970) reflecting an underlying assumption of the roles and responsibilities of families.

None the less, there has been a longstanding commitment to supporting people in need of continuing care in the community or home based care wherever possible. In the support of older people this commitment may be traced to statements in Ministry of Health Reports (Cm 1418, 1961) and in policy terms to the White Paper *Health and Welfare: The Development of Community Care* (Cm 1973, 1963). However, it is possible to date the substantive basis of community based care for older people to the Health Services and Public Health Act of 1968, which gave local authorities a general responsibility for promoting the welfare of elderly people and placed them under an obligation to establish a home help service.

From the 1970s there was a progressive withdrawal of the NHS from the provision of convalescent and continuing care for older people (Wistow, 1996). Thus the number of NHS beds specifically designated for older people fell from 55 600 to 37 500 between 1976 and 1994, a reduction of one third (House of Commons Health Committee, 1995). This made more visible the boundary between NHS-provided continuing care and that provided through social care, and led to attempts to produce more explicit eligibility criteria for the NHS care which was free at the point of delivery (Department of Health, 1995). Wistow (1996) has suggested that this represented a process of redefining the boundary between health and social care, as both acute bed numbers and hospital length of stay reduced. Increasingly, the health and social care boundary can be seen as developing into one between acute and long-term care. Alternatives to long-stay hospital care were explored in the Care in the Community Initiative (DHSS, 1983), a series of 28 projects offering care in the community to previous hospital residents. Of these, seven were for older people, three focused on those with predominantly physical frailty, and four for older people with mental health problems. The relevance of these developments lay less in the hospital closure process and more in the testing of alternative methods of providing community based support (Renshaw et al., 1988; Knapp et al., 1992).

The White Paper *Growing Older* (Cm 8173, 1981) placed a greater emphasis on the place of voluntary and informal support in the care of older people: 'Care in the community must increasingly mean care by the community' (p. 3). Despite the policy commitment to community care, the 1980s saw a substantial growth in private and not for profit residential and nursing care for older people, supported by social security funds. Access to care homes was not on the basis of care needs but financial eligibility, thereby creating a substantial new sector of care homes for older people supported by social security funds and a bias in favour of institutional rather than community based care.

The effects of this were analysed by the Audit Commission (1986) in an influential report identifying the 'perverse incentives' created by these funding arrangements and criticising the organisational failure to match resources appropriately to need in community care. The Government appointed a special adviser to report on possible solutions for community care, and this report was produced in early 1988 (Griffiths, 1988). It recommended a more coordinated approach to the funding and management of care, placing the responsibility for allocation of funds, assessment of need and coordination of care with the local authority social services department, and proposed care management to ensure a more planned and effective use of resources at the individual service user level. The majority of the recommendations were accepted by the Government in the 1989

Box 10.1   Key objectives of the 1989 White Paper *Caring for People* (Cm 849, 1989).

- To promote the development of domiciliary, day and respite services to enable older people to live in their own homes wherever feasible and sensible
- To ensure that service providers make practical support for carers a high priority
- To make proper assessment of need and good care management the cornerstone of high quality care
- To promote the development of a flourishing independent sector alongside good quality public services
- To clarify the responsibilities of agencies and so make it easier to hold them to account for their performance
- To secure better value for taxpayers' money by introducing a new funding structure for social care

---

Crown copyright. Reproduction with permission of the Controller of HMSO and the Queen's Printer for Scotland.

White Paper *Caring for People* (Cm 849, 1989) and were introduced in stages up to 1993 following the 1990 NHS and Community Care Act. The six key objectives of *Caring for People* are summarised in Box 10.1.

The policy thus addressed the need to develop community based care services within a context of targeting services upon those with the greatest need. It made a clear statement of the importance of the needs of carers to a greater extent than hitherto. Through assessment and care management, more appropriate responses to needs were to be made and a better use of resources achieved at the level of the individual user of services. The role of social services authorities was to be that of an 'enabling organisation' taking responsibility for the effective development of the local social care economy. In so doing they were expected to make maximum possible use of private and voluntary providers and thereby increase care options and choice. As Wistow and colleagues (1992) have noted, many of the ideas around the 'enabling authority' were at least implicit in documents such as the Seebohm (Cm 3703, 1968) and Barclay Reports (Barclay, 1982). Of the additional funding provided to local authorities, 85%, which had previously been part of the social security budget, had to be spent on services provided by the independent sector. Overall, the reforms were designed to achieve better value for money and, in particular, no longer provide an incentive to enter care homes.

The developments and the funding distortions that led to the policy changes were not unique to the UK. Similar events had occurred in the 1980s in Australia (Challis et al., 1995). The longstanding concern with coordination of services which had often been expressed only at the macro level between health and social care, with a focus on activities such as joint planning (Webb and Wistow, 1986), was also given a micro level focus through care management. Certainly the reforms created a reasonably coherent framework for developing community based care akin to the trend towards the reduced institutional care and enhanced home based care evident in many countries (Kraan et al., 1991; Challis, 1992). The definition of community based care moved towards a definition that included residential and nursing homes as not community based care, as distinct from the 'hospital versus community' definition that had prevailed earlier. However, there remained several anomalies to be addressed in the changes to long-term care amongst which two were particularly important:

- How would the issue of hospital discharge from acute settings be addressed in a set of reforms designed to address long-term care?
- What was to be done regarding the changing relationship between free NHS long-term care and means tested social care?

Developments in the early 1990s

During the 1990s the effects of these changes unfolded. A review of the progress and obstacles in relation to these six objectives was undertaken as one of the volumes of the Royal Commission on Long Term Care (Cm 4192-II/3, 1999; Henwood and Wistow, 1999). More detail is provided in Chapters 11 and 12 of this book and a few key issues are highlighted briefly here.

First, there did appear to be at first a stabilisation and subsequently a reduction in the numbers of publicly supported residents in care homes. Second, in part arising from the reduction in admissions to care homes, more people were remaining at home. However, the development of effective home care services was hampered by such factors as cost ceilings, fast hospital throughput, a reduction in low-level home help as a consequence of the policy of targeting and a lack of development and innovation. Third, a wider social care economy developed through the 1990s, encompassing both public and independent sector providers. Although there was a very rapid growth of independent sector care homes during the 1980s, the 1990s saw considerable growth of the independent home care sector. Fourth, there was a varied and unfocused development of assessment and care management. Assessment approaches were of very varied quality, and care management arrangements provided little evidence of the kind of intensive care management capable of offering a realistic alternative of care at home to admission to residential or nursing home care (Challis, 1999).

During the 1990s, as the momentum created by the 1990 NHS and Community Care Act was carried through the system, the role of local authority social services departments (SSDs) changed fundamentally. Interacting with individual external providers to secure specialist and niche market services had long been an important function of SSDs in discharging their statutory duties towards vulnerable people. However, initially spurred by financial incentives, directions on user choice and consultation, and other advice and guidance from central government (including the Department of Health, Social Services Inspectorate and Audit Commission), by the 1990s guiding and managing local markets for social care had become a central activity. By 1999 residential care and domiciliary care for older people were both predominantly purchased from external agencies for the first time.

One important policy development during the early 1990s was to further enhance the position of carers through the Carers (Recognition and Services) Act in 1995, which entitled the carers of vulnerable people to an assessment of their own needs. Carers' rights were later further strengthened by the Carers and Disabled Children Act 2000, which permitted the carers of adults to have an assessment even when the cared-for person refused an assessment.

Policy developments from the late 1990s

In this section, a brief discussion of modernisation is followed by a discussion of the modernisation of social care services and key related issues such as the social care workforce, the acute and long-term care interface, performance, regulation and Best Value as they relate to long-term care.

The modernisation of social care

It is possible to characterise the policies that have unfolded following the change of government in 1997 as reflecting the development of a process of modernisation. The concept of public sector modernisation is common to most of the developed world (OECD, 2003). Its ideals are intertwined with theories of governance including the importance of networks, decentralisation of government and accountability (Rhodes, 1997). In the UK, modernisation of the public sector has been a key priority of the Labour administration. It has spanned many areas of policy and administration such as education, employment and health care.

Within the wider modernisation process it is possible to identify specific areas salient to the social care and long-term care of adults. This can be identified as a response to concerns about access to, and the quality, responsiveness and appropriateness of services. Other concerns relate to variation and consistency in services and the need for more effective regulation and clearer standards. In a recent review of modernisation of social care services for adults (Challis et al., 2004) six main themes of modernisation of social care services were identified:

- Integrated health and social care
- Independence
- Consistency
- Carers
- Making sure services fit individuals' needs
- Workforce.

To these should be added the broader and non-service specific themes of performance and regulation.

Modernisation of social care services

In 1998 the White Paper *Modernising Social Services* was published (Cm 4169, 1998). It stressed three key themes in services for adults: helping people to live independently; fairer and more consistent services; and ensuring that services fit individual needs. In the White Paper other initiatives were also announced including performance measurement and regulation. Many of these themes have been developed and consolidated in later policy documents and legislation.

In the White Paper, the theme of integrating health and social care is given the priority status of bringing down the 'Berlin Wall' between health and social care (Cm 4169, 1998, p. 97). The Health Act 1999 removed legal obstacles to joint working and promoted partnership working by allowing:

- Pooled budgets – where health and social services put a proportion of their funds into a mutually accessible joint budget to enable more integrated care.
- Lead commissioning – where one authority transfers funds to the other who will then take responsibility for purchasing both health and social care.
- Integrated provision – where one organisation provides both health and social care (Cm 4818-I, 2000).

The NHS Plan moved this process further in a brief indication of the future development of integrated provision through Care Trusts, joint health and social care organisations. The NHS Plan also noted the introduction of the Single Assessment Process, detailed in Standard 2 of the *National Service Framework for Older People* (Department of Health, 2001b; 2002a), designed to provide a more standardised assessment process which improves practice and ensures that needs are fully assessed (para. 2.27). This is discussed in more detail in Chapter 11.

Current processes for determining eligibility can be seen as having their origins in the community care reforms of the 1990s. The issue of eligibility for different levels of care, be it NHS-funded continuing care or for care provided through the social services, has proved to be a major concern (Hughes et al., 1997) and guidelines for NHS Continuing Care have been subject to refinement (Department of Health, 1995; 2001a). The White Paper *Modernising Social Services* (Cm 4169, 1998), referring to the need for consistency, indicated the need for a Fair Access to Care Initiative to address variability in eligibility criteria for social care (para. 2.31). *Fair Access to Care* was published in 2002 (Department of Health, 2002a). Councils were expected to operate a single eligibility decision for all adults seeking social care support based upon a national framework and existing legislation and reflecting the degree of risk arising from needs associated with various forms of disability, impairment and difficulty. Eligibility for assistance was to be determined following assessment of an individual's presenting needs with the provision of services determined on the basis of statements of purpose, based on eligible needs (Department of Health, 2002b). The eligibility framework was divided into four bands – critical, substantial, moderate and low – which describe the seriousness of the risk to independence or other consequences if needs are not addressed.

Workforce

Two themes appear in relation to the social care workforce, both currently and over a longer period of time. These are first, the issue of recruitment and retention of staff, and second, the training of staff. Underlying this is a concern for quality and standards. As indicated in *Modernising Social Services* (Cm 4169, 1998), for the first time social care staff were to be regulated. Under the Care Standards Act 2000, the General Social Care Council (GSCC) was created to regulate and act as a registration body for different sectors of the social care workforce. Additionally, the General Social Care Council is responsible for regulating, accrediting and supporting social work education and training.

The Quality Strategy for Social Care reflects a number of elements to enhance the social care workforce standards. An employer-led body, the Training Organisation for the Personal Social Services (TOPSS – England), was created to provide a strategic lead on education, training and workforce development strategy for social care, including social work. It aims to support employers in improving standards of care provision through training and development, workforce planning and workforce intelligence. The Social Care Institute for Excellence (SCIE) was created to collect and publicise knowledge about good practice to improve quality in services.

The acute and continuing care interface

The development of long-term care services needs also to address the interface with acute care (Department of Health, Housing, Local Government and Community Services, 1993). In England, the issue of hospital discharge has continued to be of concern from the community care changes of the 1990s when receipt of new funding was made conditional upon local agreements being in place to facilitate discharge (Gostick et al., 1997), to the present day. Intermediate care (Department of Health, 2001b; 2001c) has been discussed earlier in this book. It can be seen as an important part of the interface between acute and continuing care and the government policy for the pursuit of prevention of inappropriate care provision. The targeting definition for intermediate care included 'people who would otherwise face unnecessarily prolonged hospital stays or inappropriate admission to acute in-patient care, long-term residential care, or continuing NHS in-patient care' (Department of Health, 2001c). The Community Care (Delayed Discharges) Act 2003 introduced an approach whereby financial incentives were put in place to avoid people remaining in hospital beds after their clinical need for such care was complete. At one level this can be seen as a means to provide a financial penalty since the costs of care will pass to social services when a patient is ready to leave a hospital. However, the additional central funds provided afford an opportunity to develop more appropriate discharge services, which in conjunction with intermediate care offer services appropriate to the needs of these patients. The introduction of intermediate care in the NHS Plan (Cm 4818-I, 2000) and the *National Service Framework for Older People* (Department of Health, 2001b), and the Community Care (Delayed Discharges) Act 2003 can be seen as the beginning of the emergence of a separate strategy for managing the acute/long-term care interface as opposed to the distortion of long-term care policy in the service of the acute sector (Gostick et al., 1997).

Performance

Performance measurement in social care developed through the work of the Audit Commission and Social Services Inspectorate through the 1980s and 1990s, particularly reflecting the Audit Commmission (2000) indicators and the Key Indicators Graphical System (Department of Health, 1999). In the White Paper *Modernising Social Services* (Cm 4169, 1998) the Performance Assessment Framework was announced which included indicators in five domains related to Personal Social Services performance. These were: national priorities and strategic objectives; cost and efficiency; effectiveness of service delivery and outcomes; quality of services for users and carers; and fair access. These have been subject to continuing refinement linked to the other areas of performance monitoring undertaken by the Audit Commission, the NHS Performance Assessment Framework and the standards employed by the Commission for Social Care Inspection. In 2002 the Star Rating System (Department of Health, 2002c) was introduced into social services. This assessment includes evidence from inspections and reviews, monitoring, and performance indicators, to form an overall picture of performance over time on both qualitative and quantitative aspects of performance. The star ratings summarised the Social Services Inspectorate's independent judgements of performance across all social services, on a scale of zero to three stars.

Regulation

The principal contribution of the regulatory function to long-term care is to ensure that homes, agencies, proprietors and workforce are fit for the purpose when they initially register, and continue to be so. The concept of 'fit for the purpose' encompasses both protection of vulnerable adults and providing an adequate quality of care.

During the 1980s there had been considerable development of regulatory bodies, associated with the development of the 'New Public Management' (Dunleavy and Hood, 1994). The White Paper *Modernising Social Services* (Cm 4169, 1998) introduced the widening of regulation to more services and the development of stronger national standards by which services were to be assessed. The problems with the existing approaches were adjudged to be lack of independence of the regulators (who were from local health and social services authorities); lack of coherence due to split responsibilities of different regulators; and lack of consistency between local regulators.

The Care Standards Act 2000 provided a major overhaul of the regulatory infrastructure for social care by establishing national bodies to carry forward the government's modernisation agenda. In April 2002 the National Care Standards Commission (NCSC) was set up with the responsibility for regulating care homes for adults and children, boarding schools and adoption agencies. From April 2003 the Commission gained responsibility for registering nurse agencies, domiciliary care agencies and family care centres. From April 2004 inspection of private and voluntary health care transferred to the Commission for Healthcare Audit and Inspection (CHAI) and the inspection and regulation of social care services transferred to the new Commission for Social Care Inspection (CSCI), which also incorporates functions previously undertaken by the Social Services Inspectorate (SSI) and the SSI/Audit Commission Joint Review team.

The establishment of the National Care Standards Commission and National Minimum Standards for care provision was part of a multi-pronged approach to the protection of vulnerable people and the raising of quality of welfare provision. A set of national minimum standards for care homes was issued in 2001 (Department of Health, 2001e). There were subsequent negotiations about the applicability of certain physical standards to existing homes before implementation. There are 38 standards organised into seven domains of evaluation: choice of home; health and personal care; daily life and social activities; complaints and protection; environment; staffing and management; and administration. As discussed later in Chapter 13, the introduction of these standards had a profound impact on the care home market. In 2003 national minimum standards for domiciliary care were produced (Department of Health, 2003) with 27 standards organised into five domains. These were: user focused services; personal care; protection; managers and staff; and organisation and running of the business. These standards provide a more explicit and consistent framework to regulation of services than hitherto had been in existence.

It is interesting to note the increasingly closer moving together of the various monitoring bodies in long-term care – SSI, the Audit Commission and the Care Standards Commission and their shared utilisation of the tools of performance review. The organisational fusion of these separate activities into CSCI can be seen as representing the growing proximity and overlap of their activities.

Best value

The theme of value for money continued from the 1990s as part of the modernisation developments but was given a wider focus. Best Value was introduced as a means of redressing the focus upon cost as the sole criterion by which to adjudge the services provided, which had prevailed hitherto. It introduced a balance between cost and quality. Local authorities were charged with a duty of Best Value (Cm 4014, 1998): 'to deliver services to clear standards covering both cost and quality, by the most effective, economic and efficient means available'. It is designed to secure continuous improvements in performance, and to deliver services which bear comparison to the best. Best Value applies to all local government services, including social services. The Performance Assessment system for social services is based on the Best Value regimen but includes a number of supplements that reinforce the central aims of Best Value and meet the specific demands of social services. All councils must ensure that their services are responsive to the needs of citizens, are efficient and of high quality, and provided within a clear policy framework. They must prepare annual Best Value Performance Plans, setting out their strategic objectives and corporate priorities.

Funding long-term care

A critical aspect of long-term care from the perspective of individuals is eligibility for funding. It is in the field of continuing and long-term care that the contrast between universal entitlements to health care free at the point of delivery and the means tested approach to social care is placed in sharp relief. This is an issue that has raised considerable feeling among self-funded care home residents and their relatives (Netten and Darton, 2003). The Report of the Royal Commission on Long Term Care (Cm 4192–II/3) recommended that the provision of all personal care should be made available after an assessment and paid for from general taxation. In effect this was free at the point of delivery. The Government responded in the NHS Plan (Cm 4818-II, 2000), which stated that, in England, nursing care would be made free under the NHS to everyone in a care home who needed it. In effect, this addressed the anomaly that a person in a residential home could receive nursing care from a community nurse under the NHS, whereas a similar resident in a nursing home would be contributing towards the cost of their nursing care. The provision of personal care, whether in a care home or in a person's own home would continue to be means tested (Department of Health, 2001b). Inevitably, the definition of what constitutes nursing care remains contested and, in the absence of a standard approach to definition and assessment (Carpenter et al., 2003), there is a real risk of considerable territorial variation in the interpretation of eligibility for the provision of the nursing care contribution.

The use of Direct Payments represents a fundamentally important shift in the way that long-term care services are funded. Based on an assessment of needs, the individual is allocated funds and (to a lesser or greater degree) support to organise and purchase their own services. In England, close relatives cannot be paid and the system is characterised by relatively low levels of regulation. Direct payments have been an option for younger disabled people for some time, and became available to older people in 2000. To date, take-up by older people has been slow and there is little information as yet on their effectiveness. Potentially, however, they could have a profound impact for some service users, enhancing choice and supporting more informal approaches that more closely reflect household or family production of care. There are, however, dangers of exploitation on both sides and in many instances (for example, where people have dementia) the older person themselves will not be in a position to or want to manage their own care.

Commissioning

Since the 1990s, expertise in the field of commissioning services has developed rapidly in local authorities (Wistow et al., 1996). However, there remain a number of problems and new challenges presented by the move to joint commissioning and the use of direct payments. Past practice has had a profound impact, primarily in keeping prices down and loading the risk on to the provider. In the

White Paper *Modernising Social Servcies* (Cm 4169, 1998) the key element of good commissioning was seen as moving away from a focus upon who provides services, to one where the key issue is service quality as experienced by the individual, their carers and their family (para. 1.7). The desired outcome of good commissioning was that it 'will help to ensure that services meet people's specific individual needs, and that groups with particular needs, such as people from ethnic minorities, are better served' (p. 36). The importance of joint commissioning was that it could contribute to the goals of both efficiency and integration.

National context

It is increasingly difficult to talk of a common approach to continuing and long-term care across the United Kingdom. Many of the policy initiatives discussed since 1997 are specifically relevant to England. It is noteworthy the extent to which the establishment of the Scottish Parliament and Welsh Executive has rendered greater national differences in the provision of long-term care in the UK. As an example the Single Assessment Process in Wales has some different dimensions of assessment to that in England (National Assembly for Wales, 2002). Of greater significance for individual older people is the decision in Scotland to make the provision of personal care no longer chargeable from 2002.

In Scotland charges are no longer made for personal care provided for people aged 65 and over in their own homes, and those living in care homes, who would otherwise pay their own fees, receive funding towards personal care and further funding if nursing care is also required. This latter funding is also provided to those aged under 65 (Scottish Executive, 2003). Again, with regard to the workforce, whereas in England a specific body (TOPSS) is responsible for the strategic lead, in Northern Ireland, Scotland and Wales, these functions are undertaken by the respective social care/services councils.

Future demand for long-term care

The rising number of older people in the population suggests that the number of people in need of long-term care will continue to rise, assuming that rates of dependency continue to be similar. The most helpful estimates can be derived from Comas-Herrera et al. (2003) in their work projecting demand for long-term care. Between 2001 and 2031 it is expected that the numbers of people in England over the age of 65 years will increase by 54% and those over 85 years by 81%. The numbers of dependent elders are expected to rise from approximately 2.5 million in 2001 to over 4 million in 2031. To meet this need, assuming that there were no change in patterns of dependency, would require an increase in both care home places and home care provision of between 57% and 58%.

The availability of informal care to support this vulnerable population has declined over the past 50 years, so that the proportion of older people living with an adult child has reduced from 42% in 1962 to 14% in 1986 and further to the present. This could mean increased demand for care homes and specialist housing. However, all such projections are subject to assumptions about trends in dependency and the debates about compression of morbidity. They are also subject to assumptions of fixity in 'technologies of care'. This is a conservative assumption as can be seen in the discussion in Chapter 12 on the development of shelter with care provision.

Summary

The position of carers can be seen to have moved from recognition of their burdens in the 1970s, through to a growing perception of their centrality in the caregiving process in documents such as *Growing Older* (Cm 8173, 1981), to the support of carers being one of the national objectives of social care (Cm 849, 1989; Cm 4169, 1998).

Through time it is possible to see what amounts to two separate strands of policy and strategies for care emerging: one for the acute/long-term care interface under the intermediate care strategy and a separate long-term care policy. Over time this may permit a long-term care policy to emerge that is less at risk of deflection by the needs of the acute sector.

The early phase of modernisation can be seen as one of establishing standards and a move towards greater consistency. It is noteworthy that there is an increasing focus upon the pursuit of local approaches and strategies within an overall framework. The extent to which there is room for conflict between these approaches and how they are resolved will be important in shaping the future development of long-term care services.

References

Audit Commission (1986) *Making a Reality of Community Care*. London: HMSO.

Audit Commission (2000) *Aiming to Improve: The Principles of Performance Measurement*, Management Paper. London: Audit Commission.

Barclay, P. (1982) *Social Workers: Their Roles and Tasks*. London: NISW/Bedford Square Press.

Carpenter, G.I., Perry, M., Challis, D., Hope, K. (2003) Identification of registered nursing care of residents in UK nursing homes using the Minimum Data Set Resident Assessment Instrument (MDS/RAI) and resource utilisation groups version III (RUG-III). *Age and Ageing* **32**, 279–85.

Challis, D. (1992) Community care of the elderly: bringing together scarcity and choice, needs and resources. *Financial Accountability and Management* **8**, 77–95.

Challis, D. (1999) Assessment and care management: developments since the community care reforms. In: Henwood, M. and Wistow, G. (eds) *With Respect to Old Age*, Cm 4192-II/3. London: The Stationery Office.

Challis, D., Darton, R., Johnson, L., Stone, M., Traske, K. (1995) *Care Management and Health Care of Older People*. Aldershot: Ashgate.

Challis, D., Xie, C., Hughes, J., Jacobs, S., Reilly, S., Stewart, K., Braye, C., Cambridge, P. (2004) *Social Care Services Before the Influence of Modernisation: A Review of the State of Service Delivery, Commissioning and Service Impact. Interim Report,* Discussion Paper M090. Manchester: PSSRU, University of Manchester.

Cm 849 (1989) *Caring for People.* London: HMSO.

Cmnd 1418 (1961) *Report of the Ministry of Health for the Year Ended 31st December 1960.* London: HMSO.

Cmnd 1973 (1963) *Health and Welfare: The Development of Community Care.* London: HMSO.

Cmnd 3703 (1968) *Report of the Committee on Local Authority and Allied Personal Social Services.* London: HMSO.

Cm 4014 (1998) *Modern Local Government: In Touch with the People.* London: The Stationery Office.

Cm 4169 (1998) *Modernising Social Services.* London: The Stationery Office.

Cm 4192-II/3 (1999) *With Respect to Old Age: Long Term Care – Rights and Responsibilities. Community Care and Informal Care,* Research Volume 3. London: The Stationery Office.

Cm 4818-I (2000) *The NHS Plan: A Plan for Investment, A Plan for Reform.* London: The Stationery Office.

Cm 4818-II (2000) *The NHS Plan. The Government's Response to the Royal Commission on Long Term Care.* London: The Stationery Office.

Cmnd 8173 (1981) *Growing Older.* London: HMSO.

Comas-Herrera, A., Pickard, L., Wittenberg, R., Davies, B., Darton, R. (2003) *Future Demand for Long-Term Care 2001 to 2031,* Discussion Paper 1980. London: PSSRU, London School of Economics and Political Science.

Department of Health (1995) *NHS Responsibilities for Meeting Continuing Health Care Needs,* HSG(95)8/LAC(95)5. London: Department of Health.

Department of Health (1999) *Key Indicators Graphical System.* London: Department of Health.

Department of Health (2001a) *Continuing Care: NHS and Local Councils' Responsibilities,* HSC 2001/015: LAC (2001)18. London: Department of Health.

Department of Health (2001b) *National Service Framework for Older People: Modern Standards and Service Models.* London: Department of Health.

Department of Health (2001c) *Intermediate Care,* HSC 2001/01: LAC (2001)1. London: Department of Health.

Department of Health (2001d) *Guidance on Free Nursing Care in Nursing Homes,* HSC 2001/17: LAC (2001)26. London: Department of Health.

Department of Health (2001e) *Care Homes for Older People. National Minimum Standards.* London: Department of Health.

Department of Health (2002a) *Fair Access to Care Services Guidance on Eligibility Criteria for Adult Social Care,* LAC (2002)13. London: Department of Health.

Department of Health (2002b) *Guidance on the Single Assessment Process for Older People,* HSC2002/001: LAC (2002)1. London: Department of Health.

Department of Health (2002c) *Social Services Performance 'Star' Ratings,* CI (2002)4. London: Department of Health.

Department of Health (2003) *Domiciliary Care. National Minimum Care Standards.* London: Department of Health.

Department of Health and Social Security (1983) *Health Service Development: Care in the Community and Joint Finance,* HC(83)6, LAC(83)5. London: Department of Health and Social Security.

Department of Health, Housing, Local Government and Community Services (1993) *Aged Care Reform Strategy: Mid Term Review Stage 2*. Canberra: Australian Government Publishing Service.

Dunleavy, P., Hood, C. (1994) From old public administration to new public management. *Public Money and Management* **14** (3), 9–16.

Fries, J.F. (1980) Aging, natural death and the compression of morbidity. *New England Journal of Medicine* **313**, 407–28.

Gostick, C., Davies, B., Lawson, R., Salter, C. (1997) *From Vision to Reality: Changing Direction at the Local Level*. Aldershot: Arena.

Griffiths, R. (1988) *Community Care: Agenda for Action*. London: HMSO.

Henwood, M., Wistow, G. (1999) Introduction and overview. In: Henwood, M. and Wistow, G. (eds) *Evaluating the Impact of Caring for People, with Respect to Old Age: Long Term Care – Rights and Responsibilities. Community Care and Informal Care*, Research Volume 3, Cm 4192-II/3. London: The Stationery Office.

House of Commons Health Committee (1995) *Long Term Care: NHS Responsibilities for Meeting Continuing Health Care Needs*, First Report, Session 1995–1996, HC19-I. London: HMSO.

Hughes, J., Challis, D., Gill, J., Stone, S. (1997) The eligibility lottery. *Working with Older People* **1** (3), 14–17.

Hunt, A. (1970) *The Home Help Service in England and Wales*. London: HMSO.

Knapp, M., Cambridge, P., Thomason, C., Beecham, J. Allen, C., Darton, R. (1992) *Care in the Community: Challenge and Demonstration*. Aldershot: Ashgate.

Kraan, R.J., Baldock, J., Davies, B., Evers, A., Johansson, L., Kanpen, M., Thorslund, M., Tunissen, C. (1991) *Care for the Elderly: Significant Innovations in Three European Countries*. Boulder, Colorado: Campus/Westview.

Manton, K.G. (1988) A longitudinal study of functional change and mortality in the United States. *Journal of Gerontology* **43**, S153–61.

Manton, K.G., Land, K.C. (2000) Active life expectancy estimates for the US elderly population: a multidimensional continuous-mixture model of functional change applied to completed cohorts, 1982–1996. *Demography* **37**, 253–65.

Means, R., Smith, R. (1998) *From Poor Law to Community Care*. Bristol: Policy Press.

National Assembly for Wales (2002) *Health and Social Care for Adults: Creating a Unified and Fair System for Assessing and Managing Care. Guidance for Local Authorities and Health Services*. Cardiff: National Assembly for Wales.

Netten, A., Darton, R. (2003) The effect of financial incentives and access to services on self-funded admissions to long-term care. *Social Policy & Administration* **37**, 483–97.

OECD (2003) *Public Sector Modernisation*. OECD Policy Brief. Paris: OECD. http://www.oecd.org/publications/pol_brief.

Parker, J. (1965) *Local Health and Welfare Services*. London: Allen and Unwin.

Renshaw, J., Hampson, R., Thomason, C., Darton, R., Judge, K., Knapp, M. (1988) *Care in the Community: The First Steps*. Aldershot: Gower.

Rhodes, R.A.W. (1997) *Understanding Governance*. Buckingham: Open University Press.

Sauvaget, C., Jagger, C., Arthur, A.J. (2001) Active and cognitive impairment-free life expectancies: results from the Melton Mowbray 75+ health checks. *Age and Ageing* **30**, 509–15.

Scottish Executive (2003) *Guidance for Local Authorities, the NHS and other Service Providers*. Edinburgh: Scottish Executive.

Shanas, E., Townsend, P., Wedderburn, D., Friis, H., Milhoj, P., Stehouwer, J. (1968) *Old People in Three Industrial Societies*. London: Routledge and Kegan Paul.

Townsend, P. (1964) *The Last Refuge: A Survey of Residential Institutions and Homes for the Aged in England and Wales*. London: Routledge and Kegan Paul.

Townsend, P. (1981) The structural dependency of the elderly: the creation of social policy in the twentieth century. *Ageing and Society* **1**, 5–28.

Webb, A., Wistow, G. (1986) *Planning, Need and Scarcity: Essays on the Personal Social Services*. London: Allen and Unwin.

Wistow, G. (1996) The changing scene in Britain. In: Harding, T., Meredith, B. and Wistow, G. (eds) *Options for Long Term Care*. London: HMSO.

Wistow, G., Knapp, M., Hardy, B., Allen, C. (1992) From providing to enabling: local authorities and the mixed economy of social care. *Public Administration* **70**, 25–45.

Wistow, G., Knapp, M., Hardy, B., Forder, J., Kendall, J., Manning, R. (1996) *Social Care Markets: Progress and Prospects*. Buckingham: Open University Press.

Chapter 11

Community Care: Service Delivery, Development and Evaluation

David Challis and Jane Hughes

Introduction

Concern about the fragmentation of different community services and their lack of integration at the client level so as to enable vulnerable people to remain at home was evident by the early 1980s (Department of Health and Social Security, 1982). A review of the effectiveness of social care at that time concluded:

> 'These numerous local enquiries have repeatedly thrown up similar issues in many different spheres of social care: the mismatch between needs and resources, the inadequacy of initial assessment and the lack of monitoring and review procedures leading to even greater discrepancies and inappropriate resource allocation; lack of coordination between the various services not only at the field level but at the policy level too.' (Goldberg and Connelly, 1982, p. 247)

Later studies confirmed this and identified several problems common to domiciliary services in the provision of community care. Amongst the common factors were shortage of resources, significant variation in patterns and forms of provision between agencies, low levels of help to individual cases, inflexible provision not responsive to individual needs, and a lack of coordination between services (Challis and Davies, 1986; Davies and Challis, 1986; Sinclair et al., 1990).

Community care policies in the UK were reviewed in the 1980s under the constraint of financial pressure. Although attention had been given previously to the development of coordination of care in the community and transfer of finance from health to social care, coordination was seen as essentially a 'top-down' process rather than concerned with activities at the client level (Webb and Wistow, 1986). The growth in admissions to residential and nursing home care funded by social security resources during the 1980s provided the catalyst for the explicit community care policies and reforms ushered in at the end of that decade. As noted in Chapter 10, the broad shape of community care policy in the UK has taken a remarkably similar form to that observed in many other countries (Challis et al., 1994). It involves achieving a shift in the balance of care away from institution based care, made possible by the enhancement of home based care and the development of mechanisms of coordination and care management to achieve this (Kraan et al., 1991; Challis, 1992a; 1992b).

The purpose of this chapter is to review the development of community care in England with a particular emphasis upon developments since the implementation of the community care reforms in 1993. A particular emphasis will be placed on key issues in the care pathway such as eligibility, assessment, care planning and review, as well as issues of commissioning, service organisation and information.

Eligibility

The importance of explicit criteria for eligibility can be seen to have grown with the emphasis on more careful targeting of home care services in the 1980s towards providing personal care to the more vulnerable (Social Services Inspectorate, 1987) through the development of eligibility criteria following the White Paper *Caring for People* (Cm 849, 1989), to current concerns with Fair Access to Care (Department of Health, 2002a).

The present process of determining eligibility for social care has its origins in the community care reforms of the early 1990s. The White Paper *Caring for People* (Cm 849, 1989) required local authorities to devise and publicise criteria of eligibility for assessment. It was intended that these criteria operate irrespective of point of entry into the service and subsequently their purpose was described as being to inform users 'about what sorts of people with what kinds of need qualify for what types of service' (Cm 4169, 1998, p. 23). At the outset eligibility criteria were also conceived of as a means to ration social care and thereby help local authorities to deliver services within budget (Audit Commission, 1993). Subsequently concern has been expressed about the way in which eligibility criteria are used. In particular it was noted that they were poorly constructed; incomprehensible to users and carers; of no practical assistance to staff determining eligibility for assistance; applied inconsistently within authorities; and, more generally, confusion about their purpose persisted (Association of Metropolitan Authorities, 1995; Hughes et al., 1997; Cm 4169, 1998).

Further emphasis on eligibility was prompted by three factors. First, central government required that from April 1996 health authorities set and publish criteria for NHS continuing health care services and that these be agreed with the relevant local authority (Department of Health, 1995a). Second, there was the growing evidence (particularly through legal judgements) of the financial constraints facing local authorities in funding care for people to stay at home and for placements in residential and nursing homes. Finally, there was the growing public debate about arrangements for the funding of care for older people leading to the establishment of the Royal Commission on Long Term Care (Cm 4192-I, 1999).

A study of eligibility criteria for social care in England in 1997 found evidence of marked variation across local authorities as to both the form and content of criteria and limited linkage with NHS continuing care criteria. In terms of content, local authorities used different combinations of nine key domains, but in 64% of responding authorities these included: physical health, risk, carers, activities of daily living, mental health, and instrumental activities of daily living. The lack of consistency across authorities was likely also to be reflected in variations of interpretation within authorities (Hughes et al., 1997; Challis and Hughes, 2002).

The White Paper *Modernising Social Services* (Cm 4169, 1998) made an explicit commitment to greater consistency and fair access to care services (Department of Health, 2002a). It provided for the use of a similar framework to determine eligibility across all councils so as to achieve greater consistency. It provided for an eligibility framework divided into four bands – critical, substantial, moderate and low – relating to the degree of risk to independence or other adverse consequences if needs were not addressed. However, local variation and discretion remained, reflected in the requirement that councils setting eligibility criteria should take account of 'resources, local expectations and local costs' (Department of Health, 2002a, para. 18).

There are a number of mechanisms that result in the exclusion of people from either the care management process and/or from services. At a formal or managerial level, eligibility criteria and other departmental procedures play an important part, and at an informal or bureaucratic level the discretion and interpretations of front-line staff are critical (Ellis et al., 1999; Rummery and Glendinning, 1999; Rummery et al., 1999). Variations in both these formal and informal mechanisms have been reported (Rummery et al., 1999; Challis et al., 2001) and concerns about these underpin the Government's Fair Access to Care initiative (Cm 4169, 1998). A challenge for the future will be how integrated services and organisations manage the process of eligibility determination, using a framework which reflects assumptions about priority for social care, which may not map easily to priorities for health care intervention.

Delivery, coordination and continuity

This section addresses assessment – the approach used to identify needs, care management, the planning and coordination of care around individuals, and care packages, the services which are received as a consequence of assessment and care planning processes.

Assessment

A key component of the care management process, assessment, first became a central policy concern following the community care reforms of the early 1990s

(Cm 849, 1989), when assessment and care management were identified as 'cornerstones' of the new policy. Earlier work was at the individual practice level, focused upon the content of assessment and improvement of its quality by the norms of professional practice and addressing appropriateness of placement in care homes (Brocklehurst et al., 1978; Hutchinson et al., 1984; Challis and Chesterman, 1985). The community care reforms of the early 1990s led to a very substantial investment in procedures and modes of assessment.

Early concerns were raised about the quality and reliability of these assessments (Department of Health, 1993a; 1993b; 1994; Caldock, 1994) as pro-formas and procedures appeared overly complex and time consuming. In terms of the information collected, both content and quality varied and there was a lack of reliability and validity. The most comprehensive analysis of 50 existing comprehensive assessment documents, used by social service providers across the UK, revealed that the majority were generic and under a quarter were used by both health and social services. Coverage of carer needs, depression/anxiety, cognitive impairment and behavioural patterns was very varied. Assessment of activities of daily living was reasonably consistent in content but not always structured. It was concluded from this detailed analysis that variability of assessment tools is high and their comparability and capacity to generate standardised information is low (Stewart et al., 1999).

A national survey in the late 1990s shed further light upon these observations. Health professionals were involved in coordinating assessments in at most a quarter of authorities overall. Generic assessment documents (covering more than one use group) were still in use in more than half (61%) of local authorities, a similar picture to that noted previously (Department of Health, 1993a). Specialist documentation was least likely in older people's services and most likely in mental health services (Weiner et al., 2002).

Thus variability in assessment approaches appeared to be far greater than would be attributable to the needs and circumstances of those being assessed. Whilst variability of assessment systems in the community is not uncommon in many countries (Challis et al., 1996), in the UK there was marked variation not only in the content of assessment (what information is sought about needs and how it is recorded) but also in the form (the personnel involved in conducting the assessment). This was so even for critical decisions such as whether a person should enter residential or nursing home care. This can be usefully contrasted with the Australian Aged Care Reforms where such critical decisions, such as care home placement, involve multidisciplinary Aged Care Assessment Teams (Challis et al., 1995; 1998). This cumulative evidence contributed to the development of the Single Assessment Process (Department of Health, 2002b) as part of the *National Service Framework for Older People* (Department of Health, 2001a). This offers a sense of direction as to the content of assessment much more explicitly than had occurred ten years previously when each area had invested in local developments.

The Single Assessment Process (SAP) was designed to address a number of these problems. It aimed to ensure that:

- A more standardised assessment process was in place for all areas and agencies
- Standards of assessment were raised
- Older people's needs were assessed in the round (Department of Health, 2001a, para. 2.27).

It provided for four types of assessment – contact, overview, specialist and comprehensive – and established a core set of domains (see Box 11.1) designed to provide greater consistency in assessment.

The SAP raises a number of questions about interprofessional working and about integrated information systems. It is not just cultural barriers which have to be addressed with regard to information-sharing between professional groups, but the sheer technical barriers occasioned by different electronic information systems which do not communicate one with another. Kane and Kane (2000) have noted the potential of information technology to reduce workload, improve the quality of assessment and increase the involvement of older people. However, it would seem that many of the problems identified by Philp and Dunleavy (1994), during the implementation of the 1990s community care reforms, remain to be resolved where the incompatibility of computer systems between primary care, secondary care and social care were seen as inhibiting the sharing of information and leading to duplication of assessments.

An evaluation of the impact of specialist clinical assessment by geriatricians or old age psychiatrists when admission to a care home is being considered indicated real gains compared to the usual care management assessment (Challis et al., 2004a). In this study care managers could request an assessment at home by either an old age psychiatrist or a geriatrician, as they saw most appropriate, to assist them in planning care for the most vulnerable older people. In many ways this could be seen as a test of implementing an important facet of the Australian Aged Care Reforms in the UK (Challis et al., 1995; 1998), namely access to specialist clinical assessment, as well as approximating to an effective comprehensive assessment under the SAP. The findings indicated that the process was valued particularly by care managers, improved appropriateness of placements, improved functional well-being of older people, reduced stress on carers, reduced nursing home utilisation, and had lower costs for the NHS (Challis et al., 2004a).

Box 11.1 Domains of the Single Assessment Process.

- Users' perspective
- Clinical background
- Disease prevention
- Personal care and physical well-being
- Senses
- Mental health
- Relationships
- Safety
- Immediate environment and resources

Finally, it must be emphasised that a focus upon improving the form, content and process of assessment is a necessary but not sufficient condition to achieve better identification of and response to need. The incentives for the assessors must also be addressed. For example, the Personal Social Services Research Unit (PSSRU) Intensive Care Management studies (Challis and Davies, 1986; Challis et al., 1990; 1995; 2002a; 2002b) demonstrated that practitioners were motivated to undertake more holistic assessments because control over resources permitted a wider range of responses to be made to identified needs. Conversely, if only a limited repertoire of responses is possible, there is less incentive to undertake detailed assessments. In the absence of this, practitioners will continue to have difficulty in separating 'need' from 'need for a particular service' (Parry-Jones and Soulsby, 2001). In short, the outcome of assessment must be feasible interventions.

Care management

Concern with coordination of care for vulnerable people has been long-standing in policy directives. However, much of the discussion during the 1970s and early 1980s about coordination took place at the level of inter-organisational behaviour and the degree of coordination between health and social care through planning processes, financial transfers and financial incentives (Webb and Wistow, 1986). At the field level a long-standing trend towards specialisation in the delivery of field level social care (and by implication therefore care management), was in progress through the 1980s (Challis and Ferlie, 1986; 1987; 1988).

The idea of coordination through individual care packages only really became evident as the lessons of the Kent Community Care Project and subsequent PSSRU research on intensive care management (Challis and Davies, 1980; 1986; Davies and Challis, 1986; Challis et al., 1988; 1990; 1991a; 1991b; 1995; 1997; 2002a; 2002b) were increasingly reflected in policy documents (see Box 11.2).

Box 11.2   PSSRU intensive care management studies.

Study	Setting	Target population
Kent Community Care Scheme	Social care/SSD	Residential/nursing home
Gateshead Community Care Scheme	Social care/SSD	Residential/nursing home
Gateshead Primary Health Care Scheme	SSD/primary care	Hospital/nursing home/residential care
Darlington Community Care Project	Geriatric MDT/SSD	Long stay hospital/nursing home
Lewisham Case Management Scheme	Community based old age psychiatry/SSD	Dementia diagnosis and high risk of institutional care

MDT = multidisciplinary team; SSD = social services department.

The 1983 Care in the Community Initiative (Department of Health and Social Security, 1983) reflected the ideas of care management and one of the pilot projects funded was an example of intensive care management as an alternative to long-stay hospital care for frail older people (Challis et al., 1991a; 1991b; 1995). The PSSRU intensive care management studies not only addressed care management in social care (Challis and Davies, 1986; Challis et al., 2002a) but also care management in primary care (Challis et al., 1988; 1990; 2002a), geriatric medicine (Challis et al., 1991a; 1991b; 1995) and old age psychiatry (Challis et al., 2002b). Following the endorsement of the idea of care management, the 1989 White Paper explicitly cited the PSSRU studies in Kent, Gateshead and Darlington (Cm 849, 1989, para. 3.3.3) as exemplars of assessment and care management. These studies sought to provide community alternatives to care homes, by devolving control of resources to front-line care managers so as to permit the creation of flexible and individualised care packages to enable vulnerable people to maintain their independence. The evidence was that such an approach could offer a realistic alternative to care homes and hospital care, improving the well-being of older people and their carers, in most cases at no greater and sometimes less cost. 'Greater choice and user centredness were made possible by the capacity to create flexible services, through the deployment of a very substantial devolved budget' (Challis et al., 2002a, p. 239).

Thus the PSSRU intensive care management studies suggest an increased efficiency in the provision of social care with improved outcomes at similar or slightly lower costs. The evidence could not be generalised to a broader application of the care management approach to less vulnerable individuals. Key elements associated with the outcomes demonstrated included a differentiated response to need, appropriate targeting, devolution of budgets, continuity of involvement of care manager with service user, and appropriate links with specialist health care expertise.

Care management was identified as a key change in the 1990 community care reforms, seen as providing an effective method of targeting resources and planning services to meet specific needs of individual clients/users. In *Caring for People* (Cm 849, 1989, p. 21) five stages in the case/care management process were identified:

- Identification of people in need
- Assessment of care needs
- Planning and securing the delivery of care
- Monitoring the quality of care provided
- Review of client needs.

Care management was developed by local authorities following the full implementation of the 1990 NHS and Community Care Act after 1993. The evidence from a variety of sources suggested at an early stage that care management developed in a variety of ways in different places (Department of Health, 1994). Hoyes et al. (1994) studied the impact of the community care reforms upon service users and carers in four social services authorities. A number of key themes emerged from this research. First, local authorities were struggling to develop purchasing strategies in the context of resource constraints. Second, a mixed economy of care was unlikely to provide an alternative to institutional care for service users and their carers in the short term. Third, the development of bureaucratic approaches to care management and lack of resources might result in people not receiving emotional support and counselling when identified as areas of need in their own right. Fourth, communication problems were evident throughout the care management process: both between professionals and service users with communication difficulties and between professionals themselves. Fifth, organisations often failed to give service users and carers adequate information. Sixth, in order to maintain the carers' ability to continue caring as long as possible, social services staff gave priority to the needs of carers over service users. Finally, field-workers needed more support and training in order to embrace the changes in attitudes, approaches and skills consequent on the implementation of the community care legislation.

A study of five local authorities suggested that the development of care management systems was affected by the process of separating purchasing from providing, concluding that there was evidence of care management being identified as purely a purchasing responsibility (Lewis et al., 1995; 1997). However, they noted what might be described as a bureaucratisation of social work as a consequence of the separation of the purchaser and provider roles within social services departments with a greater emphasis on procedures, documentation and the demands of burgeoning information technology systems (Lewis et al., 1996; 1997) with certain similarities to the administrative approach to care management described in Challis (1994a; 1994b; 1994c). On the basis of this five-authority study, Lewis and Glennerster (1996) suggested that an early focus upon assessment distracted authorities from the broader aspects of care management. They suggest that the generality of official guidance (Social Services Inspectorate and Social Work Services Group, 1991a; 1991b) left authorities without a clearly prescribed strategy for effective implementation.

In 1995 the Social Services Inspectorate (SSI), whilst acknowledging progress by local authorities in the introduction of assessment and care management arrangements, noted a number of features requiring action. An analysis of nine inspection reports dealing with assessment and care management revealed that there was confusion about the role of a care manager and that care plans were not always meaningful or routinely given to service users; also, it was noted that the tendency of social services departments to close less complex cases after the implementation of the care plan militated against continuity of care and the provision of social work assistance such as counselling (Department of Health, 1995b). A summary of relevant SSI findings through the 1990s is provided in Box 11.3.

A later overview of social services departments (SSD) performance (Department of Health, 2003a) noted that care management arrangements were frequently ineffective and lacked coherence. Interestingly, the suggestion that care managers

Box 11.3   Key messages from Social Services Inspectorate studies in the 1990s.

Eligibility and targeting: Confusion existed as to whether eligibility concerned eligibility for assessment, services or care management; mechanisms for achieving this equitably and efficiently were seen as required.

Assessment: There was concern about quality, lack of standardisation and differentiation of assessment according to need and need for appropriate health care inputs.

Devolution of budgets: This was seen as essential for effective care planning and services responsive to a variety of need although not always evident in practice.

Monitoring and review: There was a lack of monitoring and review with care managers excessively focused upon assessment.

Continuity of involvement of care manager: Findings indicated that continuity of contact with the same care manager was valued by service users although this was rarely achieved with most care manager involvement at the assessment stage.

Clarity of care management role: Confusion remained apparent as to the nature of the role of care manager and the content of activities which they were expected to undertake. A differentiated response was seen as necessary, with levels of care management intensity reflecting levels of need.

Management arrangements: Organisational context was an important determinant of the ability to achieve positive outcomes for service users.

Health care linkages: Close links were needed for effective assessment and for rehabilitation. These were rarely formalised either structurally or contractually.

Specialist services: Good quality care for people with dementia was seen as associated with specialist services; however, no observation was made more generally about specialist response or links with specialist health care providers for services to other older people.

Information systems: A more sophisticated use of information was required to support the link between field level activity and planning and service development.

Adapted from Challis (1999).

were spending more time in assessment related activities and less upon other core tasks of care management were confirmed in a study of time use (Weinberg et al., 2003). However, the study provided little evidence of a reduction of face to face work with service users and carers.

A major national survey of care management arrangements in England in the late 1990s concluded that there was a very marked variation in the way in which care management had been implemented across different local authorities (Challis, 1999; Weiner et al., 2002). The information could be summarised under three headings: organisational arrangements; performance of core tasks; and degree of differentiation of care management arrangements (Challis et al., 1998). Key findings are summarised in Box 11.4.

In terms of organisational arrangements fewer than half of authorities had invested in pilot work prior to the full implementation of the NHS and Community Care Act in 1993. The degree of flexibility available to front-line staff in arranging care packages through access to budgetary decisions was very limited, with only 12% of authorities providing front-line staff with this authority.

Box 11.4 Key aspects of care management in the late 1990s.

Care management features	Patterns found
Organisational arrangements Care management before 1993 Authority to purchase services	45% of local authorities (LAs) Very limited at level of front-line staff
Performance of core tasks Care management definition Staff mix Undertaking reviews	Variable and skill requirements unclear NHS staff as care managers <21% Often neglected, variable and problematic
Degree of differentiation Specialist teams Targeting of care Management Intensive care management	For older people in less than 50% of LAs Evident in 52% of LAs In only 5% of LAs and only in part

Adapted from Challis (1999); Weiner et al. (2002).

This is despite its having been identified in the Personal Social Services Research Unit (PSSRU) studies as an essential feature of effective care (Challis and Davies, 1986; Challis et al., 1995; 2002a; 2002b) and also by the Audit Commission (1997). In terms of the performance of the core tasks of care management, there was a lack of clarity in the definition and goals of care management with much variability in terms of the perception of the skill mix required for the job. In only around one fifth of local authorities were NHS staff stated to be acting as care managers for older people, exercising the same responsibilities as social services staff.

Furthermore, detailed investigation indicated that this was in fact an overestimate and that this degree of integration was in fact considerably rarer and where present was often only a pilot project (Weiner et al., 2003). One author suggested that the community care reforms of the 1990s gave social services departments the lead role in care management and thereby cemented the separation of health and social care structures despite mutual dependence (Lewis, 2001).

The process of undertaking reviews was seen as a common problem across authorities with a real expectation of their not being undertaken, particularly for individuals living in their own homes. In respect of the degree of differentiation of care management arrangements, it was found that fewer than half of local authorities provided services for older people through specialist teams, compared with nearly all in mental health. Intensive care management (ICM), targeted upon high risk individuals requiring high levels of support by staff working with small caseloads, was very rare, found in about 5% of authorities and in those it was not widespread. Furthermore, few indicators, such as small caseloads, service targeting, integration of NHS staff, or devolved budgets, likely to be associated with ICM were found in older people's services confirming the lack of differentiation in care management services (Challis et al., 2001). This is despite the fact that it is only intensive care management which has an evidence base to support its capacity to support vulnerable people at home (Challis and Davies, 1986; Challis et al., 1995; 2002a; 2002b).

Thus, despite the provision of detailed guidance on care management (Social Services Inspectorate and Social Work Services Group 1991a; 1991b), there was marked variation in the ways in which care management had developed following the 1990 NHS and Community Care Act (Challis, 1999). This may be attributable to the fact that the early guidance on care management (Social Services Inspectorate and Social Work Services Group 1991a; 1991b) provided a broad definition of care management, permitting wide variations in interpretation (Welch, 1998) and to the fact that early guidance on the implementation focused the attention of health and local authorities on a number of key tasks concerned with developing arrangements for closer collaboration. Gostick and colleagues (1997) argue that this guidance distracted local authorities from the development of other aspects crucial to the implementation of the community care reforms, including care management.

None the less, the role of care management was endorsed in *Modernising Social Services* (Cm 4169, 1998) and identified key areas for action:

- To identify individuals with social care needs who are eligible for public support.
- To assess those needs accurately and consistently.
- To review care packages as necessary to ensure that they continue to be appropriate and effective.

In short, eligibility, assessment and involvement of care managers beyond the assessment and initial allocation of services, remained important areas for action. The 1998 White Paper summarised the function of care management, stating that it was an objective for social services to involve users and carers in the process of tailoring individual packages of care. It was also a requirement 'to maximise the benefit to service users for the resources available, and to demonstrate the effectiveness and value for money of the care and support provided, and allow for choice and different responses for different needs and circumstances' (Cm 4169, 1998, p. 111). Thus the potentially conflicting concerns of cost effectiveness, choice and involvement were again cited at the end of the 1990s (Challis, 1992b). The concerns of the 1998 White Paper indicated some of the problems identified in implementation during the 1990s.

Two issues are worthy of further comment, the involvement of health care staff in care management and the degree of differentiation of care management. First, the lack of evidence of health service staff acting as care managers and their low degree of involvement in the core tasks of care management is indicative of a lack of integration of services between heath and social care. None the less, integration of health and social care provision is central to policy after 1998 (Cm 4169, 1998; Cm 4818-I, 2000) and is discussed later in this chapter. Second, recent government reports have been increasingly explicit in their recommendation of a differentiated approach to service provision. Such an approach would link levels of service user need to the skills of staff to be employed and to the assessment, monitoring and reviewing arrangements to be implemented (Department of Health, 1994; 1996; 1997a). In 1997, the SSI recommended the implementation of a system of care management for all users involving three tiers of response: administrative, coordinating and intensive (Department of Health, 1997b). The continuing importance of targeting of care management, within the modernising agenda, was made clear in the *National Service Framework for Older People* (Department of Health, 2001a) in the statement that:

> '. . . the most vulnerable older people will often require fuller assessment and more intensive forms of care management. For this reason dedicated care managers should work with the most vulnerable older people over time.' (para. 2.39)

Similarly, the Scottish Executive (2000) has recommended that care management should be redefined as 'intensive care management', which would be reserved for people with complex or frequently changing needs. The introduction of the Single Assessment Process across health and social care for older people (Department of Health, 2002b) may well reinforce the development of differentiated care management services, with different levels of care management linking to different types of assessments.

In 2002 Weiner and colleagues concluded:

> 'Clearly, for care management to contribute to the modernisation agenda, there must be a greater planned differentiation of approach to both strategy and to need. This will also require a managed implementation of differentiated care management to ensure greater proximity between policy goals and agency outcomes.' (p. 436)

This is in many ways truer at the time of writing with the development of a form of intensive case management for people with chronic diseases. This more differentiated approach to case management was outlined in the *NHS Improvement Plan* (Cm 6268, 2004). It is argued that 5% of patients with complex needs account for 42% of hospital inpatient days and that patients with long-term health problems account for about 80% of GP consultations (Cm 6268, 2004, para. 3.3). Thus the impact on the NHS and social care of supporting people with long-term conditions is significant, resulting in heavy use of secondary care services. One problem has been that care for many people with long-term conditions has traditionally been reactive, unplanned and episodic (Department of Health, 2005). The policy provides for three levels of response for patients with long term-conditions: *self management* for some 70 to 80%; *disease management* for a second group needing support to avoid complications; and a third group with complex conditions needing active *case management*. For this latter group the aim is for an NHS case manager to develop tailored care plans, to

Box 11.5 Key aspects of the NHS and Social Care Long Term Conditions Model.

(1) Identify all long-term condition patients in a local health community

(2) Stratify the patients to match care to different needs of patients
- Level 3: Case management – Identify the most vulnerable people, those with highly complex multiple long-term conditions, and use a case management approach, to anticipate, coordinate and join up health and social care.

- Level 2: Disease-specific care management – This involves providing people who have a complex single need or multiple conditions with responsive, specialist services using multidisciplinary teams and disease-specific protocols and pathways, such as the National Service Frameworks and Quality and Outcomes Framework.

- Level 1: Supported self care – collaboratively help individuals and their carers to develop the knowledge, skills and confidence to care for themselves and their condition effectively.

Adapted from Department of Health (2005).

prevent worsening of the condition, and, where possible, prevent unplanned admissions to hospital (Cm 6268, 2004 para. 3.13–5). The Department of Health has issued guidance upon the new model of care for supporting people with long-term conditions (Department of Health, 2005). It is summarised in Box 11.5.

This is an ambitious development, anticipating some 3000 new NHS case managers by March 2007. What are the potential pitfalls to successful implementation? Murphy (2004) has argued that the separation between the health care research which has underpinned this initiative and the PSSRU intensive care management studies is unfortunate, since important lessons for integrated health and social care case management are indicated therein. Furthermore she argues the need is not just for good clinical practice but also to ensure that the incentives for all the actors in the system are not perverse. Perverse incentives arising from funding availability underlay the unnecessary growth in care home admissions in the 1980s (Audit Commission, 1986). She suggests that there are risks of new perverse incentives arising from the funding arrangements for hospital care under payment by results (Department of Health, 2002c) which may encourage maximisation of admissions which runs counter to the main policy of preventing unnecessary hospital care. Of course this, like intensive care management as an alternative to nursing and residential care, depends upon effective targeting.

It will be important to observe whether, through careful and appropriate targeting, the new chronic disease case management emerges as a real alternative to hospital care, or whether some of the same concerns about implementation emerge as occurred with care management, as part of the community care reforms during the 1990s. Key issues are likely to include targeting; caseload size; access to and influence of case managers over resources; integration of health and social care practice; and the clarity and coherence of the development of the new role.

Another factor likely to influence the development of care management arrangements is the extension of direct payments to the care of older people

(Leece, 2001). This opens up the possibility of a spectrum of care management arrangements ranging from self care management on the one hand through a variety of positions such as advice and brokerage arrangements to arrangements where people with severe impairments may not be in the position to or wish to manage their own care. Given the earlier criticism of the lack of differentiation of care management according to need, this would appear to offer a constructive way forward with differentiation based upon both need and user preferences.

Care packages

The use of the concept of care packages can be traced to the early publications of the PSSRU evaluations of care management (Challis and Davies, 1980; 1986) and to the DHSS study of community care in 1981 (Department of Health and Social Security, 1981). It refers to the idea of a number of ongoing services, planned in an integrated fashion to meet the continuing needs of a specific individual. Care packages consist of home care services, day care, carer support, meals and other social care services. Ideally they would also involve health care services such as community nursing. It was in contrast to the evidence in much work that the 'care system' consisted of an uncoordinated set of different activities and that the care an individual received was largely dependent upon which service they contacted initially (Plank, 1977; Goldberg and Connelly, 1982; Sinclair et al., 1990).

By the mid-1980s there was a clear debate regarding the future development of the home help service, the largest component of domiciliary care. This took the form of whether it should be a widespread provider of relatively modest amounts of care, or whether it should provide more intensive support for fewer and more dependent older people (Goldberg and Connelly, 1982; Audit Commission, 1985; Sinclair and Williams, 1990). In an influential report entitled *From Home Help to Home Care* (Social Services Inspectorate, 1987) the Government's Social Services Inspectorate identified concern about a lack of intensity and flexibility of home care provision. Intensity was found to be sacrificed for low-level cover to a larger number of users. The service provided was predominantly domestic work rather than personal care and there was a danger of users being 'slotted' into one of a limited number of standard service responses.

A number of initiatives set in place to provide more intensive home care were developed to address these concerns (Dunnachie, 1979; Gibbins et al., 1982; Latto, 1984; Gibbins, 1984). By the late 1980s it appeared that what was needed was more intensive levels of service, planned and coordinated around the unique needs of individual older people through case or care management (Challis and Davies, 1986).

Following the community care reforms of the early 1990s it was observed that more intensive packages now were to be found (Warburton and McCracken, 1999). For example in the short period between 1992 and 1996, they cite a reduction in the numbers of households receiving home care and an increase in the amount received by those to whom it is provided. This can be seen as constituting an increase in intensity of provision at the expense of coverage. This has increased steadily through time (Department of Health, 2003b). During the 1990s there was a similar trend towards a higher proportion of care services being provided by the independent sector so that by 2002 around two thirds of contact hours were provided by independent sector agencies and a market in domiciliary care had emerged (Wistow and Hardy, 1999). None the less, it did appear that the range of services being offered in care packages was not sufficiently flexible and often did not offer a real alternative to care homes for vulnerable older people. In particular domiciliary care services could be inconsistent and unreliable and insufficiently varied in relation to the needs of individuals (Audit Commission, 1997; Department of Health, 1997a), providing for a limited range of care tasks (Harding and Beresford, 1996; Harding, 1999). One contributory factor to the lack of flexibility could be that care managers lacked flexible budgets and may have worked to relatively low cost ceilings (Audit Commission, 1997; Harding, 1999; Weiner et al., 2002). A study in Scotland concluded that there was no adequate continuum of support to provide individual choice to vulnerable older people as to whether to remain at home. Mainstream domiciliary services were inflexible in terms of both hours worked and tasks performed (Curtice et al., 2002).

Whilst there was recognition that more intensive and flexible packages of care were needed to offer vulnerable people an alternative to nursing or residential care, it was felt that there was an important balance to be achieved by also investing in services which effectively prevented decline (Browning, 1999; Harding, 1999). Some studies have emphasised the value of low level services in helping older people maintain their independence (Clark et al., 1998). Whilst the emphasis in the White Paper *Modernising Social Services* (Cm 4169, 1998) can be seen as attempting to balance these twin imperatives of preventing decline for the less vulnerable, and maintaining residential independence of the more vulnerable, it remains questionable whether, in terms of levels of service or intensity of care management arrangements, care at home has been a real alternative to long-term care for many vulnerable older people.

Services and service development

In this section two aspects of service development are considered: the processes of commissioning and integration between health and social care.

Commissioning

The idea of commissioning social care services by local authorities is not new in that some areas of service were contracted to large voluntary organisations in the 1970s and before. None the less, during the 1980s the idea of the enabling authority was made explicit by the then Secretary of State, Norman Fowler, in 1984, which included the role of local authorities taking a comprehensive and strategic view of all sources of care within their locality. As Wistow and colleagues (1992) have noted, many of the ideas around the 'enabling authority' were at least implicit in documents such as the Seebohm (Cm 3703, 1968) and Barclay reports (Barclay, 1982).

The development of this role of enabling was accepted by Griffiths (1988) who also introduced the concept of SSDs as purchasers of social care within a market of different providers. It was envisaged that they would become 'designers, organisers and purchasers of non-health care services and not primarily direct providers, making the maximum possible use of voluntary and private sector bodies to widen consumer choice, stimulate innovation and encourage efficiency' (Griffiths, 1988, para. 1.3.4). The idea of the enabling authority, and explicit separation of purchasing and providing in the White Paper *Caring for People* (Cm 849, 1989) was also influenced by the purchasing and providing arrangements in the NHS White Paper *Working for Patients* (Cm 555, 1989). Thus in *Caring for People* (Cm 849, 1989) enabling was laid down as one of the responsibilities of SSDs: 'securing the delivery of services, not simply by acting as direct providers but by developing the purchasing and contracting role to become 'enabling authorities' (para. 3.1.3). Thus, the separation of the purchaser and provider functions within social services departments was a requirement placed on local authorities by central government as part of the implementation programme for the introduction of the community care legislation.

Over half of English local authorities had introduced this division of function prior to or during 1993 (Weiner et al., 2002) and an early SSI study noted a rigid interpretation of the split (Department of Health, 1994). However, the development of a purchaser/provider split was a slow, evolutionary process (Wistow et al., 1994; Gostick et al., 1997; Lewis et al., 1997). Nevertheless, since the care of vulnerable older people constitutes the largest component of work undertaken by social services departments, the introduction of this separation has arguably had a significant impact on the delivery of services for this user group. The policy guidance accompanying the White Paper *Caring for People* stressed that the development of the enabling role of the authority should be apparent at two levels in the organisation: at the 'micro-level', in respect of the provision of services in response to individual need and at the 'macro-level', involving plans to meet strategic objectives (Department of Health, 1990).

At the 'micro-level' whilst it was noted that a needs-led approach 'presupposes a progressive separation of assessment from provision' (Department of Health, 1990, p. 25), the guidance did not include a requirement for budgetary devolution to front-line workers, with appropriate systems for financial management and monitoring. However, it has been noted that devolved budgets can provide a more flexible response to needs within a complex package of care (Audit Commission, 1996). Furthermore, devolved budgets were a feature common to the programmes of intensive care management in England. These schemes did demonstrate that it was possible to provide complex care packages for vulnerable older people in their own homes (Challis and Davies, 1986; Challis et al., 1995; 2002a; 2002b). Here, a close relationship between care managers and those providing practical care was a significant component of the service delivery system (Challis et al., 1995; 2002a) thereby illustrating the inadequacy of a rigid purchaser/provider split. It appears that commissioning at the micro-level in England was impeded by lack of effective monitoring and review (Audit Commission, 1997; Cm 4169, 1998) and lack of devolved budgets (Weiner et al., 2002) meaning that care managers were without necessary information and the resources to undertake this role. Nevertheless, this area of service development is often cited as a key element of care management systems in the literature from other countries (Moxley, 1989; Applebaum and Austin, 1990).

At the 'macro-level', the commissioning role of social services authorities in respect of community care also developed following the introduction of the community care reforms. As noted, one of the key objectives of the White Paper *Caring for People* (Cm 849, 1989) was that social services authorities should be 'enabling' agencies securing the delivery of services, not simply by acting as direct providers, but by developing their purchasing and contracting role. It was envisaged that this change would increase the use of private and voluntary providers and so increase the range of options and widen consumer choice. As the Audit Commission (2002) noted, clear goals are required for effective commissioning, including the intended balance between home based, day, out-patient, residential and hospital services, yet these essential building blocks are often not in place. Early work on the implementation of the community care changes noted that significant improvements were needed in the strategic commissioning of many local authorities, both in terms of local needs assessments and to render service provision more flexible (Gostick et al., 1997). In their review of the development of the Community Care Reforms, Warburton and McCracken (1999) noted that, with regard to commissioning, SSDs lacked adequate management information to commission and develop services, and that relationships between SSDs and independent providers were adversarial or distant, to the detriment of service quality. Consequently, SSDs were not in a position to identify whether the services they commissioned or provided offered best value. The development of effective commissioning is likely to depend upon a more informed and systematic approach to contracting than has hitherto been the case if the complex balance between cost and quality of services is to be achieved (Forder et al., 2004). This needs to take account of the differing motivations of providers as well as price (Kendall et al., 2003).

A number of initiatives have been introduced, designed to improve the commissioning of services for vulnerable adults within social services departments. In 1998, the White Paper *Modernising Social Services* outlined measures to improve service commissioning processes in the key areas of needs analysis, strategic planning, contract setting, market management and contract monitoring to help ensure that services meet specific needs. The evolution of commissioning was described as moving away from a focus upon who provides services to one where the key issue is service quality as experienced by the individual, their carers and their family (Cm 4169, 1998, para. 1.7). For older people's services it was stated that:

> 'Staff working in services for older people and their carers will be supported in their aim to deliver person-centred care across organisational boundaries by joined up processes for commissioning and delivering older people's services.' (Department of Health, 2001a, para. 2.18)

Fair Access to Care Services (Department of Health, 2002a) confirmed the duty placed on councils to have services in place to meet eligible needs, with the caveat that specialist services for groups of service users should be developed where there is justification for such.

Nonetheless, evidence suggests that choice for users and carers was much more evident in relation to residential services than domiciliary services (Ware et al., 2003). The extent to which choice, a long-standing policy objective, is available from commissioning at both the strategic/macro-level and at the micro-level of individual care packages remains a crucial area of concern to improve the quality of care (Hardy et al., 1999). Another commissioning challenge is likely to emerge from the extension of Direct Payments, with an expectation for mixed packages of care, which contain elements of services and elements of direct payments, and for commissioners to provide services, which may be used as part of Direct Payments (Commission for Social Care Improvement, 2004). This suggests the creation of a continuum of support services available ranging from intensive care management through Direct Payments, with differing levels of support available as required (Glendinning et al., 2000a; 2000b).

Service integration

There is an international concern to promote the greater integration of health and social care for older people (Johri et al., 2003; Kodner, 2003; Leichsenring and Alaszewski, 2004). In the British policy context, although the concern about bringing health and social care closer together has been a long-standing one, the pursuit of integration itself is relatively new. Strategies such as collaboration and markets have been employed previously (Hudson, 1998). In 1998 the Government committed itself to breaking down the 'Berlin Wall' that can divide health and social care to create a system of integrated care that places users at the centre of service provision (Cm 4169, 1998, p. 97). As noted in Chapter 10, the Health Act 1999 removed legal obstacles to joint working and promoted partnership working by allowing pooled budgets, lead commissioning and integrated provision. The creation of integrated health and social care organisations, Care Trusts, was made feasible in the Health and Social Care Act 2001. It is helpful to consider developments at the more macro-level of partnership working between organisations and at the more micro-level of joined up services.

At the level of partnership working, studies have been undertaken of emerging partnerships between Primary Care Trusts and social services departments.

It appeared that despite SSD representation on PCT Boards the decision making processes were dominated by GPs and the social care representatives felt marginalised. There appeared to be considerable need to build trust and effective working between agencies (Glendinning et al., 2001; 2002; Coleman and Rummery, 2003; Glendinning, 2003; Rummery and Coleman, 2003). However, few studies address the gains associated with organisational integration. Interestingly, the UK contains what amounts to a 'natural experiment', namely the different systems of health and social care in Northern Ireland and England. However, there is surprisingly little comparative work examining the apparent benefits in this. In the field of care of older people there are two studies which directly address this by comparing services in the two different settings. In the field of social care and care management it would seem that integration was associated with more integrated approaches to assessment practice and recording, greater involvement of health staff in care planning, greater differentiation within care management arrangements and more specialist approaches to care management, including dementia care (Challis et al., 2004b). Conversely, in old age mental health services the evidence would suggest that whereas integrated services are more likely to promote integrated management, the impact on joint working is much less clear (Reilly et al., 2003).

At the micro-level the Audit Commission (2002) have suggested that too often older people receive a disjointed, confused response to their needs. However, a number of developments are evident. There is evidence of work on links between care homes and specialist health care services (Baillon et al., 1996; Proctor et al., 1999; Challis et al., 2002c; Jacobs and Rummery, 2002). The long-standing area of links between social work and primary care has also re-emerged as an area for development (Ross and Tissier, 1997; Le Mesurier and Cumella, 2001; Brown et al., 2003). Multidisciplinary working in old age mental health care appears to have been more strongly developed than in other areas (Hughes et al., 2001; Challis et al., 2002b). The PSSRU intensive care management studies offer examples of integrated care management in primary care, geriatric medicine and old age psychiatry (Challis et al., 1995; 2002a; 2002b). Interestingly, in old age services there has been little development of the generic worker across home care, home nursing and other health activities. This role was commended in the Griffiths Report (Griffiths, 1988) and was a part of one of the PSSRU intensive care management studies (Challis et al., 1991a; 1991b; 1995), but since that time has only been examined occasionally (Taylor, 2001). At the individual service level, one feature has been the growth of integrated community equipment services, from 400 separate health and social services facilities in 2000, to 70% of the country being covered by integrated community equipment facilities in 2004 (Philp, 2004).

The *National Service Framework for Older People* (Department of Health, 2001a) links the successful provision of person centred care to the development of integrated commissioning and delivery of older people's services. At the time of writing there are only a small number of Care Trusts in place as integrated care organisations, although many developments have taken place under the 1999

Health Act. The precise forms of integration, which are developing, and whether these are predominantly horizontal or vertical integration (Challis, 1998; Kodner, 2003), remains less clear. However, Coxon et al. (2004) conclude that:

> '. . . since the 1950s all governments in the UK have sought to enhance collaboration and joint working in services providing support for older people. However, there is very little evidence that any of the initiatives have successfully overcome the divisive and competitive tendencies in the public sector.' (p. 486)

In the report *Better Health in Old Age*, Philp (2004) concludes that as joined up services develop, the next phase will be to link services more explicitly to levels of need, with services operating at three levels: complex care teams; a better coordinated primary care network; and stronger local strategic partnerships. This approach links to the argument for differentiated care management earlier in this chapter, and would appear to indicate an emphasis on vertical integration of care services (Challis, 1998; Kodner, 2003).

Information needs and systems to support care

The importance of good quality information to the provision of community care is widely acknowledged. In 1988, Sir Roy Griffiths made an indictment of social services department information systems, commenting that their lack of refinement would plunge most organisations in the private sector into a quick and merciful liquidation (Griffiths, 1988).

At the outset of the implementation of community care reforms of the 1990s, it was stated that the development of a mixed economy of care would require an improvement in information gathering systems (Cm 849, 1989). Research conducted shortly after the introduction of the community care reforms confirmed this. It was for example noted that the system of devolved budgets in one authority was made possible by the extensive involvement over several years in computerised information systems (Hoyes et al., 1994). However, it was often the case that information about service users' needs, the services provided, the costs of care, and information about quality and effectiveness were all held in different systems which could not be easily integrated. The scale and priority of the information task was noted by the Social Services Inspectorate (Department of Health, 1997c). Problems have been identified in promoting and managing information use across social services departments; in developing information systems which are operationally useful; in achieving the effective use of information technology; and in devising effective information sharing with other agencies (Philp and Dunleavy, 1994; Department of Health, 1997c).

The Government is committed to the development of information technology to assist integration between health and social care with the potential for both electronic referral and e-conferencing (Department of Health, 1999, 2001b; Warburton, 1999). An inspection of the use of information in social care (Rhodes,

2003) noted that information about cost and quality were not well linked, thereby impeding effective commissioning; that information systems did not support effective use of information across organisational boundaries; and that information sharing arrangements were particularly poorly developed for the SAP. It is likely that a particular challenge to the current information systems used across both health and social care is the development of the Single Assessment Process, since it demands explicit information sharing protocols and is likely to highlight problems both in information systems and in inter-agency working. Although many agencies have sophisticated computer systems in place, the evidence suggests that they are not using them to their full potential (Warburton, 1999; McNally et al., 2003; Cameron and Lart, 2003). The West Midlands Regional Single Assessment Process Group (2004) noted in their study that the extent to which cross-boundary issues were affecting successful SAP implementation was largely determined by the quality of existing inter-agency relationships and the success or otherwise of cross-boundary working on other issues.

Summary

The development of community based care has proceeded rapidly since the reforms of the 1990s. The areas discussed in this chapter – eligibility, assessment, care management and coordination, care packages, commissioning, integration and information systems – have all proved problematic to address. Each of these areas, deemed important at the time of the 1989 White Paper *Caring for People* (Cm 849, 1989), has been the subject of subsequent initiatives to address identified problems. In the development of care services the underlying issues – such as who gets services; how to identify need; how to effectively coordinate care; and what are the correct range of services – are the subject of debate internationally. These areas will need to be the subject of continuing scrutiny and concern.

References

Applebaum, R.A., Austin, C.D. (1990) *Long-Term Care Case Management: Design and Evaluation*. New York: Springer.

Association of Metropolitan Authorities (1995) *Who Gets Community Care? A Survey of Community Care Eligibility Criteria*. London: Association of Metropolitan Authorities.

Audit Commission (1985) *Managing Social Services for the Elderly More Effectively*. London: HMSO.

Audit Commission (1986) *Making a Reality of Community Care*. London: HMSO.

Audit Commission (1993) *Taking Care: Progress with Care in the Community*. London: Audit Commission.

Audit Commission (1996) *Balancing the Care Equation: Progress with Community Care, Community Care Bulletin Number 3, March 1996*. London: HMSO.

Audit Commission (1997) *The Coming of Age: Improving Care Services for Older People*. London: Audit Commission.

Audit Commission (2002) *Integrated Services for Older People: Building a Whole System Approach in England*. London: Audit Commission.

Baillon, S., Neville, P., Broome, C. (1996) A survey of the relationship between community mental health teams and residential homes for the elderly. *International Journal of Geriatric Psychiatry* **11**, 807–11.

Barclay, P. (1982) *Social Workers: Their Roles and Tasks*. London: NISW/Bedford Square Press.

Brocklehurst, J., Carty, M., Leeming, J., Robinson, J. (1978) Care of the elderly: medical screening of old people accepted for residential care. *Lancet* **ii**, 141–2.

Brown, L., Tucker, C., Domokos, T. (2003) Evaluating the impact of integrated health and social care teams on older people living in the community. *Health and Social Care in the Community* **11**, 85–94.

Browning, D. (1999) Value for money. In: Wistow, G. and Henwood, M. (eds) *With Respect to Old Age* (Cm 4192-II/3). London: The Stationery Office.

Caldock, K. (1994) The new assessment: moving towards holism or new roads to fragmentation? In: Challis, D., Davies, B. and Traske, K. (eds) *Community Care: New Agendas and Challenges from the UK and Overseas*. Aldershot: Arena.

Cameron, A., Lart, R. (2003) Factors promoting and obstacles hindering joint working: a systematic review of the research evidence. *Journal of Integrated Care* **11**, 9–17.

Challis, D. (1992a) The care of the elderly in Europe: new perspectives – social care. *European Journal of Gerontology* **1**, 334–47.

Challis, D. (1992b) Community care of elderly people: bringing together scarcity and choice, needs and costs. *Financial Accountability and Management* **8** (2), 77–95.

Challis, D. (1994a) *Implementing Caring for People: Care Management: Factors Influencing its Development in the Implementation of Community Care*. London: Department of Health.

Challis, D. (1994b) Case management. A review of UK developments and issues. In: Titterton, M. (ed.) *Caring for People in the Community: The New Welfare*. London: Jessica Kingsley Publishers.

Challis, D. (1994c) Care management. In: Malin, N.A. (ed.) *Implementing Community Care*. Buckingham: Open University Press.

Challis, D. (1998) Integrating health and social care: problems, opportunities and possibilities. *Research, Policy and Planning* **16** (2), 7–12.

Challis, D. (1999) Assessment and care management: developments since the community care reforms. In: Wistow, G. and Henwood, M. (eds) *With Respect to Old Age: Research Volume 3* (Cm 4192-II/3). London: The Stationery Office.

Challis, D., Chesterman, J. (1985) A system for monitoring social work activity with the frail elderly. *British Journal of Social Work* **15**, 115–32.

Challis, D., Davies, B. (1980) A new approach to community care for the elderly. *British Journal of Social Work* **10**, 1–18.

Challis, D., Davies, B. (1986) *Case Management in Community Care*. Aldershot: Gower.

Challis, D., Ferlie, E. (1986) Social services departments: changing patterns of fieldwork organisation I: The headquarters view. *British Journal of Social Work* **16**, 181–202.

Challis, D., Ferlie, E. (1987) Changing patterns of fieldwork organization II: The team leaders' view. *British Journal of Social Work* **17** (2), 147–67.

Challis, D., Ferlie, E. (1988) The myth of generic practice: specialisation in social work. *Journal of Social Policy* **17** (1), 1–22.

Challis, D., Hughes, J. (2002) Frail old people at the margins of care: some recent research findings. *British Journal of Psychiatry* **180**, 126–30.

Challis, D., Chessum, R., Chesterman, J., Luckett, R., Woods, R. (1988) Community care for the frail elderly: an urban experiment. *British Journal of Social Work* **18**, (Supplement), 13–42.

Challis, D., Chessum, R., Chesterman, J., Luckett, R. and Traske, K. (1990) *Case Management in Social and Health Care: The Gateshead Community Care Scheme.* Canterbury: Personal Social Services Research Unit, University of Kent.

Challis, D., Darton, R., Johnson, L., Stone, M., Traske, K. (1991a) An evaluation of an alternative to long stay hospital care for frail elderly patients: Part I The model of care. *Age and Ageing* **20**, 236–44.

Challis, D., Darton, R., Johnson, L., Stone, M., Traske, K. (1991b) An evaluation of an alternative to long stay hospital care for frail elderly patients: Part II Costs and effectiveness. *Age and Ageing* **20**, 245–54.

Challis, D., Davies, B., Traske, K. (1994) Community care: promise, ambition and imperative – an international agenda. In: Challis, D., Davies, B.P., Traske, K. (eds) *Community Care: New Agendas and Challenges from the UK and Overseas.* Aldershot: Ashgate.

Challis, D., Darton, R., Johnson, L., Stone, M., Traske, K. (1995) *Care Management and Health Care of Older People: The Darlington Community Care Project.* Aldershot: Arena.

Challis, D., Carpenter, I., Traske, K. (1996) *Assessment in Continuing Care Homes: Towards a National Standard Instrument.* Canterbury: Personal Social Services Research Unit, University of Kent.

Challis, D., Von Abendorff, R., Brown, P., Chesterman, J. (1997) Care management and dementia: an evaluation of the Lewisham Intensive Care Management Scheme. In: Hunter, S. (ed.) *Dementia: Challenges and New Directions.* London: Jessica Kingsley.

Challis, D., Darton, R., Hughes, J., Huxley, P., Stewart, K. (1998) Emerging models of care management for older people and those with mental health problems in the UK. *Journal of Case Management* **7** (4), 153–60.

Challis, D., Darton, R., Hughes, J., Stewart, K., Weiner, K. (2001) Intensive care-management at home: an alternative to institutional care? *Age and Ageing* **30**, 409–13.

Challis, D., Chessum, R., Chesterman, J., Luckett, R., Stewart, K., Chessum, R. (2002a) *Management in Social and Primary Health Care: The Gateshead Community Care Scheme.* Aldershot: Ashgate.

Challis, D., von Abendorff, R., Brown, P., Chesterman, J., Hughes, J. (2002b) Care management, dementia care and specialist mental health services: an evaluation. *International Journal of Geriatric Psychiatry* **17**, 315–25.

Challis, D., Reilly, S., Hughes, J., Burns, A., Gilchrist, H., Wilson, K. (2002c) Policy, organisation and practice of specialist old age psychiatry in England. *International Journal of Geriatric Psychiatry* **17** (4), 1018–26.

Challis, D., Clarkson, P., Williamson, J., Hughes, J., Venables, D., Burns, A., Weinberg, A. (2004a) The value of specialist clinical assessment of older people prior to entry to care homes. *Age and Ageing* **33**, 1–10.

Challis, D., Stewart, K., Donnelly, M., Hughes, J., Weiner, K. (2004b) *Care Management for Older People: Does Integration Make a Difference?* Discussion Paper 100. Manchester: PSSRU, University of Manchester.

Clark, H., Dyer, S., Horwood, S. (1998) *That Bit of Help. The High Value of Low Level Preventative Services for Older People.* Bristol: Policy Press/Joseph Rowntree Foundation.

Cm 555 (1989) *Working for Patients.* London: HMSO.

Cm 849 (1989) *Caring for People.* London: HMSO.

Cm 3703 (1968) *Report of the Committee on Local Authority and Allied Personal Social Services.* London: HMSO.

Cm 4169 (1998) *Modernising Social Services*. London: The Stationery Office.

Cm 4192-I (1999) *With Respect to Old Age: Long Term Care – Rights and Responsibilities*. London: The Stationery Office.

Cm 4818-1 (2000) *The NHS Plan*. London: The Stationery Office.

Cm 6268 (2004) *The NHS Improvement Plan*. London: The Stationery Office.

Coleman, A., Rummery, K. (2003) Social services representation in Primary Care Groups and Trusts. *Journal of Interprofessional Care* **17**, 273–80.

Commission for Social Care Improvement (2004) *Direct Payments: What are the barriers?* London: Commission for Social Care Improvement.

Coxon, K., Billings, J., Alaszewski, A. (2004) Providing integrated health and social care for older persons in the United Kingdom. In: Leichsenring, K. and Alaszewski, A. (eds) *Providing Integrated Health and Social Care for Older Persons*. Aldershot: Ashgate.

Curtice, L., Petch, A., Hallam, A., Knapp, M. (2002) *Over the Threshold? An Exploration of Intensive Domiciliary Support for Older People*. Edinburgh: Scottish Executive Central Research Unit, Health and Community Care Research Findings No. 19.

Davies, B.P., Challis, D. (1986) *Matching Resources to Needs in Community Care*. Aldershot: Gower.

Department of Health (1990) *Community Care in the Next Decade and Beyond: Policy Guidance*. London: HMSO.

Department of Health (1993a) *Monitoring and Development: Assessment Special Study*. London: Department of Health.

Department of Health (1993b) *Inspection of Assessment and Care Management Arrangements in Social Services Departments. Interim Overview Report*. London: Department of Health.

Department of Health (1994) *Implementing Caring for People: Care Management*. London: Department of Health.

Department of Health (1995a) *NHS Responsibilities for Meeting Continuing Health Care Needs*, HSG(95)8/LAC(95)5. London: Department of Health.

Department of Health (1995b) *Caring for People at Home. An Overview of the National Inspection of Social Services Department Arrangements for the Assessment and Delivery of Home Care Services*, CI(95)10. London: Department of Health.

Department of Health (1996) *Caring for People at Home – Part II. Report of a Second Inspection of Arrangements for Assessment and Delivery of Home Care Services*, CI(96)34. London: Department of Health.

Department of Health (1997a) *The Cornerstone of Care: Inspection of Care Planning for Older People, Social Services Inspectorate*. London: Department of Health.

Department of Health (1997b) *Better Management, Better Care. The Sixth Annual Report of the Chief Inspector Social Services Inspectorate 1996/97*. London: The Stationery Office.

Department of Health (1997c) *Informing Care: Inspection of Social Services Department Information Strategies and Systems (With Reference to Community Care)*, CI(97)02. London: Department of Health.

Department of Health (1999) *Information for Health*. London: Department of Health.

Department of Health (2001a) *National Service Framework for Older People*. London: Department of Health.

Department of Health (2001b) *Information for Social Care*. London: Department of Health.

Department of Health (2002a) *Fair Access to Care Services. Guidance on Eligibility Criteria for Adult Social Care*, LAC (2002)13. London: Department of Health.

Department of Health (2002b) *Guidance on the Single Assessment Process for Older People*, HSC2002/001: LAC (2002)1. London: Department of Health.

Department of Health (2002c) *Reforming NHS Financial Flows by Introducing Payment by Results*. London: Department of Health.

Department of Health (2003a) *Improving Older People's Services: An Overview of Performance*. London: Department of Health.

Department of Health (2003b) *Modern Social Services: A Commitment to the Future, 12th Annual Report of the Chief Inspector of Social Services*, CI(2003)10. London: Department of Health.

Department of Health (2005) *Supporting People with Long Term Conditions: An NHS and Social Care Model to Support Local Innovation and Integration*. London: Department of Health.

Department of Health and Social Security (1981) *Report of a Study on Community Care*. London: DHSS.

Department of Health and Social Security (1982) *Elderly People in the Community: their Service Needs*. London: HMSO.

Department of Health and Socil Security (1983) Care in the Community Circular HC(83)6. London: HMSO.

Dunnachie, N. (1979) Intensive domiciliary care of the elderly in Hove. *Social Work Service* **21**, 1–3.

Ellis, K., Davis, A., Rummery, K. (1999) Needs assessment, street-level bureaucracy and the new community care. *Social Policy and Administration* **33**, 262–80.

Forder, J., Knapp, M., Hardy, B., Kendall, J., Matosevic, T., Ware, P. (2004) Prices, contracts and motivations: institutional arrangements in domiciliary care. *Policy and Politics* **32**, 207–22.

Gibbins, F.J. (1984) High intensity community nursing. In: Evans, J., Grimley Caird, F. (eds) *Advanced Geriatric Medicine 4*. London: Pitman.

Gibbins, F.J., Lee, M., Davison, P., O'Sullivan, P., Hutchinson, M., Murphy, D., Ugwu, C. (1982) Augmented home nursing as an alternative to hospital care for chronic elderly invalids. *British Medical Journal* **284**, 330–33.

Glendinning, C. (2003) Breaking down barriers: integrating health and social care services for older people in England. *Health Policy* **65**, 149–51.

Glendinning, C., Halliwell, S., Jacobs, S., Rummery, K., Tyrer, J. (2000a) Bridging the gap: Using direct payments to purchase integrated care. *Health and Social Care in the Community* **8**, 192–200.

Glendinning, C., Halliwell, S., Jacobs, S., Rummery, K., Tyrer, J. (2000b) New kinds of care, new kinds of relationships: how purchasing services affects relationships in giving and receiving personal assistance. *Health and Social Care in the Community* **8**, 201–11.

Glendinning, C., Coleman, A., Shipman, C., Malbon, G. (2001) Progress in partnerships. *British Medical Journal* **323**, 28–31.

Glendinning, C., Coleman, A., Rummery, K. (2002) Partnerships, performance and primary care: developing integrated services for older people in England. *Ageing and Society* **22**, 185–208.

Goldberg, E.M., Connelly, N. (1982) *The Effectiveness of Social Care*. London: Heinemann.

Gostick, C., Davies, B., Lawson, R., Salter, C. (1997) *From Vision to Reality in Community Care: Changing Direction at the Local Level*. Aldershot: Arena.

Griffiths, R. (1988) *Community Care: an Agenda for Action*. London: HMSO.

Harding, T. (1999) Enabling older people to remain in their own homes. In: Wistow, G. and Henwood, M. (eds) *With Respect to Old Age: Research Volume 3* (Cm 4192-II/3). London: The Stationery Office.

Harding, T., Beresford, P. (1996) *The Standards We Expect: What Service Users and Carers Want from Social Services Workers.* London: National Institute for Social Work.

Hardy, B., Young, R., Wistow, G. (1999) Dimensions of choice in the assessment and care management process: the views of older people, carers and care managers. *Health and Social Care in the Community* **7**, 483–91.

Hoyes, L., Lart, R., Means, R., Taylor, M. (1994) *Community Care in Transition.* York: Joseph Rowntree Foundation.

Hudson, B. (1998) Circumstances change cases: local government and the NHS. *Social Policy and Administration* **32**, 71–86.

Hughes, J., Challis, D., Gill, J., Stone, S. (1997) The eligibility lottery. *Working with Older People* **1** (3), 14–17.

Hughes, J., Stewart, K., Challis, D., Darton, R., Weiner, K. (2001) Care management and the care programme approach: towards integration in old age mental health services. *International Journal of Geriatric Psychiatry* **16** (3), 266–72.

Hutchinson, P., Grimley Evans, J., Greveson, G. (1984) Linking health and social services: the liaison physician. In: Grimley Evans, J. and Caird, F. (eds) *Advanced Geriatric Medicine 4.* London: Pitman.

Jacobs, S., Rummery, K. (2002) Nursing homes in England and their capacity to provide rehabilitation and intermediate care services. *Social Policy and Administration* **36**, 735–52.

Johri, M., Beland, F., Bergmann, H. (2003) International experiments in integrated care for the elderly: a synthesis of the evidence. *International Journal of Geriatric Psychiatry* **18**, 222–35.

Kane, R.L., Kane, R.A. (2000) *Assessing Older Persons: Measures, Meaning and Practical Applications.* New York: Oxford University Press.

Kendall, J., Matosevic, T., Forder, J., Knapp, M., Hardy, B., Ware, P. (2003) The motivations of domiciliary care providers in England: new concepts, new findings. *Journal of Social Policy* **32**, 489–511.

Kodner, D. (2003) Long term care integration in four European countries: a review. In: Brodsky, J., Habib, J. and Hirschfeld, M. (eds) *Key Policy Issues in Long Term Care.* Geneva: World Health Organization.

Kraan, R.J., Baldock, J., Davies, B.P., Evers, A., Johansson, L., Knapen, M., Thorslund, M. Tunissen, C. (1991) *Care for the Elderly: Significant Innovations in Three European Countries.* European Centre, Vienna with Westview Press, Boulder.

Latto, S. (1984) *Coventry Home Help Project: Main Report.* Coventry: Coventry Social Services Department.

Le Mesurier, N., Cumella, S. (2001) The rough road and the smooth road: comparing access to social care for older people via area teams and GP surgeries. *Managing Community Care* **9**, 7–13.

Leece, J. (2001) Direct support: direct payments and older people, generations review. *Journal of the British Society of Gerontology* **11** (3), 23–5.

Leichsenring, K., Alaszewski, A. (eds) (2004) *Providing Integrated Health and Social Care for Older Persons.* Aldershot: Ashgate.

Lewis, J. (2001) Older people and the health–social care boundary in the UK: half a century of hidden policy conflict. *Social Policy and Administration* **35**, 343–59.

Lewis, J., Glennerster, H. (1996) *Implementing the New Community Care.* Buckingham: Open University Press.

Lewis, J., Bernstock, P., Bovell, V. (1995) The community care changes: unresolved tensions in policy and issues in implementation. *Journal of Social Policy* **24**, 73–94.

Lewis, J., Bernstock, P., Bovell, V., Wookey, F. (1996) The purchaser/provider split in social care: is it working? *Social Policy and Administration* **30** (1), 1–19.

Lewis, J., Bernstock, P., Bovell, V., Wookey, F. (1997) Implementing care management: issues in relation to the new community care. *British Journal of Social Work* **27** (1), 5–24.

McNally, D., Cornes, M., Clough, R. (2003) Implementing the single assessment process: driving change or expecting the impossible? *Journal of Integrated Care* **11**, 18–29.

Moxley, D. (1989) *The Practice of Case Management*. Newbury Park, California: Sage.

Murphy, E. (2004) Case management and community matrons for long term conditions. *British Medical Journal* **329**, 1251–2.

Parry-Jones, B., Soulsby, J. (2001) Needs led assessment: the challenges and the reality. *Health and Social Care in the Community* **9**, 414–28.

Philp, I. (2004) *Better Health in Old Age*. London: Department of Health.

Philp, I., Dunleavy, J. (1994) Community health assessment of elderly people – the national picture. *Health and Social Care in the Community* **2**, 117–19.

Plank, D. (1977) *Caring for the Elderly: Report of a Study of Various Means of Caring for Dependent Elderly People in Eight London Boroughs, Research Memorandum 512*. London: Greater London Council.

Proctor, R., Burns, A., Stratton Powell, H., Tarrier, N., Faragher, B., Richardson, G., Davies, L., South, B. (1999) Behavioural management in nursing and residential homes: a randomised controlled trial. *Lancet* **354**, 26–9.

Reilly, S., Challis, D., Burns, A., Hughes, J. (2003) Does integration really make a difference? A comparison of old age psychiatry services in England and Northern Ireland. *International Journal of Geriatric Psychiatry* **18**, 887–93.

Rhodes, D. (2003) *Better Informed? Inspection of the Management and Use of Information in Social Care*. London: Department of Health.

Ross, F., Tissier, J. (1997) The care management interface with general practice: a case study. *Health and Social Care in the Community* **5**, 153–61.

Rummery, K., Coleman, A. (2003) Primary health and social care services in the UK: progress towards partnership? *Social Science and Medicine* **56**, 1773–82.

Rummery, K., Glendinning, C. (1999) Negotiating needs, access and gatekeeping: development in health and community care policies in the UK and the rights of disabled and older citizens. *Critical Social Policy* **19**, 335–51.

Rummery, K., Ellis, K., Davis, A. (1999) Negotiating access to community care assessments: perspectives of front line workers, people with disability and carers. *Health and Social Care in the Community* **7**, 291–300.

Scottish Executive (2000) *Community Care: A Joint Future*. Edinburgh: The Stationery Office.

Sinclair, I., Williams, J. (1990) Domiciliary services. In: Sinclair, I., Parker, R., Leat, D. and Williams, J. (eds) *The Kaleidoscope of Care: A Review of Research on Welfare Provision for Elderly People*. London: HMSO.

Sinclair, I., Parker, R., Leat, D., Williams, J. (1990) *The Kaleidoscope of Care: A Review of Research on Welfare Provision for Elderly People*. London: HMSO.

Social Services Inspectorate (SSI) (1987) *From Home Help to Home Care: An Analysis of Policy, Resourcing and Service Management*. London: Department of Health.

Social Services Inspectorate and Social Work Services Group (SSI/SWSG) (1991a) *Care Management and Assessment: Managers' Guide, Social Services Inspectorate and Social Work Services Group*. London: HMSO.

Social Services Inspectorate and Social Work Services Group (SSI/SWSG) (1991b) *Care Management and Assessment: Practitioners' Guide, Social Services Inspectorate and Social Work Services Group*. London: HMSO.

Stewart, K., Challis, D., Carpenter, G.I., Dickinson, E. (1999) Assessment approaches for older people receiving social care: content and coverage. *International Journal of Geriatric Psychiatry* **14**, 147–56.

Stewart, K., Hughes, J., Challis, D., Darton, R., Weiner, K. (2003) Care management for older people: access, targeting and the balance assessment, monitoring and review. *Research Policy and Planning* **21** (3), 13–22.

Taylor, P. (2001) Meeting the holistic needs of older people in the community: an examination of a new generic health and social care worker role. *Local Governance* **27**, 239–46.

Warburton, R. (1999) *Meeting the Challenge: Improving Management Information for the Effective Commissioning of Social Care Services for Older People.* London: Department of Health.

Warburton, R., McCracken, J. (1999) An evidence based perspective from the Department of Health on the impact of the 1993 Reforms on the care of frail elderly people. In: Wistow, G. and Henwood, M. (eds) *With Respect to Old Age* (Cm 4192-II/3). London: The Stationery Office.

Ware, T., Matosevic, T., Hardy, B., Knapp, M., Kendall, J., Forder, J. (2003) Commissioning care services for older people in England: the view from care managers, users and carers. *Ageing and Society* **23**, 411–28.

Webb, A., Wistow, G. (1986) *Planning, Need and Scarcity: Essays on the Personal Social Services.* London: Allen and Unwin.

Weinberg, A., Williamson, J., Challis, D., Hughes, J. (2003) What do care managers do? A study of working practice in older peoples' services. *British Journal of Social Work* **33**, 901–19.

Weiner, K., Stewart, K., Hughes, J., Challis, D., Darton, R. (2002) Care management arrangements for older people in England: key areas of variation in a national study. *Ageing and Society* **22**, 419–39.

Weiner, K., Hughes, J., Challis, D., Pedersen, I. (2003) Integrating health and social care at the micro level: health care professionals as care managers for older people. *Social Policy and Administration* **37** (5), 498–515.

Welch, B. (1998) Care management and community care: current issues. In: Challis, D., Darton, R. and Stewart, K. (eds) *Community Care, Secondary Health Care and Care Management.* Aldershot: Ashgate.

West Midlands Regional Single Assessment Process Group (2004) *The Single Assessment Process and Cross Boundary Working.* London: ADSS West Midlands/Department of Health.

Wistow, G., Hardy, B. (1999) The development of domiciliary care: mission accomplished? *Policy and Politics* **27** (2), 173–86.

Wistow, G., Knapp, M., Hardy, B., Allen, C. (1992) From providing to enabling: local authorities and the mixed economy of social care. *Public Administration* **70**, 25–45.

Wistow, G., Knapp, M., Hardy, B., Allen, C. (1994) *Social Care in a Mixed Economy.* Buckingham: Open University Press.

Chapter 12

Alternative Housing and Care Arrangements: the Evidence

Robin Darton and Ann-Marie Muncer

Introduction

Internationally, demographic and cost pressures, together with rising expectations, have led to the development of new forms of housing and care services for older people. However, specialised housing in Britain dates back at least to the Middle Ages (Tinker, 1997), and a number of trade-based continuing care communities were established in the 19th and early 20th centuries (Hearnden, 1983). The postwar reconstruction of housing led to the development of sheltered housing, which still provides the majority of specialised housing for older people. The term 'sheltered housing' appears to derive from 1940s and 1950s design guidance, which recommended selecting a sheltered site (Butler et al., 1983).

Initially, sheltered housing provision grew relatively slowly, but accelerated during the 1960s and 1970s (Department of the Environment data). It was seen as part of a continuum, for people who did not need the degree of care provided in residential accommodation. However, Townsend (1962) viewed sheltered housing as an alternative to residential care for most residents, and the extent to which it should replace or be complementary to residential care has been a matter of debate (Butler et al., 1983). By the late 1990s, the overall levels of provision of sheltered housing dwellings and care home places were broadly similar (Audit Commission, 1998; Conway, 2000), although the contraction in care home capacity that began in 1997 (Laing and Buisson, 2003a) has been changing the balance of provision. Thus, two different forms of communal living for older people have existed side by side, differing in regulatory requirements and financial arrangements (Oldman, 2000).

By the early 1980s, there was a trend towards greater support to people in their own homes and towards the development of the concept of very sheltered housing (Butler et al., 1983). For example, Warwickshire County Council actively promoted very sheltered housing, which had enhanced design features and full-time warden cover, supplemented by domiciliary services (Reed et al., 1980), with the aim of supporting residents as they became more frail and reducing admissions to residential homes.

Very sheltered housing provision developed gradually but, more recently, local authorities have expressed increased interest in integrated care and housing as an alternative to care homes, particularly for physically frail older people. For example, Wolverhampton has a strategy involving the closure of local authority residential homes, and the creation of new very sheltered schemes, resource centres for community support and specialist centres for older people with mental health needs (Bailey, 2001). Such developments have been stimulated by several factors: a greater need for care and support among people in existing sheltered housing; the unpopularity of some ordinary sheltered housing schemes; poor quality local authority residential accommodation; and developments in services and buildings enabling people to age in place (Fletcher et al., 1999). Local authorities also view very sheltered housing as good value for money (Baker, 1999). Furthermore, some care homes still have shared bedrooms (Laing and Buisson, 2003a), which the moderation of the National Care Standards (Department of Health, 2003a; 2003b) is likely to perpetuate.

Local authorities such as Wolverhampton have viewed very sheltered housing as a means of replacing residential care by a more enabling housing and support model and philosophy, aimed at meeting the changing aspirations of older people (Fletcher et al., 1999). In contrast to care homes, very sheltered housing claims to encourage independent living, and some developments provide a wide range of facilities and stimulating environments (Oldman, 2000). It may be difficult for schemes to provide a substitute for care homes as well as a more independent living environment, but providers claim that very sheltered housing can counter the dependency and decline associated with living in care homes (Oldman, 2000). Very sheltered housing is intended to support ageing in place, although the degree to which schemes aim to provide a 'home for life' varies (Oldman, 2000). There is some evidence that very sheltered housing can accommodate people with dementia (Tinker, 1989), unless the lives of other residents appear to be affected by their behaviour (Oldman, 2000).

For owner-occupiers, entry to a care home frequently requires the sale of their home, whereas private sector sheltered housing, usually termed retirement housing, enables some housing equity to be retained. Private retirement housing developed rapidly during the 1980s, but it is very responsive to economic conditions, and declined sharply in the early 1990s (Dalley, 2001), before recovering gradually (Elderly Accommodation Counsel, 2003).

Sheltered housing, private retirement housing and very sheltered housing schemes have usually been developed as free-standing facilities. Continuing care communities, where the housing, personal and health care needs of residents are met on one site (Hearnden, 1983), are relatively rare in Britain, but have been developed extensively in Europe and, especially, in the United States. Another type of combined scheme is close care, where accommodation for independent living is situated adjacent to a care home.

A number of countries in western Europe have developed new forms of housing, often integrated with community based services, to provide greater support and to help maintain older people in the community (Kodner, 2003). As in the United Kingdom, earlier models of specialised housing have become unsuitable for current needs, expectations and levels of disability (Phillips et al., nd). Developments in other countries are informing new housing arrangements in the UK, for example co-housing (Brenton, 2002). However, these need to fit the specific economic and social context. For example, collective living arrangements are less popular in the UK (Heywood et al., 2002) or the USA (Folts and Muir, 2002) than in mainland Europe.

A long-standing aim of government policy has been to enable people to live independently in their own homes (Cm 8173, 1981; Cm 849, 1989; Cm 4169, 1998). This contributed to a decline in support for sheltered housing and a steep reduction in the number of new developments in the 1990s (Tinker et al., 1999; Oldman, 2000). Furthermore, relatively little attention was paid to housing issues prior to the 1990 National Health Service and Community Care Act (for example: DHSS, 1981; Audit Commission, 1986; Griffiths, 1988). The 1990 Act formalised the involvement of housing authorities in assessments for community care services, but progress was unsatisfactory (Audit Commission, 1998; Harrison and Heywood, 2000; Cameron et al., 2001).

The present Government supported the development of specialist, or extra care housing in guidance for establishing joint strategies for housing and community care (Department of Health and Department of the Environment, 1997), and reaffirmed the role of housing (Cm 4169, 1998). In 2002, plans were announced for an expansion in extra care provision (Department of Health, 2002a), and subsequently the Extra Care Housing Fund was created to develop innovative housing with care arrangements (2004b). Further guidance was published in 2003 (ODPM, 2003). However, the Government remained concerned that sheltered housing was being used to meet a shortfall in small, ordinary housing, and that the objectives for very sheltered housing were not being clarified before development began (ODPM, 2001).

Since sheltered housing provides the majority of specialised housing for older people, and is the forerunner of the majority of housing developments with more intensive care services, the next section of this chapter describes the types and levels of provision of sheltered housing. The chapter then describes more recent developments in extra care housing, before examining a number of important current issues, relating to costs and funding, and the characteristics and needs of residents and staffing. This is followed by a discussion of continuing care or retirement communities, in particular the results from the research conducted at Hartrigg Oaks in York and the studies of retirement villages developed by the ExtraCare Charitable Trust. The development of integrated care and housing and its potential as an alternative to care home provision raises a wide range of issues, and the chapter concludes with a discussion of some of the current gaps in knowledge that need to be explored.

Sheltered and very sheltered housing

Definitions

There has been considerable confusion about definitions of sheltered housing (Butler et al., 1983; Fletcher et al., 1999; Riseborough et al., 2001; Department of Health, 2003d; Laing and Buisson, 2003b).

The design guidance for postwar housing reconstruction described self-contained dwellings for able-bodied old people, and warden-supervised hostels with bed-sitting rooms, communal facilities and an alarm system (MoH and MoW, 1944; MoH, 1949; MLGP, 1951). Subsequently, recommendations were published for bedsitting-room flatlets with kitchen facilities, an intermediate form of accommodation (MHLG, 1958; 1960).

In 1969, housing designed for older people was classified into two categories: self-contained dwellings for more active older people (Category 1); and grouped flatlets for less active older people (Category 2) (MHLG, 1969). Optionally, Category 1 accommodation could include common rooms, an alarm system to communicate with a nominated person or be visible externally, and guest facilities. Category 2 accommodation was required to include self-contained accommodation for a warden, an alarm system from each dwelling to the warden and communal facilities. Consequently, there was considerable blurring between the two categories (Fletcher et al., 2001).

In 1981, all housing circulars were withdrawn (Butler et al., 1983), but the Housing Act 1985 identified specialised housing for older people as having a resident warden or the services of a non-resident warden with a call system and the use of a common room. Very sheltered housing was also termed 'Category $2^1/_2$' or 'Category 2.5', since it fell between Category 2 sheltered housing and residential care regulated under Part III of the National Assistance Act 1948 (Tinker, 1989). McCafferty (1994) distinguished an intermediate category (Category 1.5) as housing with an alarm system and warden support, but no communal facilities, and stated that categories 1.5, 2 and 2.5 corresponded to the description in the 1985 Act. However, these categories do not appear to be completely consistent with the wording of the Act.

For the purposes of the Housing Investment Programme returns (DETR, 2000a), sheltered dwellings were specially designed or adapted with either a resident warden, or an alarm system offering access to a warden with a common room close by, or conformed to the provisions of the 1985 Housing Act. However, the first two criteria appear to be sufficient to correspond directly to the Act.

Prior to the implementation of *Supporting People* (DSS, 1998; DETR, 2001b) in 2003, the Housing Corporation classified housing for older people as Category 1 accommodation, Category 2 accommodation, and housing for frail elderly people (Housing Corporation, 2003). The latter would include a warden or 24-hour emergency care and communal facilities, but could be either shared or self-contained.

Riseborough et al. (2001) argued that the distinctions between the categories were much less straightforward than suggested by McCafferty, and did not adequately define the range of provision available, and also created widespread confusion among consumers. In a separate report (Fletcher et al., 2001), it was argued that Category 1 sheltered housing could provide additional choice for older people if it was clearly presented and marketed. However, although the term 'sheltered housing' often includes Category 1 accommodation, technically it should be restricted to schemes with the services of a warden and communal facilities (Audit Commission, 1998). Variations in definitions have important implications for the statistics collected on provision (Fletcher et al., 2001; Riseborough et al., 2001; Laing and Buisson, 2003b).

Riseborough et al. (2001) proposed that sheltered housing should be defined as 'grouped housing particularly aimed at people over retirement age and at people with disabilities who are approaching retirement age' with 'a set of descriptors clarifying which design and service features are present in the scheme' (p. 12). Following the implementation of *Supporting People*, and to improve the definitions of sheltered housing, the Housing Corporation has changed its definitions of housing for older people to distinguish housing for older people with all or some specific design features, designated supported housing for older people, and general needs housing (Housing Corporation, 2004).

Private retirement housing

Private retirement housing has received very little attention in the literature (Dalley, 2001). It is usually purchased on a long lease, or less often as a freehold (Laing and Buisson, 2003b). Developers of private retirement housing include for-profit and not-for-profit organisations: the term 'private' refers to the ownership of the property (Laing and Buisson, 2003b). However, some providers offer properties for purchase or rent. Private retirement housing emphasises the property and property-related services, rather than any care and support provided, but providers are increasingly developing integrated housing and care (Laing and Buisson, 2003b).

Levels of provision

Information on sheltered and very sheltered housing was collected on the Housing Investment Programme (HIP) returns until 2000. Subsequently, however, the forms were revised in the light of changes in government policy and to reduce the burden on local authorities (DETR, 2001a). There were approximately 500 000 units of sheltered and very sheltered housing in 2000 (see Table 12.1), a slight reduction from 1997 (Tinker et al., 1999). The information for very sheltered housing relates to places rather than dwellings, and thus Table 12.1 overstates the relative provision of very sheltered housing. However, the degree of overstatement is likely to be small. In 1990, nearly 95% of category 2.5 units

Table 12.1 Sheltered and very sheltered housing provision for older people, England, 2000.

	Local authority	RSLs	Other public sector	Private sector[3]	Total
Sheltered[1]	244 475	181 614	1802	—	479 267
Very sheltered[2]	7043	12 555	532	—	20 130
Total dwellings	251 518	194 169	2334	51 376	499 397

Adapted from DETR 2000a.
[1] Sheltered housing dwellings. [2] Very sheltered places. [3] Very sheltered places in the private sector were not collected separately.

were bedsits or single-bed units (McCafferty, 1994). Thus, very sheltered housing accounted for less than 5% of social or public sector sheltered housing in 2000. Private providers accounted for 10% of the total number of units, and Registered Social Landlords (RSLs), formerly housing associations, accounted for 39%.

Until 1998/99, the Survey of English Housing provided information about the number of people living in sheltered housing, which was defined as accommodation with a warden (ONS, 2000). However, few units are likely to have a warden service but no alarm system. For example, in 1977 the figure was only 8% (Department of Environment data). In 1998/99, around 600 000 people were living in sheltered housing, 86% of whom were living in social or public sector schemes.

Difficult-to-let properties

The recommendations contained in the early design manuals were intended to minimise the burden of housework. However, bedsitting rooms with cramped facilities and communal bathrooms and toilets became difficult to let (Butler et al., 1983; Middleton, 1987; Tinker et al., 1995). Location, lack of a lift, over-provision in some areas and high rents are further reasons for schemes being difficult to let (Tinker et al., 1995; Nocon and Pleace, 1999). This problem is not confined to ordinary sheltered housing. Some very sheltered housing was created by upgrading ordinary sheltered schemes and, in 1994, Tinker et al. (1995) found that some very sheltered housing was difficult to let, possibly because of a dislike of shared facilities (Tinker et al., 1999). In 1990, 32% of very sheltered housing units were not self-contained (McCafferty, 1994). Concern about obsolescence has led to an emphasis on flexible designs that avoid future redundancy and anticipate technological and other developments (Robson et al., 1997; Fletcher et al., 1999), that is, 'future proofing' (Department of Health, 2002b).

Extra care housing

Definitions

Until recently, the umbrella term 'assisted living' was used for integrated housing and care in the UK (Laing and Buisson, 2003a), but it has been replaced by the term 'extra care housing' (Laing and Buisson, 2003b). Extra care housing covers a range of specialist housing models, and refers to a concept rather than a particular type of housing (Riseborough and Fletcher, 2003). Extra care housing was originally synonymous with very sheltered housing. More recently, however, retirement communities have incorporated extra care provision, and schemes for particular service user groups are being developed. There is no clear definition of extra care housing (Department of Health, 2003d; Laing and Buisson, 2003b), since the characteristics of extra care housing are often found in ordinary sheltered housing, and different agencies and providers have their own definitions.

Laing and Buisson (2003b) suggest that extra care housing can be recognised by several characteristics: it is for older people; the accommodation ought to be self-contained; care can be delivered flexibly, usually by a team of staff based on the premises; communal facilities and services are available; it aims to be a home for life; and it offers security of tenure. Although the previous Housing Corporation definition included non-self-contained accommodation, developers are unlikely to build shared accommodation (Laing and Buisson, 2003b). In addition, Laing and Buisson indicate that care and support staff should be available for 24-hour care, and suggest that the requirement to have integrated care means that a single agency should be providing care to most residents. The Department of Health (Department of Health, 2003d) has also suggested an additional category of enhanced sheltered housing, which has additional staffing and some specialised facilities, without remodelling the building or providing full 24-hour care.

Levels of provision

The lack of a universal definition complicates attempts to collect statistics on extra care housing. Taking a broad definition, the Elderly Accommodation Counsel identified 596 extra care schemes in England in 2003, providing around 21 000 dwellings (Department of Health, 2003c). However, some schemes did not provide 24-hour care, and it is likely that the estimated number will be reduced by the collection of more detailed information. The numbers were already lower than those reported in an earlier version of the directory (Laing and Buisson, 2003b). The majority of the schemes were free-standing, generally for fewer than 50 residents, although some were larger, and a small number of larger care villages and details of linked care homes were also included. Previous work by the Elderly Accommodation Counsel had identified 150 close care schemes, providing an estimated 1000 to 1500 units of accommodation (Laing and Buisson, 2003b).

Assisted living

In the USA, assisted living refers to housing-based long-term care for frail older people who require personal care but not usually skilled nursing care (Regnier et al., 1995; Schwarz, 2001). It developed from the mid-1980s (Regnier et al., 1995), and was providing care for a million individuals by the late 1990s (Schwarz, 2001). Regnier et al. (1995) describe two typical resident profiles for assisted living: cognitively alert but physically frail individuals; and physically able but mentally frail individuals experiencing the first stages of dementia. The lack of alternatives to nursing homes meant that such individuals had been forced into nursing home care. However, assisted living is more readily available to middle- and upper-income individuals, while those on lower incomes have to rely on subsidised housing without care or on medically-orientated long-term care institutions (Schwarz, 2001). In addition, increasing frailty and declining health may result in residents being asked to leave (Frank, 2001).

Costs and funding issues

The possibility of replacing care homes with extra care housing has focused interest on their comparative costs. Tinker et al. (1999) examined the resource costs of a variety of scenarios, but other studies have made contentious claims based on accounting costs (Oldman, 2000). There are also concerns that local authorities may develop extra care housing to transfer costs to social security funding (Laing and Buisson, 2003a). For example, housing benefit has enabled extra care housing to develop opportunistically (Oldman, 2000).

Netten and Curtis (2003) indicate that capital costs of local authority sheltered housing are higher than for residential care, but revenue costs are lower. Tinker et al. (1999) showed that the costs of care in different locations depend on the level and organisation of care: extra care housing was more expensive than private sector residential care, and for some individuals it was more expensive than local authority residential care. Most studies do not consider sufficiently all the factors associated with costs, specifically the contribution of informal carers and affordability (Oldman, 2000). Another factor is the potential impact on other forms of provision, for example savings to the health services from reduced admissions to hospital (Laing and Buisson, 2003b).

From 2003, *Supporting People* introduced new financial arrangements for state-supported tenants, in order to replace the fragmented system of funding arrangements and to overcome legal restrictions on the use of housing benefit for care services. It was also intended to remove the link between support and tenure. Personal care services would be provided separately following a social services or health assessment. However, providers have raised concerns about the impact on the warden service of disaggregating the service charge element from rents (Fletcher et al., 1999; Oldman, 2000). Further concerns have been raised about whether support for housing will be adequately recognised in a cash-limited scheme administered by local authorities, (Heywood et al., 2002). The Government's rent restructuring policy (DETR, 2000b) has also affected relative rent levels in the local authority and RSL sectors.

The Extra Care Housing Fund (Department of Health, 2004b) has enabled a number of schemes to obtain funding. However, a large number of proposals were unsuccessful (Department of Health, 2004a) and limits on funding have restricted the development of extra care housing (Fletcher et al., 1999). New funding opportunities using Public–Private Partnerships, such as the Private Finance Initiative, are being used to develop schemes, but further development of partnerships at the commissioning and development stages and innovations in construction and remodelling will be needed to match development to demand (Fletcher et al., 1999).

Extra care or very sheltered housing enables residents to safeguard their capital and to purchase a flexible package of care on the domiciliary model, rather than a fixed quantity of care as in a care home. Whereas publicly-funded residents in care homes only retain a small personal expenses allowance, income from pensions and benefits can be used to pay the rent and personal care in extra care housing and still provide a comfortable sum to live on (Oldman, 2000). Each resident has substantially more accommodation than in a care home and the privacy and independence given by self-contained accommodation. Although larger accommodation may appear to be more costly, Laing (2002) argues that the greater potential for alternative use suggests that long-term financing can be achieved at lower rates of return than for care home premises. Further investigation of the costs to all parties of extra care housing is vital before its role can be properly evaluated. More generally, the relative outcomes for residents need to be considered in making an overall judgement of relative costs.

The characteristics and needs of residents

A number of studies have collected information enabling comparisons with residential care (for example, Boldy et al., 1973; Plank, 1977; Reed et al., 1980; Baker, 1999; McCoy, nd). Providers of sheltered and very sheltered housing, mainly in the social housing sector, have also sponsored studies, principally for management purposes, which have included information about residents (for example, Fennell, 1986; Middleton, 1987; Riseborough and Niner, 1994; Bartholomeou, 1999). A small number of larger scale studies have provided more systematic comparisons of sheltered and very sheltered schemes (Butler et al., 1983; Tinker, 1989; McCafferty, 1994).

Butler et al., Tinker and McCafferty reported similar findings about the characteristics of residents in sheltered and very sheltered housing. Residents tended to be older, and were more likely to be female, to be living alone and more dependent than individuals living in ordinary housing. Equally, these characteristics also distinguished residents in very sheltered housing from those in sheltered housing, while residents in very sheltered housing were much less dependent than those in residential homes. Residents in local authority provision were more likely to have come from council housing and have been in a partly skilled or unskilled occupation than those in housing association schemes. However, it appeared that, in some cases, specialised housing was being used to respond to specific housing problems. Butler et al. and McCafferty found that sheltered housing tenants were more likely to have been living in privately-rented housing, where the standard of accommodation tended to be poorer than elsewhere, than older people as a whole. Secondly, McCafferty identified an apparent increase in the proportion of residents in sheltered and very sheltered housing with no measured dependency, as well as an increase in those with high levels of dependency.

A particular concern during the development of sheltered housing was the level of need of sheltered housing tenants and the role of the warden. In 1961, the concept of a 'balanced population' of tenants was advocated (MHLG and MoH, 1961). This was seen as necessary for tenants to provide mutual support and to reduce demands on the warden (Butler et al., 1983), although tenants have been found to provide very limited help to others (Middleton, 1987; Tinker, 1989). It was also seen as creating a fundamental contradiction about the role of sheltered housing, since the provision of additional services to people with lower levels of need was inequitable (Butler et al., 1983; Tinker, 1984; Middleton, 1987). Furthermore, although sheltered housing was developed to tackle both housing and care needs, it was usually allocated according to housing need and managed as housing provision (Butler et al., 1983; Tinker, 1984). At the same time, insufficient attention was given to the development of ordinary housing suitable for older people (Oldman, 1986; Middleton, 1987).

The development of extra care housing has reactivated the issue of a balanced community (Robson et al., 1997), since the principle of ageing in place may contradict the targeting of care towards the most frail, particularly where extra care is seen as an alternative to care home provision. In addition, if extra care housing incorporates higher levels of care than residents require, on average, it is difficult to justify on cost grounds (Department of Health, 2003d).

In the case of people with dementia, extra care housing schemes are usually able to accept people in the early stages of the disease and support people who develop dementia while they are residents (Fletcher et al., 1999). However, where the lives of other residents appear to be affected by the behaviour of residents with dementia, a move to a care home may be encouraged (Oldman, 2000). The Department of Health has also encouraged the development of pilot schemes for people with learning disabilities who can no longer be supported by their parents (Department of Health, 2003d).

Relatively little specialised housing has been developed specifically for older people in black and minority ethnic groups, in contrast to day care and home care services (Social Services Inspectorate, 1998; Fletcher et al., 1999). However, the increasing number of older people from minority groups, facing different housing and social conditions (Blakemore, 2000), has led to greater concern to develop culturally appropriate forms of provision (Fletcher et al., 1999; Department of Health, 2004b).

The development of mixed tenure schemes and schemes that provide community facilities raises questions about the acceptability of the arrangements to residents. Studies in care homes have indicated tensions between long-stay residents and short-stay residents and day centre users (Allen, 1983; Wright, 1995). The design of schemes that provide community facilities needs to incorporate the principles of progressive privacy (Fletcher et al., 1999), for example by ensuring that there is a physical barrier between public areas and areas used solely by residents and staff.

Staffing issues

A central aspect of sheltered housing is that it is supervised by a warden, and the role, training and qualifications of wardens have received extensive examination. Traditionally, the warden has acted as a caretaker of the property and as a 'good neighbour' (Butler et al., 1983; Laing and Buisson, 2003b), although the 'good neighbour' role was rarely defined, and views of the role varied considerably (Butler et al., 1983). With increasing dependency among residents, the role of the warden became more welfare-oriented and more demanding (Laing and Buisson, 2003b). At the same time, wardens have become more professionalised, with a coordinating and enabling role (Tinker et al., 1999; Heywood et al., 2002). However, relatives and wardens remain unclear about their respective roles, and the emphasis on the enabling role can lead to a reduction in direct contact between the warden and the residents (Heywood et al., 2002).

In order to reduce costs, sheltered housing schemes are increasing the use of non-resident, peripatetic wardens (Laing and Buisson, 2003b). Some providers of very sheltered housing have replaced the warden by a scheme manager who is responsible for housing, care and support, whereas others have retained the warden role, but renamed as the estate manager, and contract out care services to separate agencies (Oldman, 2000).

The integration or separation of accommodation and care raises issues relating to cost-effectiveness, registration and the delivery of care (Oldman, 2000; Heywood et al., 2002). For older people in social housing, the emphasis on residents as tenants rather than as social work clients suggests a bias towards the separation of the housing function (Tinker et al., 1999). The separation of accommodation and care, for example in schemes run by Hanover (Bartholomeou, 1999), may ensure that housing support services are given greater attention. However, there are concerns about whether this can achieve a seamless service (Oldman, 2000), particularly if there is no care team manager on site (Fletcher et al., 1999). Another reason for the separation of care is that the scheme would be registered as providing domiciliary care under the Care Standards Act 2000 (Department of Health, 2003d), whereas providing personal care would require the scheme to register as a care home (Department of Health, 2002c), with significant costs (Oldman, 2000).

Very sheltered housing usually has a dedicated team of care or support workers to provide 24-hour care services. When they are based on-site, these are usually sleeping-in staff, although some newer schemes have night staff on duty (Fletcher et al., 1999). However, some providers only offer 24-hour cover through an alarm service. The provision of 24-hour care also raises issues about the overall size of the scheme. The size of sheltered housing schemes was often based on the maximum workload that the warden could manage (Fisk, 1986), and there were criticisms that developments were over-concentrated (Fisk, 2003). Schemes in which 24-hour care is provided would need to be sufficiently large for day-time staffing to be organised efficiently without over-provision (Department of Health, 2003d).

Retirement communities

Definitions

Continuing care communities provide for a broader mix of age and dependency ranges and a wider range of communal facilities than would be feasible in a smaller development. They have been relatively rare in the UK, although a number of villages have been developed in the past 20 years. However, not all provide personal care (Laing and Buisson, 2003b). In the USA, continuing care retirement communities form part of the wider retirement community industry. The broad range of retirement communities is unique to the USA, and has been attributed to the availability of land and areas with attractive climates (Streib, 2002). Retirement communities in the USA date back to the 1920s, but substantial development followed the Second World War, ranging from complete new towns, such as Sun City in Arizona, to small retirement residences (Hunt et al., 1984). Many classifications of retirement communities have been proposed, but have frequently omitted precise definitions of what should be included in particular categories, and have ignored their dynamic nature (Hunt et al., 1984). Hunt et al. identified four types of leisure-oriented retirement community (LORCs) (Folts and Muir, 2002), which catered for predominantly healthy, often relatively young residents; and continuing care retirement centres (or communities), which catered for a mixture of healthy and frail older residents. In addition to specially-designed communities, naturally-occurring retirement communities (NORCs) can develop through the ageing of the local population or by the out-migration of younger people (Phillips et al., 2001).

In the UK, the terms 'retirement village' and 'continuing care retirement community' tend to be used interchangeably (Laing and Buisson, 2003b). However, Laing and Buisson suggest that, following US practice, the charges to residents should include insurance against future care costs for a scheme to be classed as a continuing care retirement community (Streib, 2002). There are approximately 2000 continuing care retirement communities in the USA, located in both the for-profit and the non-profit sectors (Streib, 2002). However, in the UK, only Hartrigg Oaks in York, operated by the Joseph Rowntree Housing Trust (JRHT), meets this specific definition.

Hartrigg Oaks: a continuing care retirement community

Although planning began in 1983, Hartrigg Oaks was opened only in 1998, following seven years' delay in obtaining planning permission. The development includes 152 bungalows, which can accommodate up to 247 residents, and a central building providing communal facilities and a 41-place care home (Rugg, 2000; Sturge, 2000). Residents contribute an initial capital payment or residence fee, and a monthly maintenance or community fee, and there are several payment options. The standard community fee covers care for up to 21 hours per week. Where care needs exceed this, the resident may be asked to move to the care centre (Sturge, 2000). The contract is similar to a tenancy agreement, and residents who breach it will be asked to leave. However, there is a hardship fund for residents who need financial help.

Providers managing continuing care retirement communities need actuarial estimates of health status and life expectancy, and need to predict the future finances of the community (Streib, 2002). The JRHT needed to ensure that there were groups of older people who would be able to afford the fees. Actuarial calculations of the likely mortality rates and care needs of residents were particularly important since residents would be relatively wealthy and have high survival rates. However, there was a lack of information about the needs of the target group of residents and a degree of uncertainty in making predictions for relatively small numbers of individuals (Rugg, 2000).

Internal monitoring (Sturge, 2000) and external evaluation (Rugg, 2000; Croucher et al., 2003) demonstrated that Hartrigg Oaks was popular, and enabled the development of an active community with numerous leisure interests. Some problems were identified with the design of the bungalows and the organisation of care. For example, low-level baths designed for ease of access were considered to be too institutional. Similarly, many residents disliked being associated with a retirement community, and the phrase 'Continuing Care Retirement Community' was removed from the entrance sign. More residents required support than had been anticipated, and the community fees had to be increased to cover increased staffing levels. However, the care home was little used for permanent stays, but more for respite and rehabilitative/intermediate care. Residents who were older or more frail tended to be less likely to participate in social activities, while the capacity to care for people with dementia was relatively limited and raised concerns about whether the scheme could provide a home for life.

The majority of continuing care retirement communities in the USA and Germany are not-for-profit concerns, and residents viewed the reputation of the JRHT as a non-profit organisation as an important safeguard (Rugg, 2000; Croucher et al., 2003). Only about 25% of older people were estimated to be able to afford the charges (Croucher et al., 2003), and Hartrigg Oaks is expensive until residents need the level of support that is available (Hanson, 2001). Although the level of satisfaction suggests that further schemes for people with similar income levels would be feasible (Croucher et al., 2003), there are questions about how easily the model could be replicated (Rugg, 2000). However, the high space standards, amenities and range of care services provide general lessons for all types of retirement community (Croucher et al., 2003).

Although the growth in home ownership may be expected to increase the proportion of older people who could afford the cost of developments like Hartrigg Oaks, a majority of older people are unlikely to be able to afford such schemes in the foreseeable future. Developments offering a range of tenures will be accessible to a much wider range of older people. In recognition of the growth in home ownership, some providers of rented schemes have considered developing mixed tenure schemes, for example the ExtraCare Charitable Trust (Appleton and Shreeve, 2003).

ExtraCare Charitable Trust developments

The ExtraCare Charitable Trust had 19 extra care schemes in 2003, providing 958 units of accommodation (Laing and Buisson, 2003b), and further developments are in progress. Two of the schemes were retirement villages: Berryhill Retirement Village in Stoke-on-Trent consists of 148 units, and was developed for social renting; Ryfields Retirement Village in Warrington consists of 243 units, including 70 to be sold, either outright, or by using a variety of shared equity arrangements (Appleton and Shreeve, 2003). One of the Trust's earlier schemes formed part of the strategy for replacing residential care in Wolverhampton. An independent comparison of the tenants of the scheme and a comparable community sample found that the tenants had maintained their physical and mental health and social functioning, in contrast to the deteriorating functioning among the comparison group, and were more satisfied with their lives, despite being more than three years older, on average, than the comparison group (Kingston et al., 2001). Peer support and safety and security were identified as key factors in maintaining tenants' well-being. A further study of residents of Berryhill identified greater challenges in promoting the community ethos of the Trust. The facilities and activities available encouraged participation and involvement, but for residents with physical or mental health problems the environment could exacerbate their condition and lead to greater isolation (Bernard et al., 2004). The results of this study have been used in the planning and delivery of services at Ryfields (Appleton and Shreeve, 2003).

Gaps in knowledge

The main sources of information on the provision of extra care housing are statistical returns to the Office of the Deputy Prime Minister and the Housing

Corporation, and the surveys conducted by the Elderly Accommodation Counsel. Laing and Buisson compile an annual report on extra care housing that draws on these sources of information, together with other national statistics, research reports and information obtained from providers. However, none of the sources of information give an overall picture (Laing and Buisson, 2003b). The collection of statistical information has been complicated by the variety of definitions used by different agencies, and it remains to be seen whether the new Housing Corporation definitions will help to clarify the position. The figures presented in Table 12.1 are drawn from the HIP returns for 2000, since this was the last year that this information was collected.

The national returns provide basic information about the stock of sheltered and very sheltered housing, by location and ownership. More detailed information is collected by the Elderly Accommodation Counsel on extra care housing, including information on the number of dwellings, the facilities, the support for residents, the policy on pets, the provision of meals and the types of tenure available, and is published as a directory of schemes, not as a statistical report (Department of Health, 2003c).

As noted above, three large-scale studies have been undertaken to provide systematic comparisons of sheltered and very sheltered schemes, but these are dated. In addition, a number of in-depth studies have been undertaken about individual developments, for example the monitoring and evaluation of Hartrigg Oaks and the studies of the schemes developed by the ExtraCare Charitable Trust. However, there has been no recent comprehensive evaluation of the new forms of provision and there has been no real attempt to assess outcomes and/or the quality of care (Oldman, 2000). Since extra care housing is being viewed as an alternative to care homes, comparative information is needed about both forms of provision, including information on costs and the characteristics of residents. Although more information is available about care homes and their residents, changes in care home provision (Darton et al., 2003) indicate that an up-to-date comparative study is needed. Information about residents is particularly important, because different forms of accommodation may be more suitable for different client groups, for example residents with mental health problems and members of black and minority ethnic groups.

Developments in extra care have resulted in changes in the role of the warden or scheme manager, and some providers have separated the housing and care functions. In addition, the supply of care staff is a major issue for providers of all types of care services. The advantages and disadvantages of alternative staffing arrangements and their relative costs need to be investigated, as well as more general issues of staff supply, qualifications, training and reimbursement.

Extra care housing includes a wide range of types of provision, and some schemes formerly described as very sheltered housing may have more in common with care homes than retirement villages. The developments supported by the Extra Care Housing Fund will be evaluated (Department of Health, 2003d), but these will also need to be placed in the context of extra care developments more widely. Internationally, particularly in the USA, there is a developing literature on assisted living and retirement communities, for example the volumes edited by Schwarz (2001) and Streib (2002). However, comparisons with developments in the UK need to take account of the particular economic and social circumstances of the different countries.

Extra care housing also needs to be considered in relation to housing policies more generally, and this also requires information about facilities, the characteristics of residents, costs and outcomes. Extra care housing developments that incorporate the principles of universal design, demonstrated in standards for Lifetime Homes, can provide an enabling environment in which residents can age in place (Hanson, 2001), and are examples of attempts at future proofing. The Department of Health remains concerned that extra care provision for less dependent older people is a form of over-provision. However, without a range of levels of dependency, extra care housing could become another version of a care home, with entry being delayed until few options remain for the older person. Furthermore, the ethos of extra care housing as housing would be lost.

Summary

Studies of extra care housing suggest that housing-based developments can provide greater independence and a range of activities for residents. However, compared with ordinary sheltered housing, the number of places available in such schemes is still very small. Retirement villages or communities potentially offer a very wide range of facilities, but the number of these is extremely small, and the history of Hartrigg Oaks illustrates the practical difficulties in establishing a large-scale new development. For more dependent residents, extra care schemes have been found to provide an attractive alternative form of accommodation, but the longer-term viability and limitations of such schemes for more dependent residents need to be investigated. Similarly, the social cost of extra care housing needs proper investigation. Some extra care housing developments are taking account of the implications of the growth in owner-occupation, but there are few such schemes so far, and the range of financial products and tenure arrangements available to potential residents needs much more development.

References

Allen, I. (1983) *Short-Stay Residential Care for the Elderly*. London: Policy Studies Institute.
Appleton, N., Shreeve, M. (2003) *Now for Something Different – The ExtraCare Charitable Trust's Approach to Retirement Living*. Witney: Old Chapel Publishing.
Audit Commission (1986) *Making a Reality of Community Care*. London: HMSO.
Audit Commission (1998) *Home Alone: The Role of Housing in Community Care*. London: Audit Commission.
Bailey, A. (2001) *New Agenda for Older People*. Wolverhampton: Wolverhampton City Council.

Baker, T. (1999) *'You Have Your Own Front Door'. Cambridgeshire and Peterborough Very Sheltered Housing Review.* Cambridge: Cambridgeshire County Council.

Bartholomeou, J. (1999) *A View of the Future: The Experience of Living in ExtraCare.* Staines: Hanover Housing Group.

Bernard, M., Bartlam, B., Biggs, S., Sim, J. (2004) *New Lifestyles in Old Age: Health, Identity and Well-Being in Berryhill Retirement Village.* Bristol: Policy Press.

Blakemore, K. (2000) Health and social care needs in minority communities: an over-problematized issue? *Health and Social Care in the Community* **8** (1), 22–30.

Boldy, D., Abel, P., Carter, K. (1973) *The Elderly in Grouped Dwellings: A Profile.* Publication No. 3. Exeter: Institute of Biometry and Community Medicine, University of Exeter.

Brenton, M. (2002) Choosing and managing your own community in later life. In K. Sumner (ed.) *Our Homes, Our Lives: Choice in Later Life Living Arrangements.* London: Centre for Policy on Ageing, pp. 141–60.

Butler, A., Oldman, C., Greve, J. (1983) *Sheltered Housing for the Elderly: Policy, Practice and the Consumer.* London: George Allen & Unwin.

Cameron, A., Harrison, L., Burton, P., Marsh, A. (2001) *Crossing the Housing and Care Divide.* Bristol: Policy Press.

Care Standards Act 2000 (2000 c. 14). London: The Stationery Office.

Cm 849 (1989) *Caring for People: Community Care in the Next Decade and Beyond.* London: HMSO.

Cm 4169 (1998) *Modernising Social Services: Promoting Independence, Improving Protection, Raising Standards.* London: The Stationery Office.

Cm 8173 (1981) *Growing Older.* London: HMSO.

Conway, J. (2000) *Housing Policy.* London: Routledge.

Croucher, K., Pleace, N., Bevan, M. (2003) *Living at Hartrigg Oaks: Residents' Views of the UK's First Continuing Care Retirement Community.* York: Joseph Rowntree Foundation.

Dalley, G. (2001) *Owning Independence in Retirement: The Role and Benefits of Private Sheltered Housing for Older People.* CPA Reports 30. London: Centre for Policy on Ageing.

Darton, R., Netten, A., Forder, J. (2003) The cost implications of the changing population and characteristics of care homes. *International Journal of Geriatric Psychiatry* **18** (3), 236–43.

Department of the Environment (DoE). *Report on a Survey of Housing for Old People Provided by Local Authorities and Housing Associations in England and Wales.* London: DoE.

Department of the Environment, Transport and the Regions (2000a) *2000 Housing Investment Programme: Operational Information.* London: DETR.

Department of the Environment, Transport and the Regions (2000b) *Quality and Choice: A Decent Home for All. The Way Forward for Housing.* London: DETR.

Department of the Environment, Transport and the Regions (2001a) *Housing Investment Programme (HIP) 2001: Guidance Notes for Local Authorities,* July 2001. London: DETR.

Department of the Environment, Transport and the Regions (2001b) *Supporting People: Policy into Practice.* January 2001. London: DETR.

Department of Health (2002a) *Expanded Services and Increased Choices for Older People: Investment and Reform for Older People's Social Services.* Press Release 2002/0324. London: Department of Health.

Department of Health (2002b) *Feedback on the Launch of the Housing Learning and Improvement Network on Friday, 22 November 2002 at the ICC, Birmingham.* London: Department of Health.

Department of Health (2002c) *Supported Housing and Care Homes: Guidance on Regulation.* August 2002. London: Department of Health.

Department of Health (2003a) *Amended National Minimum Standards for Care Homes*. Press Release 2003/0070. London: Department of Health.

Department of Health (2003b) *Care Homes for Older People: National Minimum Standards*. London: The Stationery Office.

Department of Health (2003c) *Extra Care Housing Directory*. Change Agent Team, Housing Learning and Improvement Network, and Elderly Accommodation Counsel. London: Department of Health.

Department of Health (2003d) *Extra Care Housing for Older People: An Introduction for Commissioners*. London: Department of Health.

Department of Health (2004a) *'Independence not Dependence' – New Extra Care Housing Places for Older People Announced*. Press Release 2004/0070. London: Department of Health.

Department of Health (2004b) *Developing and Implementing Local Extra Care Housing Strategies*. London: Department of Health.

Department of Health and Department of the Environment (1997) *Housing and Community Care: Establishing a Strategic Framework*. London: Department of Health.

Department of Health and Social Security (1981) *Report of a Study on Community Care*. London: DHSS.

Department of Social Security (1998) *Supporting People: A New Policy and Funding Framework for Support Services*. London: DSS.

Elderly Accommodation Counsel (2003) *Housing and Care Homes for Older People in England: Key Data Report 2003*. London: Elderly Accommodation Counsel.

Fennell, G. (1986) *Anchor's Older People: What Do They Think? A Survey among Tenants Living in Sheltered Housing*. Oxford: Anchor Housing Association.

Fisk, M.J. (1986) *Independence and the Elderly*. Beckenham: Croom Helm.

Fisk, M.J. (2003) *Social Alarms to Telecare: Older People's Services in Transition*. Bristol: Policy Press.

Fletcher, P., Riseborough, M., Humphries, J., Jenkins, C., Whittingham, P. (1999) *Citizenship and Services in Older Age: The Strategic Role of Very Sheltered Housing*. Beaconsfield: Housing 21.

Fletcher, P., Riseborough, M., Mullins, D. (2001) *What Future for Category 1 Sheltered Housing? Updating Ideas, Policy and Practice*. Housing Research at CURS, No. 13. Birmingham: School of Public Policy, University of Birmingham.

Folts, W.E., Muir, K.B. (2002) Housing for older adults: new lessons from the past. *Research on Aging* **24** (1), 10–28.

Frank, J. (2001) How long can I stay? The dilemma of aging in place in assisted living. In: Schwarz, B. (ed.) *Assisted Living: Sobering Realities*. New York: Haworth Press, pp. 5–30.

Griffiths, R. (1988) *Community Care: Agenda for Action*. A Report to the Secretary of State for Social Services. London: HMSO.

Hanson, J. (2001) From 'special needs' to 'lifestyle choices': articulating the demand for 'third age' housing. In S.M. Peace and C. Holland (eds) *Inclusive Housing in an Ageing Society: Innovative Approaches*. Bristol: Policy Press, pp. 29–53.

Harrison, L., Heywood, F. (2000) *Health Begins at Home: Planning at the Health–Housing Interface for Older People*. Bristol: Policy Press.

Hearnden, D. (1983) *Continuing Care Communities: A Viable Option in Britain?* CPA Reports 3. London: Centre for Policy on Ageing.

Heywood, F., Oldman, C., Means, R. (2002) *Housing and Home in Later Life*. Buckingham: Open University Press.

Housing Act 1985 (1985 c. 68) London: HMSO.

Housing Corporation (2003) *Scheme Development Standards*, 5th ed. London: Housing Corporation.

Housing Corporation (2004) *The Housing Corporation's Definitions of Housing Association Supported Housing and Housing for Older People*. Housing Corporation Regulatory Circular 03/04. London: Housing Corporation.

Hunt, M.E., Feldt, A.G., Marans, R.W., Pastalan, L.A., Vakalo, K.L. (1984) *Retirement Communities: An American Original*. New York: Haworth Press.

Kingston, P., Bernard, M., Biggs, S., Nettleton, H. (2001) Assessing the health impact of age-specific housing. *Health and Social Care in the Community* **9** (4), 228–34.

Kodner, D.L. (2003) Long-term care integration in four European countries: a review. In: Brodsky, J., Habib, J., Hirschfeld, M. (eds) *Key Policy Issues in Long-Term Care*. Geneva: World Health Organization, pp. 91–138.

Laing, W. (2002) *Calculating a Fair Price for Care: A Toolkit for Residential and Nursing Care Costs*. Bristol: Policy Press.

Laing and Buisson (2003a) *Care of Elderly People: Market Survey 2003*, 16th ed. London: Laing and Buisson.

Laing and Buisson (2003b) *Extra-Care Housing Markets 2003/4*. London: Laing and Buisson.

McCafferty, P. (1994) *Living Independently: A Study of the Housing Needs of Elderly and Disabled People*. Housing Research Report, Department of the Environment. London: HMSO.

McCoy, P.V. (no date) *Census of Residential Accommodation, 1980: Interim Report – Sheltered Housing*. Ipswich: Social Services Department, Suffolk County Council.

Middleton, L. (1987) *So Much for So Few: A View of Sheltered Housing*, 2nd ed. Occasional Papers 3. The Institute of Human Ageing. Liverpool: Liverpool University Press.

Ministry of Health (MoH) (1949) *Housing Manual 1949*. London: HMSO.

Ministry of Health and Ministry of Works (MoH and MoW) (1944) *Housing Manual 1944*. London: HMSO.

Ministry of Housing and Local Government (MHLG) (1958) *Flatlets for Old People*. London: HMSO.

Ministry of Housing and Local Government (MHLG) (1960) *More Flatlets for Old People*. London: HMSO.

Ministry of Housing and Local Government (MHLG) (1969) *Housing Standards and Costs: Accommodation Specially Designed for Old People*. Circular 82/69. London: HMSO.

Ministry of Housing and Local Government and Ministry of Health (MHLG and MoH) (1961) *Services for Old People*. Joint Circular 10/61 and 12/61. London: HMSO.

Ministry of Local Government and Planning (MLGP) (1951) *Housing for Special Purposes. Supplement to the Housing Manual 1949*. Report of the Housing Manual Sub-Committee of the Central Housing Advisory Committee under Extended Terms of Reference. London: HMSO.

National Assistance Act 1948 (11 & 12 Geo. VI c. 29) London: HMSO.

National Health Service and Community Care Act 1990 (1990 c. 19) London: HMSO.

Netten, A., Curtis, L. (2003) *Unit Costs of Health and Social Care 2003*. Canterbury: Personal Social Services Research Unit, University of Kent.

Nocon, A., Pleace, N. (1999) Sheltered housing and community care. *Social Policy and Administration* **33** (2), 164–80.

Office for National Statistics (ONS) (2000) *Housing in England 1998/99*. A Report of the 1998/99 Survey of English Housing carried out by the Social Survey Division of ONS on behalf of the Department of the Environment, Transport and the Regions. London: The Stationery Office.

Office of the Deputy Prime Minister (2001) *Quality and Choice for Older People's Housing: A Strategic Framework*. London: ODPM.

Office of the Deputy Prime Minister (2003) *Preparing Older People's Strategies: Linking Housing to Health, Social Care and Other Local Strategies*. London: ODPM.

Oldman, C. (1986) Housing policies for older people. In: Malpass, P. (ed.) *The Housing Crisis*. Beckenham: Croom Helm, pp. 174–199.

Oldman, C. (2000) *Blurring the Boundaries: a Fresh Look at Housing and Care Provision for Older People*. Brighton: Pavilion Publishing.

Phillips, J., Bernard, M., Biggs, S., Kingston, P. (2001) Retirement communities in Britain: a 'third way' for the third age? In: Peace, S.M. and Holland, C. (eds) *Inclusive Housing in an Ageing Society: Innovative Approaches*. Bristol: Policy Press, pp. 189–213.

Phillips, J., Means, R., Russell, L., Sykes, R. (no date) *Broadening Our Vision of Housing and Community Care for Older People: Innovative Examples from Finland, Sweden and England*. Kidlington: Anchor Research.

Plank, D. (1977) *Caring for the Elderly: Report of a Study of Various Means of Caring for Dependent Elderly People in Eight London Boroughs*. Research Memorandum 512. London: Greater London Council.

Reed, C.A., Faulkner, G.J., Bessell, R. (1980) *Your Own Front Door: A Study of Very Sheltered Housing in Warwickshire, 1979–80*. Warwick: Warwickshire County Council Social Services Department.

Regnier, V., Hamilton, J., Yatabe, S. (1995) *Assisted Living for the Aged and Frail: Innovations in Design, Management, and Financing*. New York: Columbia University Press.

Riseborough, M., Fletcher, P. (2003) *Extra Care Housing – What is it?* Factsheet No. 1. Housing Learning and Improvement Network. London: Department of Health.

Riseborough, M., Niner, P. (1994) *I Didn't Know You Cared! A Survey of Anchor's Sheltered Housing Tenants*. Oxford: Anchor Housing Trust.

Riseborough, M., Fletcher, P., Mullins, D. (2001) *The Case for a Common Currency: Clearer Definitions and Descriptions for Sheltered and Supported Housing*. A Discussion Paper for the Housing Corporation. Housing Research at CURS, No. 6. Birmingham: School of Public Policy, University of Birmingham.

Robson, D., Nicholson, A.M., Barker, N. (1997) *Homes for the Third Age: A Design Guide for Extra Care Sheltered Housing*. London: E & FN Spon.

Rugg, J. (2000) *Hartrigg Oaks: The Early Development of a Continuing Care Retirement Community, 1983–1999*. York: Centre for Housing Policy, University of York.

Schwarz, B. (2001) Introduction. In: Schwarz, B. (ed.) *Assisted Living: Sobering Realities*. New York: Haworth Press, pp. 1–4.

Social Services Inspectorate (SSI) (1998) *'They Look After Their Own, Don't They?' Inspection of Community Care Services for Black and Ethnic Minority Older People*. London: Department of Health.

Streib, G.F. (2002) An introduction to retirement communities. *Research on Aging*, **24** (1), 3–9.

Sturge, M. (2000) *Continuing Care Retirement Communities in the UK: Lessons from Hartrigg Oaks*. York: Joseph Rowntree Foundation.

Tinker, A. (1984) *Staying at Home: Helping Elderly People*. London: HMSO.

Tinker, A. (1989) *An Evaluation of Very Sheltered Housing*. London: HMSO.

Tinker, A. (1997) *Older People in Modern Society*, 4th ed. London: Longman.

Tinker, A., Wright, F., Zeilig, H. (1995) *Difficult to Let Sheltered Housing*. London: HMSO.

Tinker, A., Wright, F., McCreadie, C., Askham, J., Hancock, R., Holmans, A. (1999) *Alternative Models of Care for Older People*. The Royal Commission on Long Term Care (1999)

With Respect to Old Age: Long Term Care – Rights and Responsibilities. Research Volume 2. Cm 4192-II/2. London: The Stationery Office.

Townsend, P. (1962) *The Last Refuge: A Survey of Residential Institutions and Homes for the Aged in England and Wales.* London: Routledge & Kegan Paul.

Wright, F. (1995) *Opening Doors: A Case Study of Multi-Purpose Residential Homes.* London: HMSO.

Chapter 13

Care Homes and Continuing Care

Ann Netten, Robin Darton and Jacquetta Williams

Introduction

Care homes provide continuing care for the most impaired section of the older population, 4% of those over the age of 65 (Bajekal, 2002). Although many people can be maintained in their own homes and there are growing moves to develop alternative housing and care arrangements, care homes for older people still account for about 62% of public expenditure on personal social services for older people (Department of Health, 2004a).

We start by considering the supply and characteristics of homes for older people, before describing what is currently known about the characteristics and needs of residents. Funding and commissioning this costly form of care is a major concern to both individuals and governments. We discuss how care is funded and factors associated with the costs of care. Quality of care is discussed both in terms of measurable and regulated standards, and more intangible aspects of the social climate that are so fundamental to the quality of life of residents. We draw on a longitudinal study of people admitted to homes to identify health and locational outcomes and predictors of mortality. We conclude by identifying those areas where we have very limited information and where more studies are required.

Supply and characteristics of homes

In England and Wales, care homes are regulated under the Care Standards Act 2000. Prior to April 2002, nursing homes and residential care homes were regulated separately by health and local authorities and local authority managed homes were not regulated. The Care Standards Act defined a care home as an establishment that provides accommodation together with nursing or personal care, and stated that help with bodily functions must be available if required (2000, s.3). A care home must now be registered to provide personal care, or personal care with nursing care. Nursing care is defined as care that is provided, planned, supervised or delegated by a registered nurse (Health and Social Care

Act 2001, s.49). Care homes must also register their intention to provide for older people with specific care requirements, such as those who have been diagnosed as suffering from dementia, a mental illness or a terminal illness. Rehabilitation and intermediate care services may also be offered in care homes for older people, as well as to people at home or in other care settings. The policy initiative of developing intermediate care is part of the modernisation agenda to promote independence and timely and appropriate care, by supporting early discharge from hospital, preventing unnecessary hospital admission and preventing or delaying admission to long-term care (Cm 4818-I, 2000; Department of Health, 2001a).

Shifts in responsibilities for collecting statistics and changes in registration categories mean that in recent years there has been a lack of consistent and reliable data about the numbers of places in care homes. The National Care Standards Commission (NCSC) estimated that in October 2003 there were about 371 000 places in homes for older people in England, 348 000 of which were in the independent sector (Dalley et al., 2004). Laing and Buisson (2004) estimated that in April 2003 there were 464 000 places for older and physically disabled people in care homes in the UK, 418 000 of which were in independent homes. The difference between the figures for independent homes appears largely to be accounted for by the inclusion of homes in Scotland (Scottish Executive, 2003) and Wales (National Assembly for Wales, 2003), and by the inclusion of places for younger adults with physical disabilities (Department of Health, 2001b) in the Laing and Buisson figures. After adjusting for these factors, the estimated number of places in independent homes in England derived from Laing and Buisson (2004) is about 2% greater than the NCSC estimate (Dalley et al., 2004). However, for local authority homes the corresponding estimate derived from Laing and Buisson is one and a half times that estimated by the NCSC.

In 2001, 39% of places in independent homes for older people were nursing places (Department of Health, 2001b). In 2004, the proportion of places in care homes registered as providing nursing care was 53% (Laing and Buisson, 2004). However, owing to the change in registration arrangements this included all places in former dual registered homes, and the corresponding figure for 2001 was 49% (Department of Health, 2001b). Care homes often also provide general palliative care and, while the number of homes registered to provide for people diagnosed as terminally ill is currently unavailable, it has been estimated that around 20% of people die in care homes, 20% at home, 56% in hospital and 4% in hospices (House of Commons Health Committee, 2004). The number of intermediate care places located in care homes is also unknown. The Department of Health and the Medical Research Council have commissioned several projects to evaluate intermediate care services nationally, but the results are not yet available (Department of Health, 2002a). Factors identified as influencing the development of intermediate care services in care home environments include access to general practitioner and specialist medical health services, the spare physical capacity of homes and views about the desirability of providing for both short-term and long-term placements in one setting (Jacobs and Rummery,

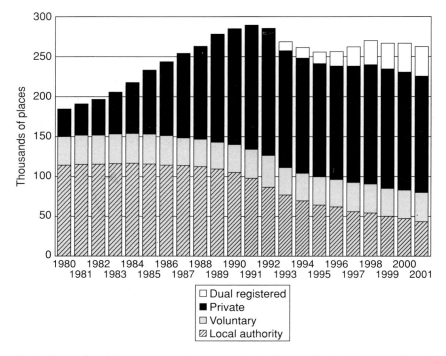

Fig. 13.1 Places for older people and younger physically disabled adults in residential homes in England, 1980 to 2001. Figure constructed using Department of Health statistics.

2002). Here we focus on what is known about the most prevalent form of care in care homes in England: personal and nursing care for older people.

While accurate data of numbers of places are difficult to establish, overall market trends are clear. As Fig. 13.1 shows, since the 1980s there has been a substantial shift away from public provision towards the independent sector. Based on central government residential and nursing home statistics, we estimate that in 1982 about 50% of care home places were in the public sector. By 2001 this had dropped to less than 9% of places, and the NCSC estimated that in 2003 only 6% of places for older people were in the public sector (Dalley et al., 2004).

Comparing Fig. 13.1 and Fig. 13.2 shows that the overall supply of care homes and places rose dramatically during the 1980s and then stabilised in the wake of the 1990 NHS and Community Care Act. Since 1998 the overall number of places available in homes, particularly those providing nursing care, has been falling (Laing and Buisson, 2003). The closure rate peaked in 2000/1 (Laing and Buisson, 2003) when 5% of independent homes closed, with rates varying regionally between 3% and 7% (Netten et al., 2002a). Despite the subsequent decline in the number of de-registrations these have continued to exceed the number of openings, and the net reduction in care home capacity is continuing. During 2002/3 the number of independent homes dropped by 6%, although the drop in places was only 1.6% (Dalley et al., 2004).

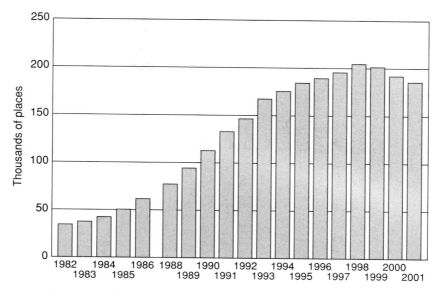

Fig. 13.2　Places in nursing homes in England, 1982 to 2001. Figure constructed using Department of Health statistics.

Home closures during 2000/1 were attributed by regulators to a combination of circumstances, including difficulties recruiting and retaining staff, staff costs, long-term payment of low fee levels by local authorities, local authority contracting arrangements and, more immediately, high property values, the anticipated costs of complying with the new care standards, and in some areas an over-supply of residential homes (Netten et al., 2002a). Providers similarly attributed closing to business failure linked to these and other factors, such as the use of residential places for 'high dependency' residents, poor relationships with regulators, loss of motivation, and a desire to retire (Williams et al., 2002; Netten et al., 2005). To some extent, voluntary closures are a feature of the market-like arrangements in the care home sector. They also present a unique risk, with consequences such as involuntary relocation that are not present with other forms of social care provision.

Drops in the number of places led to government concerns about capacity, particularly with respect to the potential knock-on implications for delayed discharges from hospital (Department of Health, 2002b). Increased funding has been made available to councils with social service responsibilities, although there is no requirement on them to spend this on the care home market (Department of Health, 2002c). However, market analysts predict that demographic changes will result in an increase in the supply of care homes from 2005 (Laing and Buisson, 2003).

One effect of recent market shifts has been the loss of smaller homes and an overall increase in home size. This is demonstrated by the relatively limited impact of recent closures on capacity compared with the proportion of homes lost, reported by the NCSC (Dalley et al., 2004). Laing and Buisson (2003) estimate that the average size of all independent homes in 2003 was 31 places, compared with 25 places in 1994. In part, this is due to the loss of nursing homes, which are generally larger. In 2003 the average size of a nursing home was 39 places, compared with 24 places in residential homes.

Factors associated with closure, and the types of home closing, point towards a further consolidation of a market already heading in that direction (Holden, 2002). Larger-scale organisations with economies of scale and scope are more able to bear the costs of regulation and to invest in raising physical standards of homes.

Characteristics of residents

Detailed data about the characteristics of residents of care homes for older people were collected in a survey funded by the Department of Health of over 11 000 residents of 600 homes conducted in 1996 (Netten et al., 2001) and from 2500 residents of 544 homes as part of the Health Survey for England 2000 (Bajekal, 2002). The latter study collected more detailed information about health status and the former focused more on funding and costs of care. In the following discussion, the results are similar in both studies unless specified otherwise. The vast majority, 98%, of residents were living in care homes on a permanent basis. The 1996 study found that short-stay residents were usually in the home for brief periods of respite care and were overwhelmingly publicly funded. Table 13.1 shows the distribution of age, gender and source of admission of permanent residents at that time.

Table 13.1 Characteristics of permanent residents by type of funding, 1996.

	Publicly-funded residents	Self-funded residents
Number of residents (65+)	6135	2050
Mean age	84	86
% Female	77	80
Source of admission (%)		
Single person household	27	43
Multi-occupancy household	14	14
Single person sheltered housing	6	4
Multi-occupancy sheltered housing	1	<1
Residential home	12	8
Nursing home	4	4
Hospital	34	25
None of these	1	1

The results are weighted to reflect the national distribution of each type of home.

Over three-quarters of all permanent residents were women. In 1996, nursing homes and local authority run residential homes had a larger proportion of men than private residential homes, but no significant differences were found in 2000. The national average age among those aged 65 and over was about 85 years, with men and those admitted to nursing homes being slightly younger than women and those admitted to residential care. Publicly funded residents were younger than self funded residents on average.

Younger people requiring continuing care, usually those with physical disabilities, formed a small proportion of residents in homes for older people. They were often there because more suitable accommodation could not be found for them. Most of these younger residents – 2% of them were under 40 in 1996 – were found in either voluntary residential homes or in the private sector. Few were in local authority accommodation.

There was a marked drop in the proportion of people admitted from hospital between 1996 and 2000. In 1996, over a third of people were admitted from hospital; this had dropped to 15% by 2000. In 1996, publicly funded permanent residents were less likely to have been admitted from single-person households and more likely to have been admitted from hospital than those who were self funded. As might be expected, a higher proportion of people in nursing homes were admitted from hospital and a lower number from single-person households.

Dependency levels in all homes increased markedly between the mid-1980s and 1990s, perhaps unsurprisingly given the policy drive to maintain people in their own homes for as long as possible. The changes were most noticeable in voluntary residential homes and nursing homes, particularly in relation to cognitive impairment (Darton et al., 2003). Table 13.2 shows levels of dependency of residents in 1996 by type of home using the Barthel Index (Mahoney and Barthel, 1965) and the Minimum Data Set Cognitive Performance Scale (MDS CPS) (Morris et al., 1994). In care homes as a whole in 1996, a fifth of residents were in the most dependent category, with a score of 4 or less on the Barthel Index, and over a quarter were severely cognitively impaired. A higher proportion of residents were dependent in nursing homes than in residential homes: 39% were in the most dependent category and 44% were classified as severely cognitively impaired. The use of different approaches to measuring dependency and disability mean that it is difficult to make direct comparisons between 1996 and 2000. The 2000 data, however, suggest that there has been an increase in overall personal care disability among residents of care homes (Bajekal, 2002).

Table 13.3 shows that in 1996 self funded residents tended to be less dependent than publicly funded residents. A subsequent study of self funded admissions to care homes confirmed that they do tend to be admitted at lower levels of dependency than publicly funded residents (Netten and Darton, 2001; Netten et al., 2002b). Based on comparative levels of dependency on admission, it was predicted that one in four self funded residents were being admitted to care homes who did not need to be (Netten and Darton, 2003). This could reflect the preferences of older people and/or their relatives (Laing and Buisson, 2003). However, the weight of previous evidence suggests that people prefer to remain

Table 13.2 Dependency of all residents by type of home, 1996.

	Residential homes			Dual registered homes	Nursing homes	All homes[1]
	Local authority	Private	Voluntary			
Total number of residents (65+)	3442	2090	2052	1279	2449	11 312
Barthel Index of ADL (ungrouped)						
Mean	13	14	14	9	7	11
Std dev	5	6	5	6	5	6
Barthel Index of ADL (grouped) (%)						
Low dependence (Score 13–20)	57	63	64	33	20	47
Moderate dependence (Score 9–12)	18	16	15	17	14	16
Severe dependence (Score 5–8)	15	12	13	23	27	18
Total dependence (Score 0–4)	10	10	8	28	39	20
Cognitive impairment[2] (%)						
Intact	28	33	35	23	14	26
Mild impairment	48	47	45	46	42	46
Severe impairment	25	21	20	31	44	28

[1] For each type of home the results are weighted to reflect the national distribution of that type of home. The data for all homes are also weighted to reflect the national distribution of home type.

[2] The measure of cognitive impairment is based on the MDS Cognitive Performance Scale (Morris et al., 1994). The categories of the scale have been grouped into three groups to facilitate comparisons with information collected in the previous surveys: intact = intact (code 0); mild impairment = borderline intact (code 1), mild impairment (code 2) or moderate impairment (code 3); severe impairment = moderately severe impairment (code 4), severe impairment (code 5) or very severe impairment (code 6).

Table 13.3   Dependency of permanent residents by type of funding, 1996.

	Publicly-funded residents	Self-funded residents
Number of residents (65+)	6135	2050
Barthel Index of ADL		
Mean	11	12
Std dev	6	6
Barthel Index of ADL (grouped) (%)		
Low dependence (Score 13–20)	45	50
Moderate dependence (Score 9–12)	16	16
Severe dependence (Score 5–8)	18	17
Total dependence (Score 0–4)	21	18
Self-care tasks (% needing assistance)		
Wash hands and face	38	34
Bath or wash all over	84	84
Dress	57	53
Cognitive impairment[1] (%)		
Intact	24	30
Mild impairment	47	43
Severe impairment	29	27

The results are weighted to reflect the national distribution of each type of home.
[1] See Table 13.2, note 2, for the definition of cognitive impairment.

in their own homes if at all possible (Warburton, 1994). Moreover, there was some evidence that self funded people were admitted earlier because of a general lack of access to support and information about options (Netten and Darton, 2003). This may be due in part to the service costs incurred by councils when a potential self funding care home resident remains in their own home.

Funding, costs and prices

The problems that individuals and society as a whole will have in financing the costs of care of older people is an issue of international concern (Pacolet et al., 2000). The degree to which the costs of care will fall to individuals themselves (directly or through insurance schemes) or be borne by the state will depend on government policies, both now and in the future. It is crucial to the understanding of the impact of such policies that we have an understanding of the factors affecting the costs and prices of care, the degree to which they take advantage of benefits already available to them and the circumstances that lead to admission to care homes.

Currently, eligibility for the vast majority of care home funding by local authorities in England is means tested. This is based on income and assets. At the time of writing, individuals whose assets are no greater than £20 000 are able to receive financial support for their care by the appropriate local authority, subject to an assessment of their care needs and weekly income (National Health Service and Community Care Act 1990; Department of Health, 2004b).

About 30% of all residents in England are self funded (Laing and Buisson, 2003). With the increase in home ownership, a larger proportion of the older population are falling into this category and having to meet the costs of their own care. Selling one's home to fund care home fees is a major commitment, and initiatives have been introduced which are aimed at increasing the flexibility and reversibility of admission to care homes. Since 2001, capital assets tied up in people's homes are disregarded for the first three months after admission (Cm 4818-I, 2000). Also, deferred payment grants were introduced in October 2001, under section 55 of the Health and Social Care Act 2001, which allow councils to offer residents who cannot or do not want to sell their own homes the opportunity to defer payment of care costs to a later date, and have a charge levied by the council on their property value (Cm 4818-I, 2000; Department of Health, 2001c).

Debate continues about which elements of long-term care should and should not be publicly funded. The Royal Commission on Long Term Care (Cm 4192-I, 1999) recommended that charges for nursing and personal care costs should be exempt from means testing. The recommendation to fund all personal care was not accepted in England, but since October 2001 residents receiving nursing care provided through care homes have been assessed and funded on the basis of three bands: high, medium and low. In 2004/5 the funding attached to these was £125 per week, £77.50 per week and £40 per week respectively. Primary Care Trusts (PCTs) have also been given the freedom to decide whether to pay a sum between the low and medium bands on an individual basis (Department of Health, 2004c). In Scotland, since July 2002, both nursing and personal care has been provided free, both in the community and in care homes (Community Care and Health (Scotland) Act 2002). This is to avoid the problem of personal care being provided free to individuals with some conditions but not others.

There is widespread resentment among older people and their relatives that they should have to run down their assets to meet, what often seem to them, excessive care home fees (Netten et al., 2002b). There is often an assumption on the part of the public that substantial profits are taken by private providers, thus raising costs and reducing quality. However, the policy of increased use of the independent sector in the provision of care was adopted with precisely the opposite intention. Local authority managed homes were considerably more costly than independently purchased care, and the objective was to use market forces to increase value for money (Cm 849, 1989).

As the major purchaser of care, local authorities have both a direct influence over the price that they pay and an indirect effect on the price paid by self-funders (Netten et al., 2002b), and they have exerted a marked downward pressure on fees. Between 1995 and 1999 there was in total just a 10% increase in the average price paid per week (Laing and Buisson, 2000).

A series of analyses based on the 1996 survey discussed above and a companion survey of admissions (Bebbington et al., 2001) were undertaken to investigate the relationship between prices, cost and mark-up (or profit) (Netten et al., 1998, 2001; Forder and Netten, 2000). Margins appeared to be low, and the convergence of prices and costs in the analyses suggested that, while surpluses were available in 1986, they had been eroded significantly over the next decade.

Dependency, using the average Barthel score (Mahoney and Barthel, 1965), was significantly associated with prices in both residential and nursing homes, as would be expected. However, the relationship between dependency characteristics and cost or price was relatively flat within home type. Most of the effect of dependency on price was associated with the differential prices paid to nursing and residential homes. Some characteristics of homes themselves were associated with price and cost variation. However, all these effects were swamped by the effect of the local labour market.

The conclusion of the analyses was that any significant further pressure on mark-up rates would raise concerns about the viability of supply in the market. Since this study, wage rates have continued to rise above the rate of prices paid to care homes. When we put this, and demands for higher standards, alongside the relatively low profit margins at the time of our 1996 study, it is clear that the financial pressures on homes have increased to the point where the dramatic rise in home closures observed in 1999 is unsurprising.

Quality of care and quality of life

Concerns about the quality of care provided by care homes have been an enduring feature of the social care literature in the United Kingdom (Townsend, 1962; Kerrison and Pollock, 2001) and internationally (e.g. Vladek, 1980; Parker, 1987). The 1989 White Paper (Cm 849, 1989) and the 1998 White Paper (Cm 4169, 1998) emphasised the importance of quality of care, and a series of reports on good practice (Centre for Policy on Ageing, 1984; 1996; Wagner, 1988; Social Services Inspectorate, 1989; Residential Forum, 1996) have made recommendations for improving quality of care. However, although high standards of care are recognised as important, quality of care should not be equated with quality of life (Davies and Knapp, 1981; Dalley, 1997). The various guides to good practice and the national minimum standards (Department of Health, 2003) make recommendations for promoting aspects of life in a care home that contribute to quality of life, for example privacy, dignity, independence, choice, rights and fulfilment (Social Services Inspectorate, 1989).

This has led to the introduction of national minimum standards for care homes in Great Britain. Legislation was introduced to establish national agencies to apply common standards to care homes in England, Wales and Scotland from 2002 (the Care Standards Act 2000 and the Regulation of Care (Scotland) Act 2001). For England, the proposed standards were published for consultation in September 1999, and published in March 2001 (Department of Health, 2001d). The standards were to apply from April 2002, unless otherwise stated, and many did not have to be met until 2007. The standards related to seven broad categories: choice of home; health and personal care; daily life and social activities; complaints and protection; environment; staffing; and management and administration.

After considerable campaigning and protest by the industry, largely about the practicability and costs of meeting the environmental standards, press coverage of closures, and a period of consultation, the Government revised some of the environment standards, mainly in terms of what was required of existing homes (Department of Health, 2002d; 2003). Revisions to standards included those relating to shared bedrooms, the floor area of single rooms, wheelchair access and living space. For example, all new homes, extensions and first time registrations are required to provide all places in single rooms, but existing homes are only required to maintain the proportion of single rooms at the level that prevailed in August 2002, instead of meeting the original requirement that 80% of places be in single rooms by 2007. However, shared rooms were still limited to double rooms.

National information about the current quality of care homes, at least in terms of the extent to which they meet the national minimum standards, is now available and should enable the performance of the industry against these standards to be tracked over time. Analysis based on the first year of national inspections established that the quality of homes varied across different standards: the quality of life standards were most frequently met by homes (by 60%)[1]; between 40–60% met the standards relating to needs assessment prior to admission, management of medication, provision of a contract, the handling of complaints, record keeping and some of the environmental standards; standards relating to information provision, producing a service user's plan, and staff supervision were met by fewer than 40% of homes (Dalley et al., 2004).

In addition to the quality of care, the social climate of a care home will be critical to the welfare and quality of life of residents. This concept incorporates how supportive people are of one another, how much conflict there is, whether people feel they can express themselves and have an impact on what goes on in the home, and whether residents are encouraged to be as independent as possible. This social climate, or atmosphere of the home, will depend on a variety of factors, including the characteristics of the residents, the characteristics of staff, the type of caring regime, and the building in which care takes place. While the specification of national minimum standards is intended to 'provide a tool for judging the quality of life of service users' (Department of Health, 2003), in practice the standards are currently focused on measurable indicators related to input and process factors, such as physical standards, which should directly or indirectly promote residents' health, welfare and quality of life. Clearly

---

[1] The quality of life standards included meeting health needs, activities in daily life, maintaining contacts with family and friends, autonomy and choice, respecting the privacy and dignity of service users and handling dying and death with sensitivity, and some of the environmental standards.

these are important; aspects of the physical environment will have an influence on quality of life. For example, availability of single bedrooms and en suite bathrooms and toilets will help residents maintain privacy. There is a need, however, to better understand how social climates of homes vary and what is associated with the social climate if we are to improve the quality of life of residents.

Ideally, residents' perspectives should be central to judgements about quality of care and social climate. However, theirs is a difficult perspective to gain because of the high proportion of people with cognitive impairment, and the problem of low expectations that can lead people to express higher levels of satisfaction than the situation often warrants. At present there is very limited information about residents' views on quality of care.

The Sheltered Care Environment Scale (Moos and Lemke, 1992) was used in our 1996 survey to identify the staff perspective on the social climate of homes. Cluster analysis was used to identify homes with a 'positive' climate: high levels of cohesion, low conflict, and so on. Characteristics of homes associated with these 'positive' climates included smaller numbers of places, lower occupancy levels and being less likely to have single bedrooms or access to all bedrooms on the level or via a lift. These results suggest that the homes identified as having a more positive social environment are those (mainly residential) care homes that are smaller, converted premises. Laing and Buisson (2003) also found that good service ratings by relatives in customer satisfaction questionnaires were not necessarily associated with high standards of physical amenity. It is striking that in the current climate it is just these smaller converted premises that are most likely to close (Darton, 2004).

Both social climate and other aspects of quality of care depend fundamentally on the staff who run the home and provide the care. The national minimum standards recognise this and include qualification requirements in an attempt to raise the quality of care provided. We have discussed above problems with implementing this from the perspective of affordability. But even more fundamental is obtaining an adequate supply of well-motivated staff. In a study of home closures, problems in recruitment were identified as a critical issue by registration and inspection managers (Netten et al., 2002a). Indeed, while there was geographical variation in concerns about the supply of care staff generally, the issue of problems in recruiting nursing staff was the most frequently cited issue underlying nursing home closures. Similarly, in the first national workforce survey conducted in 2001, the recruitment of registered nurses was identified as difficult or very difficult by over two-thirds of providers (69%), care worker recruitment as difficult or very difficult by 45%, and 50% rated recruitment of managers and supervisors as difficult (Social and Health Care Workforce Group, 2002). Turnover rates were highest among care workers, 25%, compared with 14% among nurses. This turnover rate is about twice that of care workers employed by the statutory sector (Eborall, 2003). The loss of a quarter of the care staff in a home during a twelve-month period has far-reaching implications for quality of care and training, as well as staff costs.

Length of stay and outcomes

There is very little information about the outcomes of long-term care in a residential setting. In a longitudinal study of admissions to care homes (Bebbington et al., 2001), measures of outcome were limited to changes in functional and cognitive ability, mortality, and destination (private households, other care homes or hospital). While these do not cover important aspects of welfare and quality of life, they are important both in themselves and for their implications for the long-term costs of caring for people admitted to care homes.

The study found that changes in dependency were greatest in the first six months, with survivors at six months being slightly better off on average than at the time of admission. Thereafter, there was a slow but steady decline. Improvements were most marked in those activities of daily living that relate to being in a better controlled environment, rather than any real indication that people had recovered in a way that might make them more fit to return to private households (Bebbington et al., 2001).

Between 1995 and 2000, very few people left a care home environment once admitted – the lifetime probability of returning to a private household once admitted was estimated as 11%. Of those that did, the great majority left fairly soon after admission. Rehabilitation was considered for 6% of people at the time of admission, but rarely took place. Failure to settle was given as the commonest reason for discharge back to private households, but it was evident that the majority of such people had been admitted with low levels of dependency, while for others an improvement in health was given as a reason for leaving care. Though the availability of informal care was often a factor enabling discharge, a significant number returned to live alone. This group had better survival prospects than those remaining in a care home (Bebbington et al., 2001).

Initially, mortality rates were high, especially among those admitted to nursing beds, but after about twelve months mortality settled to around 3% per month for the combined sample. Median survival for publicly funded residents on admission was 19.6 months. For those originally admitted to nursing beds it was 11.9 months, and for residential beds 26.8 months. As a few residents will live for a long while, the average length of survival was much greater than the median. Although this average cannot be calculated precisely until all have died, the best estimate was 29.7 months and almost certainly in the range 28.9–30.7 months.

The factors at admission that significantly raised subsequent mortality were, in order of significance: having a malignancy (cancer); having a low Barthel score (high dependency); old age; being a man; being admitted to a nursing home; being admitted from a hospital; having a respiratory illness; and being cognitively impaired. There was a seasonal effect, with higher death rates in winter (Bebbington et al., 2001).

It was identified above that care homes are a setting in which older people die, and palliative care is an integral part of supporting quality of life until death. As such, a 'good death' is an important outcome of the quality of care provided in care homes that is increasingly being highlighted (Hockley and Clark, 2002). The Command Paper *Building on the Best* set out a commitment to invest in training staff so that all adult patients nearing end of life have access to high quality, multiprofessional, specialist palliative care irrespective of diagnosis and are able to die in the place of their choice (Cm 6079, 2003). The extent to which this will impact on care homes is unclear since the palliative care provided by staff in care homes is regarded as generalist rather than specialist. The aims of the subsequent End of Life Care Initiative, however, include a reduction in the number of older people who are transferred from care homes to district general hospitals in the last week of life (Department of Health, 2004d). The extent to which older people's end of life in care homes is linked to a prognosis, and one that can be predicted precisely and planned, will necessarily influence the way in which palliative care can be provided and developed in care homes.

Gaps in knowledge

The lack of reliable basic data at a national level is of considerable concern when it comes to planning and policy appraisal. Moreover, since 2001, when 39% of places in independent older people's homes were nursing places, no official information has been available in the public domain about the proportion of places where nursing care is provided. The distinction is important because they are more likely to be privately run, the costs of care (and thus associated prices) are substantially higher than in care homes providing personal care, the homes are larger and residents are substantially more dependent.

The dated nature of detailed information about homes and residents is of concern given the rapidly changing context. While the Health Survey for England (Bajekal, 2002) does provide an opportunity to compare the characteristics of people in homes with those in the community, there is a lack of information about critical aspects of needs, most notably cognitive impairment, that are of immense significance in policy, planning and provision of care. Major changes in dependency levels were identified between 1986 and 1996, and the policies and incentives that led to the changes have continued since then. We also need to know more about the impact of the introduction of care standards and the use of homes for recuperative and rehabilitative care. In the past, combining short-term or day care and long-term care under the same roof was shown to be problematic for the permanent residents (Allen, 1983; Wright, 1995).

Another area where there is little information in the public domain is the provision of continuing care for younger disabled adults in care homes that primarily provide services for older people, and the multiple use of care homes in general. There is also a need for national data on the number and nature of transfers between care homes, due to 'consumer' dissatisfaction and evictions by providers, for example, as well as those due to changes in need, in order to gain a better understanding of placement change and the impact of service user 'consumer power' on the development of the market. More widely, it would be useful to identify whether and how access to services is changing over time, as new forms of housing, social and health care settings, and services are developed, either alongside or as a substitute for care homes. Information about the quantity and pattern of moves between homes, as well as the pattern of use and exit from other types of social care services would be an important part of this.

Perhaps the most significant gap in our understanding, however, relates to quality of care and outcomes, in particular from the perspective of residents. High levels of cognitive impairment among residents mean that this is a particularly challenging issue. Moreover, there is little information at a national level about the rapidly growing group of black and minority ethnic older residents.

Summary

Care homes provide continuing care for a very vulnerable group. Over the past 15 years, policy and financial incentives have led to an overwhelming dependence on independent provision for both publicly and self financed care. These incentives have also led to a reduction in the number of places and a dramatic rise in the levels of dependency of residents, although there is a lack of up-to-date data on the characteristics of homes or residents.

Concerns that capacity may not be sufficient have led to increased government funding, and some analysts predict future expansion. However, the implication of consolidation of the market is a loss of diversity in provision. Fewer and larger homes managed by corporate organisations mean reductions in choice for future residents, in terms of both type of home and location. Moreover, our analyses suggest that it is the homes most likely to close that are most able to generate the most supportive social climate.

References

Allen, I. (1983) *Short-Stay Residential Care for the Elderly*. London: Policy Studies Institute.

Bajekal, M. (2002) *Health Survey for England 2000: Care Homes and their Residents*. London: The Stationery Office.

Bebbington, A., Darton, R., Netten, A. (2001) *Care Homes for Older People: Volume 2. Admissions, Needs and Outcomes*. Canterbury: Personal Social Services Research Unit, University of Kent.

Care Standards Act 2000 (2000 c. 14) London: The Stationery Office.

Centre for Policy on Ageing (1984) *Home Life: A Code of Practice for Residential Care*. Report of a Working Party Sponsored by the Department of Health and Social Security. London: Centre for Policy on Ageing.

Centre for Policy on Ageing (1996) *A Better Home Life: A Code of Practice for Residential and Nursing Home Care*. Report of an Advisory Group convened by the Centre for Policy on Ageing and chaired by Kina, Lady Avebury. London: Centre for Policy on Ageing.

Cm 849 (1989) *Caring for People: Community Care in the Next Decade and Beyond*. London: HMSO.

Cm 4169 (1998) *Modernising Social Services: Promoting Independence, Improving Protection, Raising Standards.* London: The Stationery Office.

Cm 4192-I (1999) *With Respect to Old Age: Long Term Care – Rights and Responsibilities.* A Report by the Royal Commission on Long Term Care (Chairman: Professor Sir Stewart Sutherland). London: The Stationery Office.

Cm 4818-I (2000) *The NHS Plan: A Plan for Investment, A Plan for Reform.* London: The Stationery Office.

Cm 6079 (2003) *Building on the Best: Choice, Responsiveness and Equity in the NHS.* London: The Stationery Office.

Community Care and Health (Scotland) Act 2002 (2002 asp 5) Edinburgh: The Stationery Office.

Dalley, G. (1997) A better home life: the components of quality in continuing care. In: Centre for Policy on Ageing (ed.) *Achieving a Better Home Life: Establishing and Maintaining Quality in Continuing Care for Older People.* CPA Reports 20. London: Centre for Policy on Ageing.

Dalley, G., Unsworth, L., Keightley, D., Waller, M., Davies, T., Morton, R. (2004) *How Do We Care? The Availability of Registered Care Homes and Children's Homes in England and their Performance against National Minimum Standards 2002–03.* National Care Standards Commission. London: The Stationery Office.

Darton, R. (2004) What types of home are closing? The characteristics of homes which closed between 1996 and 2001. *Health and Social Care in the Community* **12** (30), 254–64.

Darton, R., Netten, A., Forder, J. (2003) The cost implications of the changing population and characteristics of care homes. *International Journal of Geriatric Psychiatry* **18** (3), 236–43.

Davies, B.P., Knapp, M.R.J. (1981) *Old People's Homes and the Production of Welfare.* London: Routledge & Kegan Paul.

Department of Health (2001a) *National Service Framework for Older People.* London: Department of Health.

Department of Health (2001b) *Community Care Statistics 2001. Residential Personal Social Services for Adults, England.* Statistical Bulletin 2001/29. London: Department of Health.

Department of Health (2001c) *Charges for Residential Accommodation – CRAG Amendment No. 15.* LAC(2001)25. London: Department of Health.

Department of Health (2001d) *Care Homes for Older People: National Minimum Standards.* London: The Stationery Office.

Department of Health (2002a) *National Service Framework for Older People – Supporting Implementation. Intermediate Care: Moving Forward.* London: Department of Health.

Department of Health (2002b) *Expanded Services and Increased Choices for Older People: Investment and Reform for Older People's Social Services.* Press Release 2002/0324. London: Department of Health.

Department of Health (2002c) *£200m Allocated to Councils to Further Reduce 'Bedblocking'. Delayed Discharges Reduced by 10% Since September.* Press Release 2002/0007. London: Department of Health.

Department of Health (2002d) *Care Homes for Older People and Younger Adults: Consultation Document – Proposed Amended Environmental Standards.* London: Department of Health.

Department of Health (2003) *Care Homes for Older People: National Minimum Standards,* 3rd ed. London: The Stationery Office.

Department of Health (2004a) *Personal Social Services Expenditure and Unit Costs: England: 2002–2003.* Statistical Bulletin 2004/02. London: Department of Health.

Department of Health (2004b) *Charges for Residential Accommodation – CRAG Amendment No. 21*. LAC (2004)9. London: Department of Health.

Department of Health (2004c) *Increased Nursing Care Funding for Care Home Residents*. Press Release 2004/0081. London: Department of Health.

Department of Health (2004d) *Letter to SHA Chief Executives and Directors of Performance: Building on the Best: End of Life Care Initiative*. London: Department of Health.

Eborall, C. (2003) *The State of the Social Care Workforce in England: First Annual Report of the Topss England Workforce Intelligence Unit*. Leeds: Topss England.

Forder, J., Netten, A. (2000) The price of placements in residential and nursing home care: the effects of contracts and competition. *Health Economics* **9** (7), 643–57.

Health and Social Care Act 2001 (2001 c. 15) London: The Stationery Office.

Hockley, J., Clark, D. (2002) *Palliative Care for Older People in Care Homes*. Buckingham: Open University Press.

Holden, C. (2002) British government policy and the concentration of ownership in long-term care provision. *Ageing and Society* **22** (1), 79–94.

House of Commons Health Committee (2004) *Palliative Care*. Fourth Report of Session 2003–04. Volume I. HC 454-I. London: The Stationery Office.

Jacobs, S., Rummery, K. (2002) Nursing homes in England and their capacity to provide rehabilitation and intermediate care services. *Social Policy and Administration* **36** (7), 735–52.

Kerrison, S., Pollock, A. (2001) Regulating nursing homes: caring for older people in the private sector in England. *British Medical Journal* **323**, 566–9.

Laing and Buisson (2000) *Care of Elderly People: Market Survey 2000*, 13th ed. London: Laing and Buisson.

Laing and Buisson (2003) *Laing's Healthcare Market Review 2003–2004*. London: Laing and Buisson.

Laing and Buisson (2004) *Care of Elderly People: Market Survey 2004*, 17th ed. London: Laing and Buisson.

Mahoney, F.I., Barthel, D.W. (1965) Functional evaluation: the Barthel Index. *Maryland State Medical Journal* **14**, 61–5.

Moos, R., Lemke, S. (1992) *Sheltered Care Environment Scale Manual*. Palo Alto, California: Center for Health Care Evaluation, Department of Veterans Affairs and Stanford University Medical Centers.

Morris, J.N., Fries, B.E., Mehr, D.R., Hawes, C., Phillips, C., Mor, V., Lipsitz, L.A. (1994) MDS Cognitive Performance Scale. *Journal of Gerontology: Medical Sciences* **49** (4), M174–M182.

National Assembly for Wales (2003) *Digest of Welsh Local Area Statistics 2003*. Cardiff: National Assembly for Wales.

National Health Service and Community Care Act 1990 (1990 c. 19) London: HMSO.

Netten, A., Darton, R. (2001) Formal and informal support prior to admission: are self-funders being admitted to care homes unnecessarily? In: Tester, S., Archibald, C., Rowlings, C. and Turner, S. (eds) *Quality in Later Life: Rights, Rhetoric and Reality. Proceedings of the British Society of Gerontology 30th Annual Conference, Stirling, 31 August–2 September 2001*. Stirling: Department of Applied Social Science, University of Stirling, 60–64.

Netten, A., Darton, R. (2003) The effect of financial incentives and access to services on self-funded admissions to long-term care. *Social Policy and Administration* **37** (5), 483–97.

Netten, A., Bebbington, A., Darton, R., Forder, J. (2001) *Care Homes for Older People: Volume 1. Facilities, Residents and Costs*. Canterbury: Personal Social Services Research Unit, University of Kent.

Netten, A., Bebbington, A., Darton, R., Forder, J., Miles, K. (1998) *1996 Survey of Care Homes for Elderly People: Final Report*. PSSRU Discussion Paper No. 1423/2. Canterbury: Personal Social Services Research Unit, University of Kent.

Netten, A., Darton, R., Williams, J. (2002a) *The Rate, Causes and Consequences of Home Closures*. PSSRU Discussion Paper No. 1741/2. Canterbury: Personal Social Services Research Unit, University of Kent.

Netten, A., Darton, R., Curtis, L. (2002b) *Self-Funded Admissions to Care Homes*. A report of research carried out by the Personal Social Services Research Unit, University of Kent on behalf of the Department for Work and Pensions. Department for Work and Pensions Research Report No. 159. Leeds: Corporate Document Services.

Netten, A., Williams, J., Darton, R. (2005) Care-home closures in England: causes and implications. *Ageing and Society*.

Pacolet, J.B., Hilde, R.L., Katia, V. (2000) *Social Protection for Dependency in Old Age: A Study of the Fifteen EU Member States and Norway*. Aldershot: Ashgate.

Parker, R.A. (1987) *The Elderly and Residential Care: Australian Lessons for Britain*. Aldershot: Gower.

Regulation of Care (Scotland) Act 2001 (2001 asp 8) Edinburgh: The Stationery Office.

Residential Forum (1996) *Creating a Home from Home: A Guide to Standards*. London: National Institute for Social Work.

Scottish Executive (2003) *Scottish Community Care Statistics 2002*. Edinburgh: Scottish Executive.

Social and Health Care Workforce Group (2002) *Independent Sector Workforce Survey 2001*. Provisional Report.

Social Services Inspectorate (SSI) (1989) *Towards a Climate of Confidence*. Report of a National Inspection of Management Arrangements for Public Sector Residential Care for Elderly People. London: Department of Health.

Townsend, P. (1962) *The Last Refuge: A Survey of Residential Institutions and Homes for the Aged in England and Wales*. London: Routledge & Kegan Paul.

Vladek, B. (1980) *Unloving Care: The Nursing Home Tragedy*. New York: Basic Books.

Wagner, G. (1988) *Residential Care: A Positive Choice*. Report of the Independent Review of Residential Care. London: HMSO.

Warburton, R.W. (1994) *Home and Away*. London: Department of Health.

Williams, J., Netten, A., Hardy, B., Matosevic, T., Ware, P. (2002) *Care Home Closures: the Provider Perspective*. PSSRU Discussion Paper No. 1753/2. Canterbury: Personal Social Services Research Unit, University of Kent.

Wright, F. (1995) *Opening Doors: A Case Study of Multi-Purpose Residential Homes*. London: HMSO.

Chapter 14

Interdisciplinary Working and Education in Continuing Care

Abigail Masterson and Sian Maslin-Prothero

Introduction

In the United Kingdom, since 1948 the NHS has aimed to provide a full range of health services to all on the basis of need, free at the point of delivery. In comparison social care is not a universal service and has always been means tested. However, in practice the boundaries of health and social care have always been unclear, services have varied greatly from place to place and this fluid boundary has been exploited as a means of cost shifting between services and agencies (Maslin-Prothero and Masterson, 1998).

Continuing care itself has been a key focus for such boundary disputes both in terms of definition, funding and workforce. For example, the nursing and social care literature during the late 1980s often contained discussions about whether or not a bath for an older person in the community should be described as a 'health' bath or a 'social' bath and therefore which service should be responsible for providing it and which workforce should deliver it. Indeed in 1995 the Department of Health issued guidance clarifying NHS responsibilities for meeting continuing health care needs and directed commissioning agencies to develop criteria for the purchasing of continuing care (Department of Health, 1995). It was suggested (for a nursing audience and from a nursing perspective) that continuing care includes: holistic individualised continuous assessment and collaborative patient/client care; planning focused on the achievement of self care; direct care delivery and delegation to support staff; intradisciplinary and multidisciplinary team work; prevention and health promotion; teaching patients/clients skills which may enhance their quality of life, maintain optimum functioning and prevent deterioration; evaluating care provided; and measuring outcomes (Maslin-Prothero and Masterson, 1998) – a definition that works equally well in an interdisciplinary context.

Policy trends that have and will continue to have an impact on the future shape of the health and social care workforce and thus continuing care services include: the movement of services from secondary to primary care; closer working between health and social care sectors; and government desire to break down the demarcations between different professional groups and configure the health and social care workforce differently; and, of course, a growing acknowledgement of the primacy of the client/patient in shaping service design and delivery.

Many different patient/client populations including children, people with chronic diseases such as asthma, diabetes etc., people with mental health and learning disabilities/difficulties, and older people require continuing care. It is beyond the scope of this chapter to cover all of these groups in detail so a client centred approach is adopted. The concepts of interdisciplinary working and education are considered within the context of clients with continuing care needs regardless of the lead service, agency or profession responsible for funding or delivering the service. Client/patient scenarios are used throughout to illustrate the complexities involved.

First, the policy context surrounding interdisciplinary working and education in continuing care is reviewed briefly. Second, the concept of interdisciplinary working is presented using examples from a diverse range of continuing care services including rheumatology and learning disability. Third, initiatives in interdisciplinary education at pre- and post-qualifying levels are considered. Finally, the challenges to professional self-regulation caused by the development of generic health and social care competencies are reviewed.

The policy context

The Health Act 1999 stated that NHS bodies had a statutory duty to cooperate with each other and local authorities; enabled the pooling of budgets and resources to facilitate joint working between health and social agencies and increased the arrangements for ensuring quality in service delivery. The Health and Social Care Act 2001 gave the Government powers to direct local authorities and health care organisations to pool their budgets, especially where services are failing; and reinforced their earlier commitment to interdisciplinary working and quality. Quality continuing care services depend fundamentally on the availability of an appropriately trained workforce able to perform its role effectively and efficiently. *The NHS Plan* (Department of Health, 2000a) acknowledged that:

> 'radical changes are needed in the way staff work to reduce waiting times and deliver modern, patient centred services' (para. 9.1)

It went on to describe how the traditional patterns of professional practice were effectively holding back innovation and how their plans would effectively:

> 'shatter old demarcations which have held back staff and slowed down care' (para. 9.5)

This vision of a reconfigured workforce has been echoed in all subsequent policy (see, for example, NHSE, 1999; Department of Health, 2000b; 2001a; 2001b).

In addition, the need to improve efficiency and cost effectiveness has provoked a re-evaluation of the manner in which services are delivered and has led to an examination of skill mix and the development of new roles to fill some of the gaps in provision. Furthermore, 'investment and reform in NHS staff' (Department of Health, 2001a) committed the NHS to increase its flexibility in their education and recruitment.

Government expectations expressed consistently in education policy include recognition that the skill levels to do most jobs are increasing and that health and social care staff should be lifelong learners. Education is seen as a means of supporting the implementation of service change, achieving health gain and fulfilling the personal development needs and career aspirations of practitioners. The Government believes that education should be clearly linked to competence measured by national occupational standards and that there should be greater emphasis on work based systems of learning, E-learning and distance learning. Education and training is to be employer driven and closely linked to service needs. The Government is committed to widening access, reducing attrition, and developing flexible pathways with multiple stepping on and off points. Student and patient/client involvement in curriculum development and quality assurance is expected and interprofessional provision is advocated (Department of Health, 2000b; 2002a; 2002b; Department for Education and Skills, 2003). As Horder suggests (2003, p. xiii):

'. . . change is inevitable, if only because of the increasing capability, complexity and cost of the services, alongside the needs and developing expectations of patients, clients and carers. The alternative is confusion, duplication and inefficiency.'

Interdisciplinary working

Interdisciplinary working, where professionals work towards shared client centred goals and where team members cross traditional professional boundaries to meet client need, has led to the development of a range of new roles and the demise of some older roles in continuing care. For example, in rheumatology services, when collecting data for the Exploring New Roles in Practice Project (funded by the Department of Health as part of their Policy Research Programme's Human Resources and Effectiveness Initiative) it was discovered that nurses, physiotherapists and occupational therapists in various parts of the United Kingdom were developing their roles to become 'rheumatology practitioners' (Read et al., 2001). Regardless of their original professional background they were taking on a new autonomous role as the lead practitioner in the continuing care of rheumatology patients with chronic conditions. Similarly, the development of a new specialist role, the Older People Nurse Specialist, has also been advocated as a means of comprehensively and holistically assessing and meeting older people's continuing care needs (Heath and Masterson, 2001).

On the other hand, nursing and health specialist roles in learning disability services have practically disappeared over the past decade. The White Paper *Valuing People: a New Strategy for Learning Disability for the 21st Century* (Department of Health, 2001a) set out the Government's plans for improving the lives of people with learning disabilities. These plans were built around people with learning disabilities, their families, local councils, the health service and voluntary organisations working together. Joint investment planning was seen as a practical means for bringing together the wide range of organisations that support people with learning disabilities. Also, by agencies working together in a coordinated way it was hoped that services would focus on what people with learning disabilities actually need. This policy was welcomed by both clients and professionals. Although an ostensibly positive move, its operationalisation has however coincided with a shift away from a professional to a non-professional workforce in the provision of learning disability services (Meads, 2003), and one might argue a social care takeover of these services rather than interdisciplinary working.

Case management and coordination is now predominantly managed by social workers and the majority of continuing care for people with learning disabilities now takes place in the community. The number of people entering education to become registered learning disabilities nurses is falling, and their roles and responsibilities are being taken over by social care key workers with National Vocational Qualifications (NVQs) at levels 2 and 3. Consequently responsibility for meeting continuing care needs in learning disability services has shifted from an expensive professional health care workforce to a cheaper currently unregistered social care workforce, a move that it could be argued is more about saving money than providing the most effective and appropriate care for individuals and their families.

The Government's latest annual report on learning disability *Valuing People: Moving Forward Together* (Department of Health, 2004) illustrates the different ways that the Government has tried to move the concerns of people living with learning disabilities forward, and demonstrates new ways of working and how people with learning disabilities are influencing key decisions and policy makers. Despite all these positive exhortations, people with learning disabilities and their carers were never given a choice about the wholesale transfer of their services to social care. As Manthorpe (2003) usefully points out, models of interdisciplinary working do not always meet the needs or priorities of clients/patients and interdisciplinary working can just be a way of increasing the power of the professionals. Furthermore there are still important issues that need to be addressed such as better support for people with learning disabilities from black and ethnic minority communities; as reinforced by the Healthcare Commission report (2004).

One of the barriers to interdisciplinary working in continuing care for all client groups has been that all of the different professionals involved have maintained their own patient/client records. By 2005 it is expected that electronic patient records will be created for every NHS patient and some pilots have already

been established. Staff will be able to access and update patient/client information and patients and clients will also be able to check and add information to
their own record. As Reeves and Freeth (2003) note, such developments present
health and social care staff with new opportunities for collaboration as they can
overcome the need to share the same physical space and time for collaborative
activities.

However even if professionals from the social and health sectors share patient/
client records the different 'languages' in use can still prove to be a barrier. For
example, Miller and Freeman (2003) discuss the contested concept of key worker
role. In their research with community psychiatric nurses (CPNs) and psychiatric
social workers, CPNs saw the key worker role as a coordination role whereas
social workers saw it as a coordination *and* action role. Such misunderstand-
ings had a negative impact on client care, and consequently Miller and Freeman
recommend the need for ongoing discussion at all levels in order to identify and
work through these differences in understanding.

As already identified, an outcome of the modernisation of the health and
social care services in the UK has been the increased move towards interdisciplinary working in continuing care services (Miller et al., 2001). Effective
interdisciplinary working between health and social care professionals in
such services is believed to promote improved client/patient care (Borrill et al.,
2000; 2001; Freeth and Reeves, 2002). However, for teams to work effectively,
traditional divisions between professions will need to be challenged, and ways
of working differently and collaboratively explored. This requires health and
social care professionals to become more flexible and develop a greater mutual
understanding and respect for each other (Reeves et al., 2002; Humphris and
Hean, 2004) and interdisciplinary education has been promoted as a means of
achieving this.

Interdisciplinary education

The first comprehensive framework for learning and development for all NHS
staff was launched in 2001 (Department of Health, 2001b). The framework covers
all forms of learning, from induction, adult literacy and numeracy skills and
vocational training; through to pre- and post-registration education; to continuing
professional development, management and leadership development. All NHS
staff are identified as requiring core skills in communicating effectively with
patients and colleagues; using information effectively and sensitively; understanding how the NHS and their local organisation works; working effectively
in teams; and keeping their skills and competence up to date. Universities have
been directed to regularly engage and consult with the NHS at local and national
levels concerning the review and development of curricula and programmes so
that education for health and social care staff becomes more responsive to the
needs of the NHS (Department of Health, 2000b). Interprofessional education

has thus become a key feature of social and health care education across England and common foundation programmes have been developed to enable students to switch careers and training paths more easily.

Many learned books and articles have debated the difference between inter-disciplinary and interprofessional education but, in agreement with Griffiths and Hewison (2004), there is a need to look beyond these terms and engage instead with what this approach encompasses, and so for the purposes of this chapter these terms are used synonymously to mean joint learning that people from different occupations actively engage in (Barr, 1994).

As Glen (2004, p. 1) notes, for over 30 years interdisciplinary education has been promoted as a means of implementing reforms in health and social care; indeed, 'resistance to interprofessional education has become politically unaccept-able'. Successive policy documents have emphasised the Government's com-mitment to interprofessional education pre- and post-qualification (Department of Health, 2000b; 2001b; 2002c). Interprofessional education is believed, although the evidence is scanty at best (Ovretveit et al., 1997; Hewison, 2004), to enable health and social care practitioners to deliver more client centred services and to be fundamental to successful joint working across health and social care.

Barr (2003) reports on the experience of the mid-1990s where courses were designed to prepare students for joint qualification as social workers and learn-ing disability nurses. The impetus for this change came indirectly from the Jay Committee Report (1979) which recommended the replacement of a medical model by a social model for learning disability services; and concerns by service managers that neither a nurse education or a social work education on its own would equip staff adequately for the new community services established follow-ing the closure of the large hospitals. The numbers involved have been small, the impact on practice correspondingly small and independent evaluation lack-ing; and as Barr notes, this initiative involving dual qualifications and combined professions sits uncomfortably with the contemporary notion of interprofessional education.

More recently there has been significant investment in initiatives to encourage 'common learning' in pre-registration health and social care programmes. The Department of Health is committed to the implementation of interprofessional education in all pre-registration health and social care programmes across all higher education institutions in England. There are four leading-edge sites iden-tified to lead the way in interprofessional learning. These are: the Universities of Portsmouth and Southampton, the University of Sheffield, King's College London and the University of Newcastle. At the Universities of Portsmouth and Southampton, 'common learning' is the mechanism through which students are enabled to learn about interprofessional working. This theme runs throughout their pre-registration education and involves students from 11 health and social care professional groups working together on a variety of different projects. Such projects include mapping local services, working as a team, developing shared and collaborative learning strategies, and client/patient focused case studies. This process is facilitated by social and health care professionals drawn from practice and education (Health Care Innovation Unit, 2004).

Davies (2000) suggests that when incorporating new models of collaboration it is not what people have in common but their differences that make collaborative work more powerful than working separately. Through working together there needs to be an acknowledgement that all participants bring equally valid knowledge and expertise from their professional and personal experience. Beattie (2003) when discussing the future of health and social care alliances highlights the importance of abandoning stereotypical thinking and moving towards new, flexible and open deployments of power and renegotiating boundaries and institutional identities.

Prior to 2000 the bulk of interprofessional education took place in the post-qualifying sector, and questions have been raised about the right place to introduce interprofessional education. Glen (2004) summarises the arguments thus: introducing interprofessional education post-qualification is better because by then students have sufficiently developed the experience and the confidence required to draw upon their learning with other professional groups. Alternatively, interprofessional education is only effective if delivered before qualification when students have not been socialised into their own profession and developed the negative attitudes that are often formed in this socialisation process. There are many examples of universities that have developed post-qualifying, interprofessional programmes that bring together members of different occupational groups to debate and discuss issues relating to their interdisciplinary work and to further collaboration. One such course is the Anglia Polytechnic University (2004) MSc in Interdisciplinary Childhood and Youth Studies. These programmes aim to enable students to develop new perspectives, knowledge and skills through the sharing of experiences. Also, to advance practice by increasing interdisciplinary understanding and cooperation and ultimately to improve outcomes for clients and patients. Interprofessional education is also developing across Europe, and Goble (2003) describes a number of initiatives in Sweden and France. The European Network for the Development of Multiprofessional Education in health sciences (EMPE) was set up and supported by the WHO in the 1990s. EMPE was incorporated into *The Network: Towards Unity for Health* in 2001 and continues to be supported by the World Health Organization (TUFH, 2004).

Despite all these initiatives the majority of professionals, regardless of care setting, continue to work in uni-professional silos once qualified, and in many of the universities where interprofessional learning takes place this does not include medicine. At the assistant professional level however, new qualifications such as foundation degrees and NVQs in care have been developed in domains that have previously been the remit of registered professionals and are crossing traditional professional boundaries. Foundation degrees are intended to help education providers supply the high-quality graduates needed to address the shortage of intermediate level skills such as those required by assistant practitioners, as well as making higher education more affordable, accessible and appealing to a wider range of students – thereby widening participation in HE and stimulating lifelong learning (HEFCE, 2000). The Government envisages that a significant proportion of the future resource available to expand higher education will be focused on foundation degrees (Department for Education and Skills, 2003). Many foundation degrees aim to produce an assistant practitioner who can work across health and social care. Often providers of continuing care services have been developed in the design of such programmes and are supporting their workforce to undertake these courses. Both foundation degrees and NVQs are vocationally based programmes where the acquisition of competence is key.

Competence

Health professionals have historically resisted the notion of cross-professional competency based assessment systems as they challenge the whole concept of a profession as having control of a unique and distinct body of knowledge (Masterson, 2002). However, previous research (Dowling et al., 1998) identified the ad hoc nature of the training and preparation provided to many nurses and allied health professionals working in new roles and in new ways. The majority of postholders in the rheumatology example cited earlier (Read et al., 2001) received some form of further training. However the extent of this varied: most was in-house, and tailored to the post itself rather than being generic and transferable. For instance, the physiotherapist working as the rheumatology practitioner received training from the consultant who led the team and was then only assessed on completing specific procedures such as joint injections rather than other core skills such as information giving. In other words the training these postholders received was focused on the acquisition of particular clinical skills rather than assessment of the individual's competence in performing the complete role.

One way to overcome this 'local' approach to training would be to develop nationally set competency based assessment systems (Cameron and Masterson, 2003). Work currently being undertaken by Skills for Health, the Sector Skills Council for Health, and Topss England – the strategic workforce development body for social care – may help. They are in the process of developing a variety of national occupational standards and competencies for the health and social care workforce. For example, in relation to mental health, Skills for Health (2005) has developed a set of Occupational Standards as given in Box 14.1.

These competencies cross traditional service, sector and professional boundaries and focus on 'what' needs to be done rather than 'who' should do it, which may be why thus far National Occupational Standards have not been eagerly adopted by the professions.

Box 14.1　National Occupational Standards for Mental Health E (MH_E Units).

MH_E1	Contribute to the development, provision and review of care programmes
MH_E2	Contribute to the assessment of individuals needs and the planning of packages of care
MH_E3	Contribute to the monitoring and review of care packages
MH_E4	Plan and agree service responses which meet individuals' identified needs and circumstances
MH_E5	Co-ordinate, monitor and review service responses to meet individuals' needs and circumstances
MH_E6	Work with individuals with mental health needs to negotiate and agree plans for addressing those needs
MH_E7	Contribute to the planning, implementation and evaluation of therapeutic programmes to enable individuals to manage their behaviour
MH_E8	Respond to crisis situations
MH_E9	Maintain active continuing contact with individuals and work with them to monitor their mental health needs

Source: Skills for Health (www.skillsforhealth.org.uk).

Regulation

Professional self-regulation is a contract between the public and a profession. It allows the professions to regulate their own members in order to protect the public from poor or unsafe professional practice. This notion of public protection by the professionals feels rather paternalistic in the light of a better educated public that is increasingly less tolerant of professional power (Engel and Gursky, 2003). New role and service developments such as those described earlier in relation to rheumatology and learning disabilities also pose a challenge to traditional conceptions of professional regulation. In fact the regulatory implications of new role development have challenged the regulatory body for nursing, midwifery and health visiting – the Nursing and Midwifery Council (NMC) and its predecessor the United Kingdom Central Council for Nursing, Midwifery and Health Visiting (UKCC) for the past decade. At what stage does a new role such as that of the rheumatology practitioner or the case manager in learning disability or mental health services become so distinct from the individual's previous professional background and training that a new or additional layer of regulation is required? Should that regulation be profession-specific or cross professions? Early attempts to regulate different levels of practice in nursing have been firmly tied to the acquisition of higher levels of education. However, extensive work with patient representative groups on behalf of the UKCC highlighted that the public expects that regulation should be on the basis of competence rather than achievement of educational qualifications (UKCC, 2001).

A key part of a professional's identity is their observance of their professional code of conduct; each of these codes refers to the importance of effective interprofessional team working. However, as Hewison (2004) notes, this commitment contradicts each code's fundamental focus on the uniqueness of their individual contribution. Some commentators have suggested that there should be a pan-professional code to assure the public that, whoever the professional was, their aims were the same; however, Wall (2003, p. 77) suggests that:

> 'Such a code will be generalised to such an extent that it would suffer from the platitudes found in many an organisation's mission statement . . .'

Each health and social care regulatory body also has different standards and processes but the relatively newly established Council for Healthcare Regulators has been urged to streamline the processes of regulation across member professions. Nevertheless, the majority of the continuing care workforce is currently unregulated although at the time of writing the Department of Health has just completed a consultation on the future regulation of health care assistants.

Summary

There is no doubt that the boundaries between health and social care are constantly shifting and the way the health and social care workforce works and learns is currently undergoing tremendous change. Continuing care services are delivered to a wide range of different patient and client groups in a variety of health and social care settings many of which sit on the border of health and social care. It has been shown that interdisciplinary working has led to the development of new roles and the demise of older roles in continuing care and has coincided with a move from services being mainly controlled by a regulated professional health workforce in institutional settings to services being delivered in patients' or clients' own homes by an unregulated social care workforce. Interdisciplinary education has been advocated as a means of supporting and encouraging interdisciplinary working yet there is little evidence to date to support this and considerable disagreement about whether or not such education should occur pre- or post-qualification for maximum effect. The Government's desire for a competent and flexible workforce poses a significant challenge to traditional concepts of the nature of the professions. Despite the rhetoric of patient or client led services in continuing care there is little evidence of patients/clients and their carers being involved as partners in discussions about the desirability or otherwise of interdisciplinary working and learning in these services.

References

Anglia Polytechnic University (2004) *MSc in Interdisciplinary Childhood and Youth Studies.* http://www.anglia.ac.uk/health/prospectus/courses/postgrad MScInterprofessionalPractice.htm (accessed 06.07.04).

Barr, H. (1994) NVQs and their implications for interprofessional collaboration. In: Leathard, A. (ed.) *Going Interprofessional: Working together for Health and Welfare*. London: Routledge, pp. 90–108.

Barr, H. (2003) Unpacking interprofessional education. In: Leathard, A. (ed.) *Interprofessional Collaboration: From Policy to Practice in Health and Social Care*. Hove: Brunner-Routledge, pp. 265–79.

Beattie, A. (2003) Journeys into third space? Health alliances and the challenge of border crossing. In: Leathard, A. (ed.) *Interprofessional Collaboration: From Policy to Practice in Health and Social Care*. Hove; Brunner-Routledge, pp. 146–57.

Borrill, C., West, M., Shapiro, D., Rees, A. (2000) Team working and effectiveness in health care. *British Journal of Health Care Management* **6**, 364–71.

Borrill, C., West, M., Dawson, J., Shapiro, D., Rees, A., Richards, A., Garrod, S., Carletta, J., Carter, A. (2001) *Team Working and Effectiveness in Health Care: Findings from the Health Care Team Effectiveness Project*. University of Aston, Human Communications Research Centre, Universities of Glasgow and Edinburgh, Psychological Therapies Research Centre, University of Leeds. Aston: University of Aston.

Cameron, A., Masterson, A. (2003) Reconfiguring the clinical workforce. In: Davies, C. (ed.) *The Future Healthcare Workforce*. Basingstoke: Palgrave Macmillan, pp. 68–86.

Davies, C. (2000) Getting health professionals to work together. *British Medical Journal* **320**, 1021–2.

Department for Education and Skills (2003) *The Future of Higher Education*. London: DfES.

Department of Health (1995) *NHS Responsibilities for Meeting Continuing Care Needs*. HSC 95/8 LAC 95/5. London: Department of Health.

Department of Health (2000a) *The NHS Plan: A Plan for Investment, A Plan for Reform*. London: Department of Health.

Department of Health (2000b) *A Health Service of All the Talents: Developing the NHS Workforce*. Consultation document. London: Department of Health.

Department of Health (2001a) *Valuing People: A New Strategy for Learning Disability for the 21st Century*. London: Department of Health.

Department of Health (2001b) *Working Together, Learning Together: A Framework for Lifelong Learning for the NHS*. London: Department of Health.

Department of Health (2002a) *HR in the NHS Plan – More Staff Working Differently*. London: Department of Health.

Department of Health (2002b) *Learning from Bristol: The Department of Health's Response to the Public Inquiry into Children's Heart Surgery at the Bristol Royal Infirmary 1984–1995*. London: The Stationery Office.

Department of Health (2002c) *Liberating the Talents: Helping Primary Care Trusts and Nurses to Deliver the NHS Plan*. London: Department of Health.

Department of Health (2004) *Valuing People: Moving Forward Together – the Government's Annual Report on Learning Disability*. London: Department of Health.

Dowling, S., Doyal, L., Cameron, A. (1998) *Challenging Practice*. Bristol: Policy Press.

Engel, C., Gursky, E. (2003) Management and interprofessional collaboration. In: Leathard, A. (ed.) (2003) *Interprofessional Collaboration: From Policy to Practice in Health and Social Policy*. Hove: Brunner-Routledge, pp. 44–55.

Freeth, D., Reeves, S. (2002) Evaluation of an interprofessional training ward: pilot phase. In: Leiba, T. and Glen, S. (eds) *Multi-Professional Learning for Nurses: Breaking the Boundaries*. Basingstoke: Palgrave, pp. 116–38.

Glen, S. (2004) Interprofessional education: the policy context. In: Glen, S. and Leiba, T. (eds) *Interprofessional Post-qualifying Education for Nurses: Working Together in Health and Social Care*. Basingstoke: Palgrave Macmillan, pp. 1–15.

Goble, R. (2003) Multi-professional education in Europe: an overview. In: Leathard, A. (ed.) *Interprofessional Collaboration: From Policy to Practice in Health and Social Care*. Hove: Brunner-Routledge, pp. 324–34.

Griffiths, M., Hewison, A. (2004) How to work with other professionals: multiprofessional and collaborative working. In: Hyde, J. and Cook, M.J. (eds) *Managing and Supporting People in Health Care*. Edinburgh: Baillière Tindall, pp. 35–57.

Health Care Innovation Unit (2004) *Common Learning*. http://www.hciu.soton.ac.uk/commonlearning.htm (accessed 06/07/04).

Healthcare Commission (2004) *State of Healthcare*. London: Healthcare Commission.

Heath, H., Masterson, A. (2001) *Developing an Older People's Specialist Nurse: A Feasibility Study* (Unpublished). London: Royal College of Nursing/Help the Aged.

Hewison, A. (2004) *Management for Nurses and Health Professionals*. Oxford: Blackwell.

Higher Education Funding Council for England (HEFCE) (2000) Foundation Degree Prospectus. Bristol: HEFCE.

Horder, J. (2003) Foreword. In: Leathard, A. (ed.) *Interprofessional Collaboration: From Policy to Practice in Health and Social Care*. Hove: Brunner-Routledge, pp. xiii–xiv.

Humphris, D., Hean, S. (2004) Educating the workforce: building the evidence about interprofessional learning. *Journal of Health Service Research and Policy* **9** (1), 24–7.

Jay Committee (1979) *Report of the Committee of Enquiry into Mental Handicap Nursing and Care*. London: HMSO.

Leathard, A. (ed.) (2003) *Interprofessional Collaboration: From Policy to Practice in Health and Social Policy*. Hove: Brunner-Routledge.

Manthorpe, J. (2003) The perspectives of users and carers. In: Leathard, A. (ed.) (2003) *Interprofessional Collaboration: From Policy to Practice in Health and Social Care*. Hove: Brunner-Routledge, pp. 238–48.

Maslin-Prothero, S., Masterson, A. (1998) Continuing care: developing a policy analysis for nursing. *Journal of Advanced Nursing* **28** (3), 548–53.

Masterson, A. (2002) Cross-boundary working: a macro-political analysis of the impact on professional roles. *Journal of Clinical Nursing* **11**, 331–9.

Meads, G. (2003) New primary care policies: from professions to professionalism. In: Leathard, A. (ed.) *Interprofessional Collaboration: From Policy to Practice in Health and Social Care*. Hove: Brunner-Routledge, pp. 133–45.

Miller, C., Freeman, M. (2003) Clinical teamwork: the impact of policy on collaborative practice. In: Leathard, A. (ed.) *Interprofessional Collaboration: From Policy to Practice in Health and Social Care*. Hove: Brunner-Routledge, pp. 121–32.

Miller, C., Freeman, M., Ross, N. (2001) *Interprofessional Practice in Health and Social Care*. London: Arnold.

NHS Executive (NHSE) (1999) *Agenda for Change*. Leeds: NHS Executive.

Ovretveit, J., Mathias, P., Thompson, T. (eds) (1997) *Interprofessional Working for Health and Social Care*. Houndmills: Macmillan.

Read, S., Doyal, L., Vaughan, B., et al. (2001) *Exploring New Roles in Practice: final report*. Sheffield: School of Health and Related Research, University of Sheffield.

Reeves, S., Freeth, D. (2003) New forms of technology, new forms of collaboration. In: Leathard, A. (ed.) *Interprofessional Collaboration: From Policy to Practice in Health and Social Care*. Hove: Brunner-Routledge, pp. 79–92.

Reeves, S., Freeth, D., McCrorie, P., Perry, D. (2002) 'It teaches you what to expect in future' interprofessional learning on a training ward for medical, nursing, occupational therapy and physiotherapy students. *Medical Education* **36** (4), 337–45.

Skills for Health (2005) *Standards for Mental Health – E. National Occupational Standards*. www.skillsforhealth.org.uk.

Towards Unity for Health (TUFH) (2004) *The Network: Towards Unity for Health.* www.the-networktufh.org (accessed 11 October 2004).

United Kingdom Central Council for Nursing, Midwifery and Health Visiting (UKCC) (2001) *Report of the Higher Level of Practice Pilot and Project.* London: UKCC.

Wall, A. (2003) Some ethical issues arising from interprofessional working. In: Leathard, A. (ed.) *Interprofessional Collaboration: From Policy to Practice in Health and Social Care.* Hove: Brunner-Routledge, pp. 69–78.

Part 3
Involvement of Carers and Consumers

Chapter 15

Carers and Caregiving in the Context of Intermediate and Continuing Care

Diane Seddon and Catherine Robinson

Introduction

Drawing on the existing policy, practice and research literature, this chapter considers carers within the context of intermediate and continuing care. It describes the key challenges that carers face in their daily lives, as well as recent policy initiatives designed to support carers in their caring role. The importance of working in partnership with carers to deliver intermediate and continuing care is illustrated by reference to contemporary research.

The challenges of caregiving

There are approximately 6.8 million carers in the United Kingdom caring for individuals with a wide range of health and social care needs (Maher and Green, 2002). Just over one-quarter of carers devote in excess of 20 hours per week to caring and over one-fifth have been involved in caring for ten years or more (Maher and Green, 2002). Carers are of strategic importance in supporting individuals living in the community (Pearlin et al., 2001) and in continuing care settings (Seddon et al., 2002a). A broad range of policy initiatives, including the National Strategy for Carers (Department of Health, 1999), the Carers and Disabled Children Act 2000 and the Carers (Equal Opportunities) Act 2004 have been introduced to support carers in their caring role. Less clear, however, is the extent to which carers are considered to be pivotal in the delivery of intermediate and continuing care.

Intermediate care is a concept that has been used to describe a broad range of short-term services at the interface between primary and secondary health care and between health and social care (Petch, 2003), for example rapid response schemes, hospital at home schemes and reablement schemes (see Chapters 1, 5 and 8). The goals, type of support and the service user groups for whom intermediate care is made available differ considerably (Stevenson and Spencer, 2002). The *National Service Framework for Older People* outlines the importance of intermediate care to three different care pathways: the prevention or management of crises, post-hospital rehabilitation and the avoidance of inappropriate admissions into nursing or residential care homes (Department of Health, 2001). Although framed within a person centred approach, there is little explicit recognition of carers or the effects of caring in the intermediate care literature and the emphasis is placed on the relationships between professionals and individuals in need of intermediate care services.

Research evidence confirms that caring can have profound implications for carers' lives, affecting their physical and mental health (Almberg et al., 2000; Maher and Green, 2002), employment opportunities (Phillips et al., 2002; Seddon et al., 2004a) and financial status (Holzhausen and Pearlman, 2000). Caring can affect an individual's ability to maintain personal and social relationships (Beeson et al., 2000; Wenger et al., 2002) and carers are known to be amongst the most socially isolated groups in the United Kingdom (Department of Health, 1999). A plethora of instruments have been developed to measure the stresses and strains of caregiving, for example the Carers Assessment of Difficulties Index (Nolan et al., 1996). An alternative to the largely fixed-choice instruments has recently been developed by Williams et al. (2002); the Carer Generated Index (CGI) underscores the importance of enabling carers themselves to specify those aspects of their lives that are most affected by caring.

Whilst caring for someone can be an extremely stressful experience, it may also prove to be a satisfying experience that presents carers with opportunities for personal growth and development (Nolan et al., 1996). Less attention has been paid to the positive aspects of caring, how these interact with the stresses of caring and how they influence carers' coping strategies (Schulz and Williamson, 1997). However, conceptual models of caregiving have been developed (Bowers, 1987; Nolan et al., 1996), which help to capture the complex, multidimensional nature of carer experiences. These models also highlight the emotional and psychosocial, as well as the practical and instrumental, aspects of caregiving (Keady and Nolan, 2003). The CGI mentioned previously allows both the positive and negative outcomes of caring to be considered.

A number of factors influence the ways in which carers respond to the challenges of caregiving. These factors include: the socio-cultural context of caregiving, which includes the values and beliefs of the carer and care recipient; the structural context of caregiving, including the nature and level of support the carer is involved in providing; and the interpersonal context of caregiving, that is, the nature and quality of the relationship between the carer and care recipient. They also include the temporal context of caregiving, including the timing of caring in the life course and the ways in which the caring experience unfolds over time (Dilworth-Anderson 2001).

Policy context

The commitment to developing systems of support for carers has been described as one of most 'striking developments' in the policy arena (Moriarty and Webb,

2000) and is underpinned by a broad range of social policies that emphasise the importance of carers, those they are involved in caring for, and health and social care professionals working together (Department of Health, 1998; 1999). This parallels the general shift towards more participative and inclusive ways of working with service users (Bernard and Phillips, 2000) and the move away from paternalistic practices (Barnes, 1999).

The National Strategy for Carers (Department of Health, 1999) was launched in February 1999 and it aims to:

- Empower carers by giving them greater control over the range, nature and timing of services.
- Mobilise community support to carers and give them some respite.
- Respond to the diversity of caregiving contexts, for example the needs of minority ethnic carers and young carers.

Comprising three strategic elements (information, support and care), it recognises the need to stimulate greater diversity and flexibility of provision. The priority action areas underpinning the Strategy are: care for carers, information, local support, young carers and carers in employment. The Strategy builds upon a number of initiatives, for example health improvement programmes, which aim to encourage carers and those they care for to become more involved in the planning and provision of services.

A key component of the Strategy was the introduction of the Carers Special Grant. The Government set aside £140 million over three years in Special Grants to enable local authorities to make suitable provision for carer breaks. The Carers Special Grant has been established to stimulate innovation in the provision of flexible, responsive services for carers. This direct provision for carer services is the first time that resources have been specifically allocated to address carers' support needs.

The Strategy and subsequent legislation recognises the importance of developing carer services that are focused on the outcomes that carers would like to see, where outcomes are defined in terms of: information and advice to carers; modifications to care packages that are in place to support the care recipient; the provision of carer services; and, sign-posting carers to community services such as carer centres. The focus on carer outcomes requires innovation at strategic and practice levels and flexible working between partner agencies, as set out in *Modernising Social Services* (Department of Health, 1998) and enshrined in the Health and Social Care Act 2001. At a strategic level, commissioners of services need to identify existing services that support carers and, in consultation with carers and local carer organisations, to prioritise areas for future service development. At practice level, assessors need to demonstrate initiative and flexibility in purchasing services for carers and in the provision and management of direct payments to carers. However, what constitutes a positive outcome in the context of carer support remains a conceptual challenge (Nolan et al., 2003).

Reflecting upon the assumptions that inform patterns of service provision, a number of authors have suggested that professional interventions with carers are premised upon a set of implicit and only partially validated models. For example, Twigg and Atkin (1994) suggest that health and social care agencies may view carers as resources, co-workers or co-clients. When agencies view carers as resources, they make assumptions about their availability and duties. Services are structured in light of these assumptions, responding only to shortcomings in the informal care network. In contrast, when carers are viewed as co-workers, they are encouraged to work in parallel with health and social care agencies. The focus of service intervention shifts towards a cooperative and enabling role; the aim being to maintain the carer in their caring role whilst acknowledging the importance of their health, well-being and independence. When carers are viewed as co-clients they are fully integrated into the policy and practice agenda of health and social care agencies. Services are designed to relieve carer stress and maximise carer independence and choice.

Asserting the need for a more explicit relationship between carers and health and social care agencies, Nolan et al. (1996; 2003) propose a model of carers as experts, the aim being to enhance carers' skills and support them throughout their caring role. Essentially, the carers as experts model conceptualises caregiving as a series of inter-related practical, cognitive and emotional components in which it is necessary for the carer to become skilled if they are to offer effective care. This model builds upon the growing body of research evidence that suggests that family carers are highly skilled and are capable of planning, brokering, supervising and providing direct care. Over time, many carers become experts in managing their caring commitments, building upon past experiences and developing successful coping strategies (Nolan et al., 1996). The failure of professionals to recognise and validate carers' expertise is known to increase their levels of distress and guilt about using services. Indeed, services that often form a key component of intermediate and long-term care packages may be rejected or deemed inappropriate.

Carer experiences of services and support

Services are known to be most effective when they are easily accessible, flexible, individualised and coordinated (Arksey et al., 2002). However, carer experiences of service provision are highly variable; services are not always perceived as helpful (Qureshi et al., 2000; Wenger et al., 2002) and carers sometimes have concerns about the quality of services put in place for the care recipient (Pickard, 1999).

These concerns relate to protecting the dignity and self-esteem of this person and promoting their independence. Carers encounter difficulties in accessing timely and flexible support (Clark et al., 2003). Problems of access relate to the limited and partial information on local services, especially at the point of discharge from hospital, when carers' needs are often overlooked (Warner and

Wexler, 1998; Smagt-Duijnstree et al., 2000). Indeed, a recent process evaluation of a community reablement scheme found that carers and older people were unfamiliar with the aims of the reablement scheme, were confused about the time-limited nature of the intervention and were critical of the lack of clear written information (Robinson et al., 2002).

Anomalies between the charges levied against social care provision and health care, provided free at the point of delivery, led to further confusion for both carers and the older people. Problems of access also relate to the considerable variation in local authority provision to support carers, which has been described as a 'lottery of location' (Social Services Inspectorate, 1998, s.3.1.13). Carers living in rural areas experience particular difficulties in accessing services; small centres of population do not provide a practical and cost-effective basis for supportive interventions (Department of Health, 1999). Many carers report that services are inflexible, in terms of their hours of availability and capacity to respond to sudden needs, as well as unreliable and unresponsive (Braithwaite, 2000; Qureshi et al., 2000; Seddon et al., 2004a). Predominantly instrumental in focus (Banks, 1999; Seddon and Robinson, 2001), many services fail to take account of carers' emotional needs (Wellwood et al., 1995) and other commitments, for example their employment commitments (Seddon et al., 2004a). Carers question the extent to which services are able to meet their changing needs (Seddon and Robinson, 2001) and provide continuity of care for the person they are involved in looking after (Robinson et al., 2002).

Echoing carers' concerns, health and social care professionals report that budgetary constraints encourage a service-led rather than needs-led approach to arranging short-term and long-term packages of care (Seddon and Robinson, 2001). They concede that carers are treated in the aggregate rather than individually and are channelled into pre-existing services with the person they are involved in caring for.

The provision of services for carers, heralded by the launch of the Carers Special Grant, was meant to enable innovative, needs-led approaches to supporting carers who have a broad range of caring commitments. This includes those carers supporting individuals in need of short-term intermediate care and those carers supporting individuals with more complex long-term health and social care needs. However, to date, there is limited evidence to suggest that the Carers Special Grant has encouraged the development of more flexible and responsive services for carers, although the Grant has extended the supply of *existing* services in England (Banks and Roberts, 2001) and in Wales (Seddon et al., 2003a). Although local authorities report that carers value the extension of existing services, the Carers Special Grant has failed to realise its full potential in developing new and innovative services to meet carers' identified needs (Seddon et al., 2003a). Both carers and staff have raised concerns about the sustainability of services funded by the Carers Special Grant and the capacity for future innovation (Seddon et al., 2003a). Charging carers for services that are provided under auspices of the Carers Special Grant is variable and in some local authorities these charges may be reimbursed. Decisions about reimbursement of payments are often deferred until the end of the financial year and are not guaranteed. This makes it difficult for carers to plan ahead and in some instances deters the take-up of services.

The development of innovative services has been restricted by a lack of conceptual clarity over the aims, objectives and intended outcomes of carer support (Nolan et al., 2003). Recently, there have been calls for improved dialogue between carers and service providers to help ensure that the aims and objectives of interventions are consistent with carer expectations (Zarit and Leitsch, 2001) and the outcomes consistent with carer views on what constitutes quality care (Lundh et al., 2003). This improvement in communication between carers and service-providing organisations has been formalised in consultation exercises. Consultation with carers is considered in detail below.

Qureshi et al. (2000) suggest health and social care services should enhance the quality of life of both carers and those they are involved in caring for, recognise and support the carer in their caring role, engage with carers as partners in the care process and acknowledge carers' expertise. Similarly, Askham (1998) emphasises the importance of embracing a more holistic view of carer support and developing short-term and long-term interventions that assist carers to take up or decline the caring role, continue in or relinquish the caring role. Establishing the most effective way to support carers in various care settings continues to evoke debate in the academic and practice communities, with little empirical work evaluating service outcomes from the perspectives of carers (Cooke et al., 2001; Zarit and Leitsch, 2001). This is specifically addressed in two ongoing studies related to the National Strategy for Carers, which will be completed during 2006. The first study, funded by the Welsh Assembly, focuses on the effects of the Carers Strategy in Wales (Seddon et al., 2002b). A parallel study, funded by the Department of Health, focuses on the effects of the Carers Strategy in England (Seddon et al., 2003b). Both studies adopt a multi-method approach in considering the perspectives of carers and those for whom they care and in measuring changes in carers' health and quality of life. The assessment of carer need and the inter-relationship between carers and health and social care professionals are also addressed in these studies and the issues are discussed in more detail below.

Working in partnership to deliver intermediate and continuing care

Partnerships and partnership working are part of the policy and practice rhetoric and frame the research literature related to intermediate care and to carers. There is considerable emphasis in the carer literature on the relationship between carers and health and social care professionals. The emphasis in the intermediate and continuing care literature is on the inter-relationships between health and social care professionals and between the service user and the professionals. Nevertheless the accumulating knowledge base in relation to carers is pertinent to the successful planning and implementation of intermediate and continuing care services.

Carers have been described as *the* most important members of the multi-disciplinary partnership (Wolfe, 1996) and are crucial to the provision of inter-mediate and continuing care. However, translating the commitment to this partnership into practice is not without its problems and the potential for reci-procity between carers and health and social care professionals has not been fully realised (Adams and Clarke, 1999; Qureshi et al., 2000). It has been argued that the power differential between carers and health and social care profes-sionals frames the interaction between the two (Paterson, 2001) and that dif-ferences across value systems serve as barriers to effective partnership working (Davies, 1992; Tamm, 1999; Lundh et al., 2003). Addressing this power imbal-ance requires both carers and health and social care professionals to re-evaluate their role in the multidisciplinary care partnership and to explicitly acknowledge the skills and competencies that each possess. In particular, health and social care professionals need to value and respect carers' emotional and practical know-ledge (Ward-Griffin, 2001; Seddon et al., 2002a).

Bereton and Nolan (2003) talk about the partnership between carers and services and describe some of the barriers to effective partnership working. In relation to services, carers are often the initiators but are less often in control of the process and outcomes of partnerships. This is particularly relevant to time-limited intermediate care services. Completion and withdrawal of these services may leave a carer feeling isolated, particularly if the service has been with-drawn abruptly (Bereton and Nolan, 2003; Robinson et al., 2002). This feeling of isolation may be heightened if those planning and delivering the service failed to engage with the carer in the first instance to ascertain their needs, in addition to the needs of the care recipient.

Less attention has been paid to disengagement from services than to the ways in which services are accessed. In the case of carers, disengagement can occur for several reasons: the service may have been time-limited, for example rehabilita-tion or reablement services, or the care recipient may have been admitted into nursing or residential care or may have died. Following the admission into a care home, carers continue to feel a strong sense of responsibility towards their relative; often they make a purposeful contribution to the individuals' continuing care which is an essential complement to the practical and technical care pro-vided by care home staff (Seddon et al., 2002a). Having relinquished their role as the primary provider of practical care, carers are keen to share their unique insights and expertise with staff and become involved in monitoring the quality of care delivered. However, carers' contribution and expert knowledge are often overlooked by staff.

How health and social care professionals, including individuals involved in intermediate care, engage, interrelate and disengage from carers warrants more careful consideration. Engaging the views of carers is paramount to the plan-ning, delivery and termination of effective services. Carer perspectives are also an important part of the user centred approach to holistic assessments that inform intermediate and continuing care packages (Robinson et al., 2002). Formal consultation with individual carers and carer groups has become an important part of the dialogue between carers and health and social care planners. Consultation with carers is considered in detail below.

Consultation

Consultation exercises are an important feature in public services, as agencies strive to identify and meet the needs of the users of the services provided. For example, consultation with individual carers and carer groups was a requirement of the Carers Special Grant. The ring-fenced nature of the resource demanded focused consultation exercises to determine best use of the grant. Similarly, consultation with all stakeholders has been described as the first step in the development of intermediate care services in a local community (Stevenson and Spencer, 2002). Carers should be considered one of the key stakeholders, although it is unclear to what extent they feature in the planning, delivery and continued development of intermediate and continuing care services.

The best ways of consulting carers is not prescribed in policy or guidance documents. A recent study (Seddon et al., 2003a) provides some insights into the process of consulting with carers. Emphasising the developmental nature of consultation, staff described the incremental strengthening of the processes of consultation as experience was gained and the importance of setting aside adequate time. A multifaceted approach to consulting with carers that is flexible and which draws upon a broad range of collective and individual consultation methods is becoming increasingly common (Seddon et al., 2003a). The most frequent methods of consultation are through meetings, focus groups and postal surveys (Carers UK, 2001). Our ongoing research in Wales suggests that consultation on a one-to-one basis via the carer assessment process is limited, as separate carer assessments are not an established feature of care management practice (Seddon et al., 2003a; 2004b).

Carers and staff have identified both strengths and weaknesses of consultation processes. These relate to inclusiveness (that is, the range of carer groups involved), the extent to which carers are actively engaged in the process and the particular methods utilised. Local authorities are particularly keen to reach a wide audience. However, recent evidence suggests that, in the main, consultation is limited to those individuals and carer groups that are already regular contributors to consultation exercises (Carers UK, 2001). Although local authorities have made concerted efforts to engage with carers, the extent to which carers are *actively* involved is questionable, given that the process is not made explicit to them and feedback is often limited. Indeed, many carers who have been involved in consultation are unaware that they have been consulted with (Seddon et al., 2003a). In a recent survey, over one-third of carers felt that the process of consultation was poor or very poor (Carers UK, 2001). Similarly, carers in Wales who have been involved in consultation activities describe their experiences in negative terms and question the extent to which their views have helped to shape the development and implementation of local carer strategies (Seddon et al., 2004b).

Health and social care professionals and carers have identified ways in which consultation might be facilitated and potential barriers addressed. For example, organisations need to consider the practical arrangements for consultation; the provision of transport and respite care may enable carers who otherwise would be excluded from the process to take part (Carers UK, 2001). Similarly, the choice of an accessible venue and a convenient time to hold meetings is important. Recent research suggests that greater use could be made of established community resources. A creative approach might include the use of the mobile library service and church groups to reach out to individuals or groups of carers. Harding and Oldman (1996) pointed out that often carers feel anxious about becoming involved in consultation events and that they may feel at a disadvantage in the presence of professionals. Clear guidance, together with support and reassurance, should be given from the outset to facilitate carer involvement and ensure clarity of expectations (Banks and Cheeseman, 1999).

Summary

The importance of carers in supporting individuals living in the community is widely recognised and undisputed. It seems clear from the evidence presented in this chapter that agencies with responsibility for planning and delivering intermediate and continuing care should be mindful of the contribution carers make to supporting individuals with health and social care needs. Concerted efforts should be made to ensure that carers are engaged with as partners in the planning of services and in the delivery of individual intermediate and continuing care programmes. It is important that the goals and outcomes of interventions are consistent with carer expectations and needs. Recognising and validating carers' skills is crucial to the successful delivery of support both to carers and the person they are involved in caring for.

References

Adams, T., Clarke, C.L. (1999) (eds) *Dementia Care: Developing Partnerships in Practice*. London: Baillière Tindall.

Almberg, B., Grafstrom, M., Krichbaum, K., Winblad, B. (2000) The interplay of institution and family caregiving: relation between patient hassles, nursing home hassles and caregivers' burnout. *International Journal of Geriatric Psychiatry* 15, 931–9.

Arksey, H., O'Malley, L., Baldwin, S., Harris, J., Mason, A., Golder, S. (2002) *Literature Review Report for the National Co-ordinating Centre for NHS Service Delivery and Organisation R&D*. York: Social Policy Research Unit.

Askham, J. (1998) Supporting caregivers of older people: an overview of problems and priorities. *Australian Journal of Ageing* 17 (1), 5–7.

Banks, P. (1999) *Carer Support: Time for a Change of Direction*. London: King's Fund.

Banks, P., Cheeseman, C. (1999) *Taking Action to Support Carers: A Carers Impact Guide for Commissioners and Managers*. London: King's Fund.

Banks, P., Roberts, E. (2001) *More Breaks for Carers? An Analysis of Local Authority Plans and Progress Reports on the Use of the Carers Special Grant*. Executive Summary February 2001. London: King's Fund.

Barnes, B. (1999) *Public Expectations: From Paternalism to Partnership, Changing Relationships in Health and Health Services*. Policy Futures for UK Health No. 10. London: Nuffield Trust.

Beeson, R., Horton-Deutsch, S., Farran, C., Neundorfer, M. (2000) Loneliness and depression in caregivers of persons with Alzheimer's disease or related disorders. *Issues in Mental Health Nursing* **21**, 779–806.

Bereton, L., Nolan, M. (2003) Seeking partnerships between family and professional carers: stroke as a case in point. In: Nolan, M., Lundh, U., Grant, G. and Keady, J. (eds) *Partnerships in Family Care: Understanding the Caregiving Career*. Maidenhead: Open University Press, pp. 50–68.

Bernard, M., Phillips, J. (2000) The challenge of ageing in tomorrow's Britain. *Ageing and Society* **20** (1), 33–54.

Bowers, B.J. (1987) Inter-generational caregiving: adult caregivers and their ageing parents. *Advances in Nursing Science* **9** (2), 20–31.

Braithwaite, V. (2000) Contextual or generic stress outcomes: making choices through caregiving appraisals. *The Gerontologist* **40** (6), 706–17.

Carers and Disabled Children Act (2000).

Carers (Equal Opportunities) Act (2004).

Carers UK (2001) *Give Us a Break*. London: Carers UK.

Clark, C., Chaston, D., Grant, G. (2003) Early interventions in dementia: carer-led evaluations. In: Nolan, M., Lundh, U., Grant, G. and Keady, J. (eds) *Partnerships in Family Care: Understanding the Caregiving Career*. Maidenhead: Open University Press, pp. 33–49.

Cooke, D., McNally, L., Mulligan, K., Harrison, M., Newman, S. (2001) Psychosocial interventions for caregivers of people with dementia: a systematic review. *Ageing and Mental Health* **5** (2), 120–35.

Davies, L. (1992) Building a source of caring for caregivers. *Family and Community Health* **15** (2), 1–9.

Department of Health (1998) *Modernising Social Services*, CM 4169. London: HMSO.

Department of Health (1999) *Caring about Carers: A National Strategy for Carers*. London: Department of Health.

Department of Health (2001) *National Service Framework for Older People*. London: Department of Health.

Dilworth-Anderson, P. (2001) Family issues and the care of persons with Alzheimer's Disease. *Ageing and Mental Health* **5** (supplement 1), S49–S51.

Harding, T., Oldman, H. (1996) *Involving Service Users and Carers in Local Services: Guidelines for Social Services Departments and Others*. London: NSIW.

Health and Social Care Act (2001).

Holzhausen, E., Pearlman, V. (2000) *Caring on the Breadline: The Financial Implications of Caring*. London: Carers National Association.

Keady, J., Nolan, M. (2003) The dynamics of dementia: working together, working separately, or working alone? In: Nolan, M., Lundh, U., Grant, G. and Keady, J. (eds) *Partnerships in Family Care: Understanding the Caregiving Career*. Maidenhead: Open University Press, pp. 15–32.

Lundh, U., Nolan, M., Hellstrom, I., Ericsson, I. (2003) Quality care for people with dementia: the views of family and professional carers. In: Nolan, M., Lundh, U., Grant, G. and Keady, J. (eds) *Partnerships in Family Care: Understanding the Caregiving Career.* Maidenhead: Open University Press, pp. 72–89.

Maher, J., Green, H. (2002) *Carers 2000.* London: The Stationery Office.

Moriarty, J., Webb, S. (2000) *Part of their Lives: Community Care for Older People with Dementia.* Bristol: Policy Press.

Nolan, M., Grant, G., Keady, J. (1996) *Understanding Family Care: A Multidimensional Model of Caring and Coping.* Buckingham: Open University Press.

Nolan, M., Keady, J., Grant, G., Lundh, U. (2003) Introduction: why another book on family care? In: Nolan, M., Lundh, U., Grant, G. and Keady, J. (eds) *Partnerships in Family Care: Understanding the Caregiving Career.* Maidenhead: Open University Press, pp. 1–12.

Paterson, B. (2001) Myth of empowerment in chronic illness. *Journal of Advanced Nursing* **34** (5), 574–81.

Pearlin, L., Harrington, C., Powell-Lawton, M., Montgomery, R., Zarit, S. (2001) An overview of the social and behavioural consequences of Alzheimer's Disease. *Ageing and Mental Health* **5** (Supplement 1), S3–S6.

Petch, A. (2003) *Intermediate Care: What Do We Know about Older Peoples' Experiences?* York: Joseph Rowntree Foundation.

Phillips, J., Bernard, M., Chittenden, M. (2002) *Juggling Work and Care: The Experiences of Working Carers of Older Adults.* Bristol: Policy Press.

Pickard, S. (1999) Co-ordinated care for older people with dementia. *Journal of Inter-professional Care* **13** (4), 345–54.

Qureshi, H., Bamford, C., Nicholas, E., Patmore, C., Harris, J. (2000) *Outcomes in Social Care Practice: Developing an Outcome Focus in Care Management and Use Surveys.* York: University of York, Social Policy Research Unit.

Robinson, C., Seddon, D., Hill, J. (2002) Community reablement: perspectives of older people and their carers. *Signpost* **7** (1), 17–19.

Schulz, R., Williamson, G. (1997) The measurement of caregiver outcomes in AD research. *Alzheimer's Disease and Related Disorders* **11** (Supplement 6), 1–6.

Seddon, D., Robinson, C. (2001) Carers of older people with dementia: assessment and the carers act. *Journal of Health and Social Care in the Community* **9** (3), 151–8.

Seddon, D., Jones, K., Boyle, M. (2002a) Committed to caring: carer experiences following the admission of a relative into nursing or residential care. *Quality in Ageing* **3** (3), 16–26.

Seddon, D., Robinson, C., Russell, I., Woods, R. (2002b) *A Study of the Effects of the Carers' Strategy in Wales on the Needs of Carers and the Services that they Receive.* Funded by the Wales Office of Research and Development for Health and Social Care on behalf of the National Assembly for Wales. Cardiff: National Assembly.

Seddon, D., Robinson, C.A., Jones, K., Reeves, C., Boyle, M. (2003a) *An Analysis of the Carers Special Grant Scheme and Consultation Processes Used for the Carers Special Grant.* Final Report to the Wales Office of Research and Development for Health and Social Care. Bangor: University of Wales Bangor.

Seddon, D., Robinson, C., Cheung, W., Gaze, S., Jones, K., Phillips, J., Russell, I., Williams, J., Woods, R., Youren, A. (2003b) *The Modernisation of Social Care Services: A Study of the Effectiveness of the National Strategy for Carers in Meeting Carer Needs.* Project funded by the Department of Health.

Seddon, D., Robinson, C., Bowen, S., Boyle, M. (2004a) Supporting carers in paid employment: developing a needs-led approach. *Quality in Ageing* **5** (1), 14–23.

Seddon, D., Reeves, C., Tommis, Y., Robinson, C., Russell, I., Woods, R., Boyle, M. (2004b) *A Study of the Effects of the Carers Strategy in Wales*. Progress Report to the Wales Office of Research and Development for Health and Social Care. Bangor: University of Wales Bangor.

Smagt-Duijnstree, M., Harners, J., Abu-Sead, H. (2000) Relatives of stroke patients: their experiences and needs in hospital. *Scandinavian Journal of Nursing Sciences* **14**, 44–51.

Social Services Inspectorate (SSI) (1998) *A Matter of Chance for Carers?* London: Department of Health.

Stevenson, I., Spencer, L. (2002) *Developing Intermediate Care: A Guide for Health and Social Services Professionals*. London: King's Fund.

Tamm, M. (1999) Relatives as a help or hindrance: a grounded theory study seen from the perspective of the occupational therapist. *Scandinavian Journal of Occupational Therapy* **6**, 36–45.

Twigg, J., Atkin, K. (1994) *Carers Perceived: Policy and Practice in Informal Care*. Buckingham: Open University Press.

Ward-Griffin, C. (2001) Negotiating care of frail elders: relationships between community nurses and family carers. *Canadian Journal of Nursing Research* **33** (2), 63–81.

Warner, C., Wexler, S. (1998) *Eight Hours a Day and Taken for Granted?* London: The Princess Royal Trust for Carers.

Wellwood, I., Dennis, M., Warlow, C. (1995) Patients' and carers' satisfaction with acute stroke management. *Age and Ageing* **20**, 519–24.

Wenger, G.C., Scott, A., Seddon, D. (2002) The experience of caring for older people with dementia in a rural area: using services. *Journal of Aging and Mental Health* **6** (1), 30–38.

Williams, J.G., Bayer, A.J., Cheung, W.Y., Ford, D.V., Gaze, S.A., Jackson, S., Russell, I.T., Youren, A.M. (2002) *Quantifying the Effect of Caring on Carers' Quality of Life*. Final report to the Wales Office of Research and Development. Swansea: Clinical School, University of Wales Swansea.

Wolfe, C. (1996) The burden of stroke. In: Wolfe, C., Rudd, T. and Beech, R. (eds) *Stroke Services and Research*. London: Stroke Association.

Zarit, S., Leitsch, S. (2001) Developing and evaluating community based intervention programmes for Alzheimer's patients and their caregivers. *Ageing and Mental Health* **5** (Supplement 1), S84–S98.

Chapter 16

Patient and Public Involvement in Service Design and Evaluation

Bie Nio Ong and Geoff Wood

Introduction

As several Western countries have done, the British Government has recast its 21st-century public policies within a 'Third Way' vocabulary, in which the role of citizens appears to be enhanced and alternative approaches to delivering services are being developed (Tritter et al., 2003). While the issue of patient and public involvement is not new – and the plethora of literature in this field dating back to the 1960s attests to this – the context and language has changed considerably as a result of the 'modernisation' agenda in the public sector. Rather than reviewing this considerable body of literature (see, for example, Rifkin et al., 2000), the focus in this chapter is on a number of issues that are relevant to the theme of this book.

The territories of intermediate and continuing care pose particular challenges, in that defining boundaries between the voices of patients and carers as users of health and social care, their social networks and relevant interest groups (e.g. Age Concern, Alzheimer Society) cannot always be easily drawn. The complexity surrounding receiving and providing care is derived from the interplay between these different voices, but also because of the involvement of a wide range of service providers. Furthermore, judgements about the quality of care and desired outcomes will need to be negotiated between the various stakeholders, and finding the appropriate balance between lay and professional perspectives is a key challenge. Thus, our discussion will address these issues, and in particular, attempts to outline possible ways to embed meaningful patient and public participation in processes where it can influence the delivery and evaluation of intermediate and continuing care.

Defining involvement

Recently, Contandriopoulos (2004) has argued that the so-called classical literature on public participation in health care suffers from a number of weaknesses: first, its normative approach; second, its idealistic (or at times naive) stance; and third, its argument as to the intrinsic desirability of participation. This critical assessment raises questions as to the social and symbolic construction of legitimacy and the political efficacy of public participation. Therefore, it is necessary to disentangle the desirability of patient and public involvement (and its added value), the role that is played by patients and the public, and the actual forms that lay influence can take. A number of considerations are worth mentioning.

First, one has to clarify the distinction between the role of citizens, who are concerned with the 'common good', collective provision and pooling risks, and that of consumers (patients and carers) who are essentially self-interested and focus on personal rights and services. Citizens and consumers can be engaged at individual or aggregate/collective levels and this also determines the basis for the legitimacy of their involvement (Lomas, 1997; Callaghan and Wistow, 2002). Thus, clarity as to the role people are asked to play when being involved in decision making processes is essential. Examples have demonstrated that, in particular, distinctions between individual, programme and health system level can assist in a clearer delineation between types of involvement (Litva et al., 2002).

Second, tension exists between the policies of choice and equity; the first being based upon a consumerist ideology that is driven by individualist notions of need, while the latter focuses upon comparative need, leading to a possible unequal distribution of provision in order to achieve equal outcomes. Rowland and Pollock (2004) demonstrate that these two policy strands do not sit happily alongside each other in the case of intermediate and continuing care. The steady reduction of both NHS and social services capacity, coupled with the new NHS financial regime based upon 'average length of hospital stay' create a situation whereby older people may be 'forced into accommodation which is inappropriate and does not serve their needs' (p. 5). They conclude that the right to choose might cause delays in hospital discharge, and consequently this choice is considered as an obstacle to efficiency in the NHS. People in need of intermediate or continuing care are thus squeezed in two ways: first, exercising choice becomes difficult in the face of limited provision and constraining individual choice, and second, few incentives exist to give priority in resource allocation at the care group and population level. The involvement of users in decisions about the care of individuals or care groups is hampered because of the inherent tensions between the different policy strands.

Third, Primary Care Trusts (PCTs) are charged with health improvement, and this demands serious engagement with individuals and groups within communities. The literature on social capital emphasises the importance of releasing capacity in social networks, communities and voluntary organisations, and critically assessing statutory organisations' relationships with those networks (Woolcock, 1998). The social capital framework offers a more systematic approach to 'soft measures' that assess the impact of policies on people's quality of life, changing relationships and networks that contribute to individuals' and communities' well-being. However, short-term programmes run counter to the building of trust and sustainable relationships.

It is important to develop creative ways of integrating community involvement in core decision making (and not just paying lip-service to policy directives). This needs organisational champions who are prepared to take risks, to push boundaries and who will carry others with them. Discussed below is the role that 'older people champions' play in PCTs as a strategy for influencing policy and practice. Moreover, it is important to free up grassroots staff to build on the trust that they often foster at local levels. They have the capacity to overcome institutional barriers to joint working between organisations, and between organisations and communities. Intermediate and continuing care present the challenge to make this a reality, and allow users and carers to influence the scope and nature of services.

Fourth, current understanding about responsibility and accountability appears to suffer from a 'tyranny of transparency' (Strathern, 2000). Ostensibly power has been devolved to more local levels, but tight performance measurement has the effect of eroding trust in professionals and public sector managers (O'Neill, 2002). In parallel, the idea of user involvement as located within democratic accountability has shaped much of the thinking behind government policies over the past decade without achieving any commonly agreed definition as to its purpose and implementation. From the perspective of service providers, therefore, the lack of trust emanating from the top is exacerbated by the bottom-up pressure to share power with users and carers. Tritter et al. (2003) state that 'many NHS staff remain unconvinced that the benefits of user involvement will outweigh the costs' (p. 343).

Fifth, in his book reviewing public health policy, David Hunter (2003) argues that the NHS has been focused on managing health care rather than on managing health. He proposes that re-emphasising the notions of quality of life and well-being might advance critical thinking about the contribution that health and social care make to health gain. Furthermore, the short-term political imperatives of increasing access and capacity do not necessarily address people's primary needs, or are not necessarily in harmony with the sort of outcomes from intermediate and continuing care that patients, carers and the public value. User involvement in setting the broader public health agenda for older people continues to be an underdeveloped territory.

Challenges and tensions in receiving and giving care

The relatively recent emergence of the term 'intermediate care' and the lack of precision as to what it actually entails in practice has been pointed out in an evaluation of the costs and outcomes of intermediate care (Martin et al., 2004). In theory, the fact that intermediate care aims to restore people to independence should enhance opportunities for user involvement in care decisions. However, the specific policy and management context, the relationships between users and professionals, and potential conflicting needs of patients and their carers need to be considered. These factors will shape involvement differently at the level of individual users and carers or communities. When considering continuing care, the picture becomes even more complex as differential sources of power are more marked with users who are generally in a position of greater dependency on informal and/or formal carers, and requiring support across organisational boundaries. While policy initiatives such as the Single Assessment Process should provide users with increased influence are being introduced, major cultural and operational shifts have to take place for this to become reality.

The difficulty in offering a coherent discussion of user, carer and public influence in the territories of intermediate and continuing care lies in the fact that multiple tensions are present. For example, in a BBC opinion poll in March 2004 (BBC, 2004), the public placed free personal care for dependent elderly people at the top of the health and social care agenda. However, in the programme discussing the same poll results, the care of individual cancer sufferers was also prioritised, illustrating the perennial problem of comparing life-threatening diseases with chronic conditions. The public as citizens pronounce improving quality of life as a priority, but when it comes to allocating scarce resources, individual needs for life-saving treatments gain the upper hand. The second dilemma lies in balancing user preference with the needs of informal carers. Both at the level of individual cases and in terms of local policy, contradictions arise and the danger of marginalising either the patient or the carer voice is ever present. The role of voluntary organisations as advocates in furthering the thinking and practice of user or carer influence is particularly important when developing locally sensitive services. A third issue relates to the sheer variety of intermediate care which according to Martin et al. (2004) can be viewed on the one hand as a reflection of bottom-up innovation, or on the other as unmanaged diversity that could lead to poor clinical outcomes and inefficiency. In the first instance, user and carer influence may contribute to the innovation process and responsiveness to local needs; in the latter case, users and carers may be unable to influence the quality of care and be powerless to seek alternative provision.

While similar issues emerge in the continuing care arena two specific aspects need to be considered: first, there has been very little input of patients in need of continuing nursing care at home or in residential care settings (Andrews et al., 2003), so decisions on standards and levels of care have been left to professionals and family members. User influence tends, as a result, to be superseded by social networks' influence. Second, the level of assessed care needs is directly related to the level of financial support available. This often results in differences of opinion between assessors and family members and tensions between 'exaggerating' and 'minimising' care levels needed. It could be argued that 'hands-on' professionals need to feel that they can influence organisational policies in order to allow carers the space to make their views known. Thus, a much wider cultural question has to be addressed, namely the democratisation of care organisations, which are able to foster both staff and user/carer influence.

Judging the quality of care

Limited work has been carried out on user involvement in evaluation, that is, in formulating user-derived outcomes. The work by Entwistle et al. (1998) demonstrates the complexity in terms of effects and perspectives, and in particular, opinions as to what effects are valued lead inevitably to tensions between different stakeholders. Several years on Crawford and colleagues (2002) state that the evidence base for demonstrating the effect of patient involvement on the use and quality of services is lacking. A recent review by Carr (2004) similarly stresses that monitoring involvement is ad hoc, and generally focuses on processes rather than outcomes. Evaluations in intermediate and continuing care tend to be done by professionals and managers, and often performance management indicators are used that are based upon throughput and activity rather than user or carer definitions of quality of life.

The dominant methods for measuring outcomes such as randomised controlled trials and controlled studies are not necessarily the most appropriate ones in the case of intermediate and continuing care. It could be argued that qualitative methods, including the use of narrative based criteria offer more scope for understanding improvements in the quality of life of users and carers (Kelson, 1995). Similarly, the Expert Patient Programme is based upon the assumptions that patients themselves are experts in living with chronic illness, and that this experiential expertise can be used in managing and evaluating care. Particularly within the context of shifting towards a health improvement model in Primary Care Trusts, sharing power with patients, the wider public and partner organisations becomes very relevant when evaluating outcomes in intermediate and continuing care (Callaghan and Wistow, 2002).

The methodological challenge of assessing the impact of intermediate and continuing care on people's quality of life lies in moving from the individual experience to generalisation in terms of service development and policy. Moreover, balancing equity in improving quality of life linked to standards of care (Department of Health, 2004) with flexible responses to individual need requires sophisticated evaluation across individual, care group and societal levels. At present, this battery of tools does not exist and user, carer and public influence in their development is crucial if these instruments are to be responsive to the actual experience of receiving and giving care.

Meaningful influence

Whilst policy and practice is encouraging to patient and public influence on services for older people, meaningful influence over the level and type of care offered is often an aspiration rather than a reality. As discussed above, the focus on processes rather than impact deflects from a fundamental debate as to the 'added value' of patient and public involvement: how one demonstrates influence on decision-making.

At the level of care for individuals it is important to consider the structural context of continuing care as social care provided by the state that is not free and final contributions to those costs which are related to income or savings of the client. Nursing care provided by the state is, as all NHS services, free at the point of delivery. The differences of opinion about what is social care and what is nursing care have often been central to arguments between the caring agencies and those receiving care precisely because of economic considerations. Involvement in decision making can be equally limited because of rules which require clear demarcations between social and nursing care, while the two types of care are not necessarily experienced by users and carers as separate entities.

In reality, assessors appear to be committed to arrive at the best solutions possible within the boundaries of set criteria and procedures. The actual assessment processes in continuing health care and intermediate care see assessors and providers of services fully embracing the notions of inclusion of the 'user/ patient' and their carers or social network in the assessment process. Moreover, ample opportunity is given to individuals or carers to add to or appeal against assessment decisions, but fundamental structural constraints make that influence to change decisions fairly circumscribed.

At the level of working with user and carer groups, or the general public, a number of mechanisms have increasingly been used so that they can influence the levels and types of care provided. Primary Care Trusts have a particular responsibility to connect with key stakeholders, and in the case of intermediate and continuing care these can be subdivided into the following:

- 'Well' older people: They can be involved by gathering together a group of older/retired people and asking them to contribute to the redesign or restructuring of services. Tapping into existing networks such as social clubs, groups brought together through voluntary organisations and neighbourhood networks can help to attract interested individuals. This type of grouping works well as a cultural link between 'younger' service planners or providers and older people, even though they are currently not in need of services. These groups, with encouragement, can become confident and vociferous but their actual experience of care can be limited.

- Older people in receipt of services: Facilitated group discussions, interviews focusing on people's experiences – rather than filling in survey questionnaires – and other more informal and qualitative approaches tend to be most productive. Encouragement of this group of people to speak about the services might be complicated by possible confusion of the individual users and/or feelings that future services may be compromised by expressions of dissatisfaction. Clarity about the use of their experiences for planning purposes is important so that people feel that the feedback they provide is suitably anonymised.

- Voluntary organisations and interest groups: Local branches of voluntary sector organisations, such as Age Concern, the Stroke Association, or the Alzheimer's Society, are vital to the debate on patient and public influence in their role of advocates. However, they are themselves often engaged in the provision of social care to specific client groups or carers. The dual position as 'champions' of service user views and care providers creates tensions, and, therefore, they might not necessarily be the most appropriate conduit for user and carer influence.

- The general population: Surveys of the whole patient/user body can be helpful in examining broader patterns of needs or attitudes. However, it may be necessary to stratify samples or target sections of the population as there may be bias towards older people as they are more likely to be receiving health care than a younger group. The evidence about response rates is inconclusive as studies have reported both reduced response and higher levels of response in older people. Thus, careful sampling will help the analysis so that survey results can feed into organisational decision making, alongside the above qualitative findings and clinical and cost-effectiveness evidence.

The different roles and levels of involvement are illustrated with an example relating to people with Alzheimer's disease in Box 16.1.

Box 16.1 Example of user and public influence in Alzheimer's disease policy and management.

	Individual	Programme	Health system and policy
Individual user	User influence will decrease over time as Alzheimer's disease adversely affects self determination	User influence if involved in specific groups that focus on service redesign, implementation or needs assessment	Little influence as broader policy objectives are set centrally
Carer(s)	Carer and user needs may or may not be complementary (resulting in congruence or conflict of needs)	Carer influence if involved in specific groups that focus on service redesign, implementation or needs assessment	Little influence as broader policy objectives are set centrally
Client group(s) (voluntary organisations)	Advocacy, support, advice to individual user and/or carers	Formal representation in service redesign; delivery of services; advocacy and campaigning	Limited influence, but may be invited to feed back on national and local policy objectives
General public	Limited interest, unless in exceptional high profile cases	Interest as potential users in the availability of services. May have an interest in development and/or service quality issues	Limited influence, but may be invited to feed back on national and local policy objectives

Two further routes for user or public influence need to be mentioned. First, the public sector, including health and social care providers, has been encouraged to set up networks of so-called older people's champions, who have varying remits, to consider how the general decision making of an organisation reflects the needs of older populations. This system, which theoretically should prove very useful, presently appears to be weighed down with the uncertainty of the champion's role, the overlap between agencies and the varied responses and support given by statutory and voluntary agencies. The older people's champion role has to mature before an assessment can be made about its potential to influence policy and planning in intermediate and continuing care. Second, locally all statutory and voluntary agencies can meet to discuss issues of care and caring. This has proven to be a promising platform for 'breaking down barriers' between agencies and a useable route of information dissemination. Again, further assessment is needed as to its added value in terms of strengthening user and public influence in policy and collaborative working.

Summary

User and public involvement in health and social care is now considered an essential part of running public services, but many conceptual and implementation issues remain unresolved. The tensions between individual benefit and the common good, between users and carers, and between users, carers and professionals cannot always be resolved because of different perspectives, conflicting policies and so on. Furthermore, it has been argued that lack of clarity exists as to what role users and the public are asked to adopt, and at what level they are expected to be involved in decision making.

Within the arenas of intermediate and continuing care, some of these tensions are further accentuated because of the structural constraints, the often immediate pressure to find appropriate care, and the degree of user dependency. The collective voice of users and carers is increasingly being heard, but their influence at the early stages of policy making at national or local levels requires considerable development. Voluntary organisations are capable of acting as advocates, yet sometimes experience a conflict of interest if they are also providers of care.

Particular initiatives such as the single assessment process offer an approach that places the user at the centre of care planning and delivery which should create space for real user and carer influence. The cultural shifts required will take some time, and empowering staff (assessors and care providers) is equally important, because only when staff feel that they can influence their own organisation will they gain the confidence to listen to users and carers. Devolution of decision making and fostering an innovative culture within public sector organisations go hand in hand with stimulating user and public involvement. The challenge for intermediate and continuing care is that this approach needs to take place simultaneously across a number of organisations – in particular

NHS and social services – each with their own decision making and account-ability structures.

Specific examples of creating avenues for user and public influence have been discussed, but these need to be embedded within a wider context of organisa-tional change. Furthermore, if they are to have an impact beyond a locality, contradictions between different policy strands need to be addressed (Rowland and Pollock, 2004).

In conclusion, user and public involvement in the public sector requires fur-ther conceptual development and linking with other important initiatives such as tackling inequalities in health, community engagement and social capital release, and real partnership working. The specific nature of intermediate and continuing care demands that attention should be paid to involving vulnerable people, understanding complex – and possibly contradictory – needs, and the importance of creating longer-term relationships with users and carers based upon trust. New methods of engagement may need to be explored that are sensitive to capturing the experiences of living with and adapting to illness and disability, and thus widening the focus from health and social care to enhancing the quality of life of users, carers and communities. Their input in designing and evaluating services can complement clinical and managerial expertise in that they can contribute their expertise of 'having experience' (Prior, 2003) to the wider planning and implementation processes. Knowledge to date, however, shows that user, carer and public influence operate at different levels, and tend to be most effective at the individual and programme level, rather than influencing health systems and policy as these are subject to macro-political imperatives.

References

Andrews, J., Manthorpe, J., Watson, R. (2003) Involving older people in intermediate care. *Journal of Advanced Nursing* **46** (3), 303–10.

BBC Radio 4 (2004) *Today* programme. News item on NHS funding, March.

Callaghan, C., Wistow, G. (2002) *Public and Patient Participation in PCGs: New Beginnings for Old Power Structures*. Nuffield Portfolio Programme Report, no. 19. Leeds: Leeds University.

Carr, S. (2004) *Has Service User Participation Made a Difference to Social Care Services?* Social Care Institute for Excellence. Bristol: Policy Press.

Contandriopoulos, D. (2004) A sociological perspective on public participation in health care. *Social Science and Medicine* **58**, 321–30.

Crawford, M., Rutter, D., Manley, C., Weaver, T., Bhui, K., Fulop, N., Tyrer, P. (2002) Systematic review of involving patients in the planning and development of health care. *British Medical Journal* **325**, 1263–8.

Department of Health (2004) *Standards for Better Health: Health Care Standards for Care under the NHS – a Consultation*. London: Department of Health.

Entwistle, V., Sowden, A., Watt, I. (1998) Evaluating interventions to promote patient involvement in decision-making: by what criteria should effectiveness be judged? *Journal of Health Services Research and Policy* **3** (2), 100–107.

Hunter, D. (2003) *Public Health Policy*. Cambridge: Polity Press.

Kelson, M. (1995) *Consumer Involvement Initiatives in Clinical Audit and Outcomes*. London: College of Health.

Litva, A., Coast, J., Donovan, J., et al. (2002) 'The public is too subjective': public involvement at different levels of health-care decision-making. *Social Science and Medicine* **54**, 1825–37.

Lomas, J. (1997) Reluctant rationers: public input to health care priorities. *Journal of Health Services Research and Policy* **2**, 103–11.

Martin, G., Peet, S., Hewitt, G., Parker, H. (2004) Diversity in intermediate care. *Health and Social Care in the Community* **12** (2), 150–54.

O'Neill, O. (2002) Trust and transparency. *Reith Lectures*, 4. London: BBC.

Prior, L. (2003) Belief, knowledge and expertise: the emergence of the lay expert in medical sociology. *Sociology of Health and Illness* **25**, 41–57.

Rifkin, S., Lewando-Hunt, G., Draper, A. (2000) *Participatory Approaches in Health Promotion and Health Planning – A Literature Review*. London: Health Development Agency.

Rowland, D., Pollock, A. (2004) Choice and responsiveness for older people in the 'patient centred' NHS. *British Medical Journal* **328**, 4–5.

Strathern, M. (2000) The tyranny of transparency. *British Educational Journal* **26** (3), 309–21.

Tritter, J., Barley, V., Daykin, N., Evans, S., McNeill, J., Rimmer, J., Sanidas, M., Turton, P. (2003) Divided care and the Third Way: user involvement in statutory and voluntary sector cancer services. *Sociology of Health and Illness* **25** (5), 429–56.

Woolcock, M. (1998) Social capital and economic development: towards a theoretical synthesis and policy framework. *Theory and Society* **27**, 151–208.

Chapter 17

Implications for Policy and Practice: the Future

Brenda Roe and Roger Beech

Introduction

The aim of this chapter is to provide an overview and summary of intermediate and continuing care already presented, confirming what we know in relation to policy, practice and research, and identifying any gaps in our knowledge. Intermediate and continuing care form part of the 'continuum of care', which also includes self-care, acute care and end of life care. There are temporal, spatial and gender aspects to care; its type, where it takes place, by whom and for how long. Now more than ever it is important to involve the public, patients and carers in the evaluation and development of new and existing services rather than it being left to the providers and commissioners. Care is both given and received and has an interactive dynamic. Consequently it is important to look at care from the perspectives of the providers and its recipients (Twigg, 2000). Health and social care is about bodywork and can involve technology such as thermometers, stethoscopes, catheters, wound dressings and other devices familiar to health care (Sandelowski, 2000) as well as bathing, washing and personal care involving excreta and bodily emissions (Twigg, 2000). The sociology of the body and personal care are neglected areas, but personal care comprises the basis of care packages needed to keep older people and younger disabled people living at home (Twigg, 2000). 'Care closer to home' is the policy underpinning intermediate and continuing care in the community.

What we know

Intermediate care services have been developing since the early 1990s in the UK and often they have been developed piecemeal, scheme by scheme, as and when finances became available. Until recently there had been little or no consideration of a whole system approach to their development or operation. Notable exceptions are the work of Foote and Stanners (2002) and Forte and Bowen (1997).

Intermediate care is not a universal term recognised within health services around the world, consequently it is difficult to compare schemes and services between countries. The Department of Health policy on intermediate care recommends a range of provisions to avoid hospital admission and promote early discharge along with specific targets (Department of Health, 2001). Hospital at home schemes are the most well established (Shepperd and Illiffe, 2004), with more recently focus being on rehabilitation and supported discharge along with short-term placements in care homes, use of day hospitals and palliative care (Young, 2002a; 2002b). Referrals to intermediate care are coordinated at one central point by one individual to ensure overall coordination of staff and care packages. Intermediate care is restricted to six weeks duration, when either people return to independent living or they require continuing care. Little attention has been paid to the continuum of care, where intermediate care stops and continuing care commences, and this was one of the reasons for this book being developed. The six week duration of intermediate care is a somewhat arbitrary figure, although one local evaluation has found that over a three month period one-third of clients required up to two weeks of care, one-third up to four weeks of care and the remaining clients up to six weeks or slightly over (Roe, 2001a; 2001b).

Similarly, continuing care is coordinated by one individual, as part of a care or case managed approach involving community care or institutional care. This is particularly important, as care packages can be complex. The advent of the single assessment process (SAP) is also common to both intermediate and continuing care so that duplication of effort and multiple assessments by a variety of individuals collecting similar information does not take place. Although in its infancy, once SAP is established and the data are transferred on to computerised information systems this will also assist with coordination of care and with its evaluation and development by providing collated whole systems information.

Intermediate care as a policy is still in its infancy (10 to 14 years) compared with continuing and community care (20 to 30 years), consequently services are still in their early development stages. Having recommended adopting a whole systems approach, the focus is on establishing the scope of services to be offered for each locality, and the capacity in relation to services, staff and clients. Potential approaches, illustrated by case studies, include using performance indicators and utilisation review to audit the use of acute beds by looking at clinical records to provide baseline information for planning and identifying if avoidable bed usage is occurring. The utilisation review can also provide information on the care needs of potential users and help with the planning, scope and development of intermediate care services (see Chapter 2). Other approaches for the planning and capacity of services include the Balance of Care approach using various instruments such as the Appropriateness Evaluation Protocol (AEP) and the Intensity, Severity and Discharge (ISD) instrument as outlined in Chapter 3, which may be useful planning and development procedures. A further case study illustrated in Chapter 4 demonstrates the importance of operational services management, coordination, monitoring, evaluation, audit and staff development in intermediate care.

Evidence for the cost-effectiveness of intermediate care is being established, although there is a dearth of information available. In the meantime economic issues can be explored by comparing actual running costs of different schemes and comparing the costs of various inputs, outputs and outcomes of schemes (see Chapters 8 and 9). The costing of continuing care is different as it is at fixed rates and is means tested depending upon individuals and where their care takes place and for how long (see Chapters 11, 12, 13 and 14).

Inter-agency working, staff development and interdisciplinary working and training are key features of both intermediate and continuing care. There is general recognition of the difficulties of recruiting and retaining people working in health and social care, with a shortage of nurses, therapists and care staff. This pressure has led teams to look at different ways of working and what skills and competencies are common to all and which are specific to a particular discipline. A variety of different in-house and higher education courses and training are being developed with a focus on adult learning with different and appropriate teaching focused on preferred styles of adult learning, such as verbal, experiential and visual. It is also about transfer of skills between professionals, core competencies for health and social care and specific competencies in relation to therapies or treatments.

As with intermediate care, continuing care offers a variety of simple and complex care packages in people's homes and care homes. Despite the numbers of care home places declining in the UK (10 000 places within 2003–4 and a total of 89 000 since 1996 with some growth in the sector), the demand for care is estimated to triple in coming years (Charter, 2004), and spending on long-term care for older people is projected to increase to £53.9 billion by 2051 to meet demographic pressures and rising costs (Wittenberg et al., 2004). An emerging area is for alternative housing and care arrangements for older people in the form of extra care housing, assisted living, retirement communities and congregate housing such as Hartrigg Oaks, York (Sturge, 2000; Croucher et al., 2003) and Berryhill, Stoke on Trent (Bernard et al., 2004). While there has been a large expansion of the assisted living and retirement community sectors in the USA it may not be possible to transfer their findings to UK communities and populations. Assisted living and retirement communities may not be widely accessible to a large number of older people, as they are expensive (Croucher et al., 2003).

However, in Berryhill the retirement community predominantly included residents from the working class and was of clear benefit to its population, who were highly satisfied with the community, its facilities, and the safety and security offered by staff on site. Despite having poor health status, residents felt their health had improved since moving in and was maintained over time. Keeping fit and volunteering were highly valued by residents, and autonomy, security and sociability were also highly valued. Berryhill provided a positive environment in which to age. Friendship, companionship and support were there in times of illness. Intergenerational links were promoted and maintained (Bernard et al., 2004).

Assisted living and retirement communities are proliferating in the UK and may well be the way of the future ageing 'in situ' as opposed to moving into care homes. Continuing care for vulnerable people is provided in care homes. The reduction in care home places has been a direct consequence of independent provision at home, that is publicly funded and self financed. Care closer to home is being interpreted as care in the home by carers, family or providers and not in institutions. There has been a reduction in places but a rise in levels of dependency of residents. There is still a lack of current information on residents' characteristics and needs on which to base the commissioning of home places and provision of care. There are concerns about future capacity in this sector of continuing care.

Intermediate and continuing care take place in the context of individuals who self care to a greater or lesser extent and who also have carers, either family or neighbours. The role and needs of carers and caregiver networks is being recognised with an increasing body of evidence becoming available. Financial support, respite care, resources and emotional support are critical for carers but can differ depending on the needs of the person being cared for: those with frailty and physical needs compared with people with mental health needs such as dementia where the needs may be very different. This confirms the importance of needs assessment for individuals and carers. Agencies, both public sector and voluntary, with responsibility for planning and delivering services should appreciate the extent of health and social care provided by carers and support them in this endeavour, provide them with respite care, and tailor services to meet their needs and support them, along with the people they care for. Involving carers in the audit and evaluation of services is also important.

Present policy is about involving both consumers and the public in the evaluation, justification and development of services for intermediate and continuing care. There is evidence that this is being undertaken at both national and local levels through audit, satisfaction surveys and user group feedback and consultation, although improvements in targeting groups and methods of engagement are needed.

What we don't know and need to know

Despite a proliferation of intermediate care services we are unclear as to their cost-effectiveness; robust evidence on their costs and outcomes is required. More details are needed on the characteristics of users of schemes and the nature of the care that they receive. 'Intermediate care' is not a universal term and access to services and their provision varies across the UK. Petch (2003) has recommended three key areas be addressed in relation to diversity and quality, which include equity of provision and access, services responsive for black and ethnic minority elders and scrutiny of geographical variation particularly in relation to rural and remote areas.

The focus of intermediate care is to prevent hospital admission and facilitate hospital discharge to avoid any delay. In 2003 the British Government introduced reimbursements from local councils to NHS Trusts who could not discharge patients because community care arrangements could not be made (CSCI, 2004). A study of seven councils looked at the impact of this reimbursement policy in practice and they have identified areas where we need to have a better understanding of what is going on. For example, time of discharge on its own does not guarantee quality outcomes. Also, hospital is not the place for people to make life-changing decisions. Continuity of care between hospital and community is highly valued and once again access to intermediate care and rehabilitation varies across the country. The emergency admission of older people into hospitals continues to rise and this needs to be better understood. Prevention of hospital admission and post-hospital care can be undermined where there are shortfalls in community health services. Rates of hospital readmissions varied across the seven councils and, again, why this is so needs to be understood.

Outcomes of services and care need to be a focus, not just discharge targets. Inter-agency working and partnerships varied and were seen as improving with the reimbursement scheme bringing health and social services together with a joint purpose. Council run and independent home care services are fragile. How costs, fees and outcomes relate needs to be better understood and made explicit in contracts. People first and outcomes should take priority over systems and processes. The Commission for Social Care Inspection (CSCI, 2004) recommends:

- A holistic, cross-organisational approach to planning and delivering services for older people.
- Greater focus on person centred care management.
- More robust, deliverable joint commissioning strategies designed to support independent living.
- More flexible, responsive provider market.
- More follow-up to assess longer-term outcomes for older people leaving hospital.
- Revised regulatory framework that better meets modern needs and pressures.

It remains to be seen whether the new chronic disease management will provide an alternative to hospital care for continuing care and the management of long-term conditions. Specific issues that remain unclear are targeting of service, case size, case managers' access and influence over resources, and the integration of health and social care practices, along with the development of new roles. Commissioning of services and care management arrangements as a consequence of direct payments to older people will also play a part in the continuum of care and the spectrum of care management arrangements.

What we don't do but could: 'Mind the Gap'

Intermediate and continuing care form part of a 'care continuum' provided by health and social services. The policies, services and schemes for intermediate care within the UK appear to have been developed separately from those of continuing care, which has its base over a longer period of time within community care. A six-week cut-off for the provision of intermediate care has been recommended for services (Department of Health, 2001), although there does not appear to be an empirical basis for this time limit. Where intermediate care stops and continuing care begins is not clear, nor has there been national discussion or debate on this or related issues to inform policy development. It is evident from the perspective of authors and chapters within this book that a whole systems approach to service development and delivery is required. This approach to care has been well argued and implemented by Foote and Stanners (2002) and colleagues in their pioneering work on integrating care for older people taking into account their changing needs for short term care, continuing care and end of life. This project commenced before the present day policies on intermediate care and clearly demonstrates not only a systems approach but also an understanding of the continuum of care and the need to integrate care across sectors and services for the benefit of users and carers. More recent work in the UK led by Evercare in nine pilot centres has been developing systems and practice, based on their USA model, of preventing deterioration of chronic illness in older people by adopting a population based approach to 'at risk' older people and individual nurses case managing, screening and educating older people about self care and management (Department of Health, 2004; Evercare, 2004). This screening and secondary prevention approach is useful in preventing older people being hospitalised and empowers them to continue caring for themselves. It is also an example of an intervention early on in the care continuum, pre-emptive, which can have direct benefits to older people, and again is part of an integrated whole systems approach to care. However, when 'importing' schemes, such as Evercare, it is important their local implementation is tailored to the needs of the local population and makes allowance for the configuration of existing services for health and social care (Mayor, 2004).

Local evaluations have demonstrated that palliative care is an important feature of intermediate care providing short-term and intensive treatment and support for people with terminal and chronic conditions, and their carers (Young, 2002a; 2002b; Roe et al., 2003; Beech et al., 2004). However gaps in provision have been noted due to care being limited to five days per week during day times for some schemes, a lack of medical support, inadequate technical skills of nurses related to intravenous medicine administration and support, and their inability to be able to prescribe medicines from the *Nursing Formulary* (Roe, 2001a; 2001b; Roe et al., 2003). Such gaps or limitations provide opportunities for developing services and the skills of practitioners. Palliative care is not just a feature of intermediate care but is also a consideration for continuing care, and clearly demonstrates the importance of a joined-up approach to the 'continuum of care' and how intermediate and continuing care relate to each other.

There is acknowledgment that intermediate care takes account of equity and diversity (Petch, 2003; Martin et al., 2004) and this argument can also be applied to continuing care. As well as the omissions illustrated above in relation to more technical nursing care, medical support and palliative care, there has been insufficient consideration and provision of intermediate care for people with mental health needs or dementia (Roe, 2001a, b; Department of Health, 2002; Roe et al., 2003) or from ethnic minorities and rural communities (Petch, 2003). Such omissions and considerations are not only pertinent to intermediate care provision but also for continuing care, hence further support for a whole system perspective on the 'care continuum'. Defining the role of commissioners and providers as well as the structure, content and process of services for all aspects of care is essential rather than an individual focus on either intermediate care or continuing care in isolation. This is essential if we are to ensure that systems and services are accessible, equitable, and available and sensitive to diverse populations.

End of life issues and care are not only a feature of palliative care (Payne and Ellis Hill, 2001) and consequently intermediate care but also of continuing care (Froggatt, 2001; Foote and Stanners, 2002; Enes et al., 2004). In a systematic review Davies (2005) has found unmet needs among older people in relation to pain relief, preference of place of care, information and communication, and palliative care. Care pathways, such as the Liverpool End of Life Care Pathway, are available for recognising and diagnosing dying and for assisting with all aspects of care planning and bereavement (Ellershaw and Wilkinson, 2003). End of life care pathways are predominantly used in hospice settings and palliative care but are less integrated into intermediate and continuing care, and their inclusion and implementation would be a positive development. This may also help to allay the clinical confusion and suspicion that is emerging on the prescription and administration of diamorphine, particularly in the UK since the Harold Shipman case (McFerran, 2004). Physician assisted dying and the involvement of nurses already occurs in Belgium (Bilsen et al., 2004) and palliative care nurses' views on euthanasia are available (Verpoort et al., 2004). End of life care is an important but often neglected aspect of the care continuum and is an essential consideration for intermediate and continuing care.

Empirical evidence

More evidence on the merits of intermediate care schemes is needed but there is some robust evidence on the benefits of hospital at home schemes and early discharge from hospital. These schemes maintain clinical outcomes and reduce acute hospital stays for patients at lower or equivalent costs. Whether they can prevent hospital admissions is not known. Patients and carers have positive attitudes to the hospital at home schemes. There are many schemes that constitute intermediate care and generally robust evidence to guide their development is lacking. Local evaluations are available but cannot be generalised. Realistically randomised controlled trials would be difficult to undertake as many schemes have already been developed in line with national policy. What we do have is evidence from local evaluations, which needs to be synthesised and the conclusions and recommendations disseminated.

Despite having a longer history within policy and practice, continuing care and its provision in the community continues to evolve, also with a variety of providers, locations, financial arrangements and resources. It seems that housing based developments, such as extra care housing, can provide a range of activities and independence for residents. However, the number of places available in such schemes is very small. Retirement communities or villages provide a range of facilities and benefits but their availability is limited. Their long-term viability and provision for dependent residents needs to be investigated. The social costs remain unknown, as do the benefits and consequences of financial arrangements of owner occupation, rental and part rental/ownership. Retirement communities and extra care housing have been compared with traditional sheltered housing but are being developed with the focus on integrated care and housing as an alternative to care homes.

Where domiciliary care is no longer suitable, care homes traditionally provide continuing care for vulnerable people. Similar to intermediate care, policy and financial incentives have resulted in a variety of local schemes and providers of publicly and self financed continuing care. This has resulted in a reduction of places in care homes and an increased dependency of existing residents. There is a lack of national data within the UK on the characteristics of homes and residents.

Despite increased government funding, consolidation of the market in care homes may mean fewer but larger corporate homes, resulting in a reduction of choice for future residents in relation to type of home or location. Care homes able to provide continuing care and a supportive social climate are needed.

Care in the community, whether intermediate or continuing, is largely provided by informal carers. This has been recognised within policy and practice and involving carers in the provision, evaluation and development of services is essential. Providing respite care for carers so that they can continue in their role is recognised as vital. Agencies should ensure that carers are involved in the planning and delivery of services and that their expectations and needs are considered when goals and outcomes of care are considered. Carers are often experts within their unique situations and so their skills should be recognised and valued.

Involving users and the public in the evaluation and development of health and social care has been recognised. Methods for doing this are developing and their collective voices are being heard at the local level of service provision. Their involvement in the early stages of policy development at national and local levels needs development. How their views can be sought in relation to addressing inequalities in health, community participation, social capital and partnerships needs further conceptual thinking. The nature of intermediate and continuing care means that users of these services may be vulnerable people with complex conditions over a longer time frame. Having adapted to living with chronic conditions, their views on services, place and nature of care required are essential as they live with and adapt to their own unique experiences. User and public involvement to date has mainly been at the individual or local programme level; how they can influence health systems and policy at the macro-level remains to be addressed. Involving users and carers in direct treatment decisions, and the development of care and services, varies between countries (Schoen et al., 2003). Paternalistic practices in primary care and public health still dominate within the UK. Continued focus and development of user and public involvement and engagement at macro- and micro-levels for policy and services development as well as direct care is still required (Schoen et al., 2003; Coulter and Rozansky, 2004).

As intermediate and continuing care are developing in line with policy directives and local requirements so too are the roles of health and social care providers who deliver this care. There is a recognised shortage of doctors, nurses, therapists, carers and social workers and, as such, new ways of working, whether multidisciplinary or interdisciplinary, education and training are being developed so that core competences are recognised, skills are transferred and unique roles or practices are recognised. The traditional concept of the professions is being challenged and dual professional qualifications are being considered. As evidenced in this book, interdisciplinary education in intermediate and continuing care working using adult teaching and education techniques is being advocated as a way of supporting interdisciplinary working. It is unclear whether this is borne out in reality and whether such education should be pre- or post-professional qualification. The views of patients, carers and the public in relation to interdisciplinary education and working for intermediate and continuing care have not been sought.

Implications for research, practice and policy

It is clear that consideration should be given to the 'continuum of care' in relation to policy and development and how preventive, acute, intermediate, continuing, palliative and end of life care relate to each other. What they constitute and where they are delivered in the overall health and social care system needs to be considered, so that there is a balance and range of services, and that care is integrated, so that the needs of clients and carers are taken into account along with their preference for where their care should take place. Further research on the types, location, outcomes and costs of intermediate and continuing care is required so that the most efficient and cost-effective services and care are delivered. Conclusive evidence on saving hospital admissions by case management of older at risk people and those with chronic conditions is lacking (Carvel 2004; Hutt et al., 2004; Mayor, 2004). Providing intermediate care schemes does not necessarily translate into preventing hospital admissions and freeing up beds. More emphasis should be placed on keeping people well and healthy, that is, 'upstream' services such as falls prevention or screening rather than on providing intermediate or continuing care when people become ill, which is currently the point at which they access services.

It is widely acknowledged that a proliferation of intermediate care schemes has taken place and that there are no standard definitions for what these different schemes constitute. Comparing schemes and developing a body of evidence is therefore difficult. Greater focus should be made on the needs of patients, care requirements, and where this should take place in relation to outcomes and costs for both intermediate and continuing care, rather that what a scheme or service constitutes and provides. Audit and evaluation research could address these issues where we are unable to undertake randomised controlled trials. Involvement of users, carers and the public in research, policy and service development is paramount. More robust information on demography, clients' needs, outcomes and economic merits of intermediate and continuing care policies and practice are required. Having already invested in intermediate and continuing care we need to learn lessons from what we do well and to involve users and carers in research, audit and evaluation. Adopting a whole systems approach to the continuum of care seems a sensible way forward as care needs vary across the life course. Care and services need to be integrated so that the needs of populations and users are the drivers, not the services or providers themselves. Providing a range of services and a balance of care within a whole system is key. Doing so also requires a workforce that is skilled, knowledgeable, and able to work with and across professional disciplines, and which is appropriately regulated.

Commissioning and the integration of services and care within whole systems is required and is the focus of health and social care for older people in a number of countries (Leichsenring and Alaszewski, 2004). Integration of health and social care takes the form at the macro-level with partnerships between organisations and at the micro-level with joined-up services. Only a small number of Care Trusts that are integrated care organisations exist in the UK. As yet, it remains unclear whether integration and the form it takes are predominantly horizontal or vertical (Challis, 1998; Kodner, 2003). Vertical integration appears to be recommended within current policy with complex care teams, better coordinated care networks and strong local partnerships (Philp, 2004). Information systems and technology that support integrated services and care require further development to ensure they perform at their full potential.

Summary

The debate and evidence on intermediate and continuing care, policy and practice will continue to evolve. Of paramount importance are the populations and needs of the people served as well as costs to individuals and economies. We hope this book has gone some way into furthering this objective.

References

Beech, R., McDowell, S., Wood, G. (2004) Investigating services for palliative care in Central Cheshire PCT. *Clinical Governance Bulletin* **5** (4), 7–9.

Bernard, M., Bartlam, B., Biggs, S., Sim, J. (2004) *New Lifestyles in Old Age. Health, Identity and Well-Being in Berryhill Retirement Village*. Bristol: Policy Press.

Bilsen, J.J.R., Vander Stichell, R.H., Mortier, F., Deliens, L. (2004) Involvement of nurses in physician assisted dying. *Journal of Advanced Nursing* **47** (6), 583–91.

Carvel, J. (2004) Doubts cast on US style health plan. *The Guardian* 30 November. http://society.guardian.co.uk/nhsplan/story/0,7991,1362394,00.html (accessed 02/12/2004).

Challis, D. (1998) Integrating health and social care: problems, opportunities and possibilities. *Research Policy and Planning* **16** (2), 7–12.

Charter, D. (2004) Elderly lose 10 000 places in care homes. *The Times* 7 September, 2.

Commission for Social Care Inspection (CSCI) (2004) *Leaving Hospital – The Price of Delays*. London: CSCI.

Coulter, A., Rozansky, D. (2004) Full engagement in health (Editorial). *British Medical Journal* **329**, 1197–8.

Croucher, K., Pleace, N., Bevan, M. (2003) *Living at Hartrigg Oaks. Residents' Views of the UK's First Continuing Care Retirement Community*. York: Joseph Rowntree Foundation.

Davies, E. (2005) *What Are the Palliative Care Needs of Older People and How Might They Be Met? Health Evidence Network*. Copenhagen: World Health Organization Europe.

Department of Health (2001) *National Service Framework for Older People*. London: Department of Health.

Department of Health (2002) *National Service Framework for Older People – Supporting Implementation. Intermediate Care: Moving Forward*. London: Department of Health.

Department of Health (2004) *New Health Programme Trial to Improve Older Patient Care*. London: Department of Health.

Ellershaw, J., Wilkinson, S. (2003) *Care of the Dying: A Pathway to Excellence*. Oxford: Oxford University Press.

Enes, S.P.D., Lucas, C.F., Aberdein, N., Lucioni, J. (2004) Discharging patients from hospice to nursing home: a retrospective case note review. *International Journal of Palliative Nursing* **10** (3), 124–30.

Evercare (2004) *Implementing the Evercare Programme: Interim Report*. http://www.natpact.nhs.uk/uploads/Advancing%20the%20National%20Health%20Service%20interim%202-04%20final.doc (accessed 26/1/2005).

Foote, C., Stanners, C. (2002) *Integrating Care for Older People. New Care for Old – A Systems Approach*. London: Jessica Kingsley Publishers.

Forte, P., Bowen, T. (1997) Improving the balance of elderly care services. In: Cropper, S. and Forte, P. (eds) *Enhancing Health Services Management*. Milton Keynes: Open University Press, 71–85.

Froggatt, K. (2001) Palliative care in nursing homes: where next? *Palliative Medicine* **15**, 42–8.

Hutt, R., Rosen, R., McCauley, J. (2004) *Case-Managing Long-Term Conditions. What Impact Does it Have in the Treatment of Older People*. London: King's Fund.

Kodner, D. (2003) Long term care integration in four European countries. A review. In: Brodsky, J., Habib, J. and Hirschfield, M. (eds) *Key Policies in Long Term Care*. Geneva: World Health Organization.

Leichsenring, K., Alaszewski, A.M. (2004) *Providing Integrated Health and Social Care for Older Persons*. Aldershot: Ashgate.

Martin, G.P., Peet, S.M., Hewitt, G.J., Parker, H. (2004) Diversity in intermediate care. *Health and Social Care in the Community* **12** (2), 150–54.

Mayor, S. (2004) Evidence is weak for case management for the elderly. *British Medical Journal* **329**, 1306.

McFerran, A. (2004) Careless talk jails nurses in the shadow of Shipman. *The Sunday Times* 3 October, News Review 10.

Payne, S., Ellis Hill, C. (2001) *Chronic and Terminal Illness. New Perspectives on Caring and Carers.* Oxford: Oxford University Press.

Petch, A. (2003) *Intermediate Care. What Do We Know About Older People's Experiences.* York: Joseph Rowntree Foundation.

Philp, I. (2004) *Better Health in Old Age.* London: Department of Health.

Roe, B. (2001a) *Evaluation of Intermediate Care Services: Pilot.* Keele: Centre for Geriatric Medicine, Keele University. (Unpublished report submitted to Cheshire Community Healthcare NHS Trust.)

Roe, B. (2001b) *Evaluation of Intermediate Care Services: Continuation.* Keele: Centre for Geriatric Medicine, Keele University. (Unpublished report submitted to Cheshire Community Healthcare NHS Trust.)

Roe, B., Daly, S., Shenton, G., Lochhead, Y. (2003) Development and evaluation of intermediate care. *Journal of Clinical Nursing* **12**, 341–50.

Sandelowski, M. (2000) *Devices and Desires. Gender, Technology and American Nursing.* Chapel Hill: University of North Carolina Press.

Schoen, C., Osborn, R., Huynh, P.T., Doty, M., Davis, K., Zapert, K. et al. (2003) Primary care and health systems performance: adults' experiences in five countries. *Health Affairs (Millwood)* 2004, Oct. 28, 10.1377/htltaff.w4.487.

Shepperd, S., Illiffe, S. (2004) *Hospital at Home Versus In-patient Hospital Care.* (Cochrane Review) In: The Cochrane Library, Issue 4. Chichester: John Wiley.

Sturge, M. (2000) *Continuing Care Retirement Communities in the UK. Lessons from Hartrigg Oaks.* York: Joseph Rowntree Foundation.

Twigg, J. (2000) *Bathing – The Body and Community Care.* London: Routledge, 1–17.

Verpoort, C., Gastmans, C., Dierckx de Casterle, B. (2004) Palliative care nurses' views on euthanasia. *Journal of Advanced Nursing* **47** (6), 592–60.

Wittenberg, R., Comas–Herrera, A., Pickard, L., Hancock, R. (2004) *Future Demand for Long-term Care in the UK: A Summary of Projections of Long-term Care Finance for Older People to 2051.* York: Joseph Rowntree Foundation.

Young, J. (2002a) The evidence base for intermediate care. *Geriatric Medicine* **32** (10), 11–14.

Young, J. (2002b) Review of research evidence. In: Department of Health *National Service Framework for Older People – Supporting Implementation. Intermediate Care: Moving Forward.* Appendix. London: Department of Health.

Index